Advanced nursing practice

Advanced nursing practice

Edited by Gary Rolfe and Paul Fulbrook

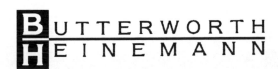
BUTTERWORTH
HEINEMANN

OXFORD   BOSTON   JOHANNESBURG   MELBOURNE   NEW DELHI   SINGAPORE

Butterworth-Heinemann
Linacre House, Jordan Hill, Oxford OX2 8DP
225 Wildwood Avenue, Woburn MA 01801-2041
A division of Reed Educational and Professional Publishing Ltd

A member of the Reed Elsevier plc group

First published 1998
Reprinted 1999
Transferred to digital printing 2001

British Library Cataloguing in Publication Data
Advanced nursing practice
  1. Nursing practice
  I. Rolfe, Gary   II. Fulbrook, Paul
  610.7'3

Library of Congress Cataloguing in Publication Data
Advanced nursing practice/edited by Gary Rolfe and Paul Fulbrook
  p.m.
  Includes bibliographical references and index
  1. Nursing   2. Nurse practitioners   3. Nursing – Philosopohy
  4. Nursing – Research   5. Nursing – Study and teaching
  I. Rolfe, Gary   II. Fulbrook, Paul
  610.73–dc21

ISBN 0 7506 3404 9

Printed in Great Britain by Antony Rowe Ltd, Eastbourne

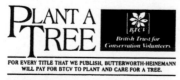

www.bh.com

For Lyn and her passenger

G.R.

To my critical care nursing colleagues in the BACCN for their inspiration,
to Jamie with love,
and to Miriam for being herself

P.F.

Contents

Contributors

John W. Albarran MSc, PG Dip Ed, BSc (Hons), RN, Dip N
Senior Lecturer in Critical Care Nursing, Faculty of Health and Social Care
University of the West of England
Bristol
UK

Phil Barker PhD, RN, FRCN
Professor of Psychiatric Nursing Practice
University of Newcastle,
UK

George Castledine
Professor of Nursing and Community Health
Health and Social Care Research Centre
University of Central England

Maureen Coombs RGN, DN (Lond), BSc (Hons), PG Dip Ed, MSc
Senior Nurse
Service Delivery Unit Manager
Intensive Care Unit
John Radcliffe Hospital
Oxford Radcliffe Hospital Trust
Oxford
UK

Pat Elliott MSc, BEd, RGN, ONC, DN, RCNT, Cert Ed
Advanced Nursing Practitioner
Worcester Community Healthcare Trust
UK

Sue Frost MPhil, BA, Cert Ed, RGN, RNT
Dean of Human and Health Sciences
University of Huddersfield
Huddersfield
UK

Paul Fulbrook MSc, BSc (Hons), PGDE, RGN, DPSN
Senior Lecturer
Centre for Research
School of Health Studies
University of Portsmouth
Portsmouth
UK

Ingrid Goodman MSc RGN
Project Officer
Royal College of Nursing Institute
London
UK

Margaret Holgate MSc, BA (Hons)
Project Manager, Integrated Care Pathways Pilot Project, Nursing Directorate
Churchill Hospital
Oxford Radcliffe Hospitals Trust
UK

Dean David Holyoake MSc, PG Dip, BA, Dip CPC (SMIC),
Dip Child Psychol, RMN
Mental Health Nurse
Birmingham
UK

Melanie A. Jasper MSc, B Nurs, BA, PGCEA, RGN, RM, RHV,
NDN Cert
Principal Lecturer
Centre for Research
School of Health Studies
University of Portsmouth
Portsmouth
UK

Chris Johns RMN, RGN, MN, PhD
Reader in Advanced Nursing Practice
University of Luton
UK

Kim Manley MN, BA, RGN, Dip N, RCNT, PGCEA
Course Director MSc in Nursing
Royal College of Nursing Institute
London
UK

Susan M. Read PhD, RGN, RHV
Senior Lecturer (Research)
Department of Acute and Critical Care Nursing
University of Sheffield School of Nursing and Midwifery
Sheffield
UK

Marie Roberts-Davis RGN, RHV, BA (Hons), MA
Subdean (Postgraduate Affairs)
University of Sheffield School of Nursing and Midwifery
Sheffield
UK

Gary Rolfe PhD, MA, BSc, RMN, PGCEA
Principal Lecturer
Centre for Research
School of Health Studies
University of Portsmouth
UK

Julie Scholes RGN, Dip N, DANS, MSc, DPhil
Senior Lecturer (Research)
Centre for Nursing and Midwifery Research
University of Brighton
Brighton
UK

Barbara Stilwell FRCN, BSocSc, RGN, RHV
Training Director
Expanded Programme on Immunization
World Health Organisation
Geneva
Switzerland
Formerly Director of Practice Development
Royal College of Nursing Institute
UK

Preface

The idea for this book arose from a symposium entitled 'Perspectives on Advanced Practice' held at the University of Portsmouth in the Spring of 1996. The context in which the symposium was planned and delivered was as a contribution to the United Kingdom Central Council for Nursing, Midwifery and Health Visiting's (UKCC) ongoing deliberations about the nature of advanced practice and, in particular, the knowledge and skills required by the nurse practising at this level. The pronouncements of the UKCC at this time were vague and non-commital, and the symposium was, to some extent, a gathering of researchers and educationalists with a vested interest in anticipating what the role of the advanced practitioner might look like.

Shortly after the symposium took place, the UKCC conducted a listening exercise in which many of the symposium speakers took part, and concluded that:

> It was felt that there are neither agreed definitions of advanced practice nor criteria against which standards for advanced practice can be set. It was also clear that most nurse practitioner graduates fill the requirements of specialist, rather than advanced, practice. For these reasons, it was felt that the UKCC, while fully supporting the notion of advancing practice, should avoid setting explicit standards but should consider how specialist practice could embrace nurse practitioners and clinical nurse specialists (UKCC, 1997).

This conclusion was in part disappointing, mainly because many of us had been holding back from educational and practice developments until the UKCC had clarified the situation, and we felt that valuable time had been lost; but it was also encouraging and liberating not to be tied down by over-restrictive guidelines about what does and does not constitute advanced practice. Indeed, there is some doubt about whether developments of this sort can and should be imposed from above in a planned and rational exercise, or whether they emerge spontaneously from the community of practitioners and academics. As the philosopher Richard Rorty pointed out, change rarely comes from a reasoned examination of the pros and cons of a position:

> The method is to redescribe lots and lots of things in new ways, until you have created a pattern of linguistic behaviour which will tempt the rising generation to adopt it, thereby causing them to look for appropriate new forms of nonlinguistic behaviour (Rorty, 1989).

By redescribing the world as we would like it to be, we establish language patterns that facilitate the existence of that world. Books do not change behaviour, no matter how persuasive they might be, but they can contribute towards establishing the climate for change. Only when practitioners start to use the new *language* of advanced practice does the *reality* of advanced practice become a possibility.

This book therefore does not attempt to present a single coherent argument for a new model of advanced practice, neither is it a cookbook of recipes for advanced practice nor an attempt by a group of academics to dictate to nurses what they ought to do. Rather, it is a collection of personal views and perspectives, some founded on research studies, some on theoretical frameworks and models, and others on what might be termed 'wishful thinking'. Some of these perspectives stand back and take a broad view of advanced practice, whereas others move in close to examine a particular aspect through a microscope. Some gaze at advanced practice full-on, while others take a decidedly sideways view. It is up to each practitioner, however, to take what he or she finds useful and to discard the rest.

In this sense, we are largely in agreement with the UKCC that it makes no sense to label a particular activity as advanced, and that we should avoid setting explicit standards. However, part of the *raison d'être* of the UKCC is 'of public protection through professional standards' (UKCC, 1997). We can see, then, why the rejection of standards must, for the UKCC, entail the rejection of the role itself, since for them, a professional role can be defined only through standards of practice.

As educationalists, researchers and practitioners, however, we are in a slightly more fortunate position, since we are able to explore and describe new roles in terms of processes, skills and knowledge, rather than in terms of outcomes. That is not to say, of course, that outcomes are not important, but rather that the inability to set measurable outcomes should not necessarily restrict new developments. As Michael Faraday was reported to have replied to someone who was questioning the usefulness of electricity: 'What use is a newborn baby?' While advanced practice is, perhaps, no longer a newborn baby, it has not developed much further than the toddler stage of taking its first faltering steps, some of which are described in this book.

We should not fall into the trap, then, of asking what use is advanced practice, but rather we must continue the process of describing what it is and what it might become, so that we might, as Rorty claimed, begin to establish a language within which the reality of advanced practice can be developed.

In the following 'Introduction', George Castledine initiates that process in three ways: first, in his assertion (which runs somewhat counter to the UKCC's latest pronouncement) that 'advanced nursing practice remains a distinct sphere of nursing in its own right'; secondly, by offering a distinctly *personal* perspective based on an extensive and long-standing involvement in the development of advanced practice; and, thirdly, by throwing down the challenge of his seven criteria, roles and functions of the advanced nurse practitioner, which are picked up and developed by most of the writers in this book. Castledine has therefore produced a template for what follows. Each of these three themes (the distinctiveness of advanced practice, the personal perspective, and the development of his criteria) is expanded into a patchwork of approaches to advanced practice, which, we believe, add up to far more than merely the sum of their parts.

References

Rorty, R. (1989). *Contingency, irony and solidarity*. Cambridge: Cambridge University Press.
United Kingdom Central Council for Nursing, Midwifery and Health Visiting. (1997). Advancing professional practice, *Register*, **19**, 5.

Introduction

Developments in the role of the advanced nursing practitioner: a personal perspective

George Castledine

In the definitive document 'The future of professional practice – the Council's standards for education and practice following registration' (United Kingdom Central Council for Nursing, Midwifery and Health Visiting (UKCC) 1994), the UKCC states that advanced nursing practice is 'concerned with adjusting the boundaries for the development of future practice, pioneering and developing new roles responsive to changing needs and with advancing clinical practice, research and education to enrich professional practice as a whole'. As someone who was particularly involved in influencing the Council's final decision on this matter, you would probably expect me to support the idea of a nurse working in such a role. However, I would probably be one of the first to point out that we 'fudged' the issue somewhat and left nursing and midwifery to contemplate on the possibilities.

In Paragraph 61 of the Post-Registration Education and Practice report (UKCC 1994), the point is made that advanced nursing practice 'is not an additional layer of practice to be superimposed on specialist nursing practice', but it is an 'important sphere of professional practice' (UKCC, 1994). The reasons behind this statement are that, although one would usually expect advanced nursing practitioners (ANPs) to be developing practice in this way, there is always the possibility that any other professional nurse working in another role could become an innovator and discover something that takes the profession forward. Perhaps what the UKCC should have done was to make a clearer distinction between nursing work that results in a new discovery with implications for nursing practice, and the practice of nursing care that demands higher levels of expertise, knowledge and skill. Some nurses working in research and innovation may well discover something new, but this does not make them an ANP, but more of an inventor, discoverer or researcher in nursing care development. The 'sphere' of advanced nursing practice referred to by the UKCC therefore includes innovations and discoveries from nurses at all levels and roles within the profession. Advanced nursing practitioners, on the other hand, are:

> specially prepared nurses who are working in roles which demand a lot of nursing experience, education at Masters degree level, and nursing skills that contribute to meeting the complex needs of vulnerable people and the need to be continuously questioning the fundamentals and boundaries of nursing (UKCC, 1994).

The first time I ever came across an ANP was during my early days in Manchester. At that time, in the early 1970s, the Salmon Report (Salmon, 1966) had recommended a new management career structure for nurses. This consisted of nursing officers and senior nursing officers. Many senior nursing sisters and charge nurses were encouraged to apply for these more management orientated roles, but unfortunately the preparation they received for fulfilling such new roles was very variable, and there were some very experienced practical nurses who were probably insufficiently prepared for the job.

At Manchester Royal Infirmary, however, the Chief Nursing Officer decided to try an experiment in developing clinical nurse specialists. This resulted in three expert nurses keeping their former clinical bases and taking on the role of a specialist practitioner. Ruth Martin was an expert in neurosurgical nursing, who acted as a nursing consultant and expert role model. Not only did she work on her own ward but also visited other wards in the hospital where neurosurgical patients were lodged. On occasions, she visited the local rehabilitation centre and communicated with GPs, and, while on the visits, she taught nurses and junior medical staff and carried out medical procedures such as lumbar punctures and ventricular taps! She was not highly educated, but had a long history of practical nursing experience, and she convinced me that there should be a clinical career structure for nurses; that has been my aim over the past 20 years.

Manchester University was the first to develop a masters programme for clinical nurses, but it was rarely taken up, the reason being that education and management were perceived as more important, and certainly as areas where nurses could more easily develop their careers.

Since the late 1970s, there have been various moves to encourage the development of ANPs. In the early 1980s, I carried out a survey into the role and function of specialist nurses (Castledine, 1982), the results of which showed that we still had a considerable way to go before we caught up with the North Americans. There were approximately 350 nurses working in some form of specialist way in the early 1980s, some of whom were simply general nurses working in a particular specialist medical field. The most common areas where specialist nurses failed to meet similar criteria to their American colleagues were in the academic requirements for their role: only two of the 353 had a masters degree in nursing; the amount and type of nursing research they were involved in was extremely limited; and many were not working autonomously and were confined to the traditional barriers of a ward or department.

More recently, a survey carried out in Birmingham (McGee et al., 1996) found that the number of specialist nurses had increased dramatically over the previous 15 years, and that there now seemed to be two types of clinical nursing expert emerging: a clinical nurse specialist and an ANP. Although no one is really sure what the criteria and role of an ANP should be, there are some indications that what we have emerging is a very experienced and educated nurse who acts in a similar way to a medical consultant. This would give us three domains of nursing practice in this country: first, general professional nursing practice; secondly, specialist nursing practice; and thirdly, advanced nursing practice.

As generalists, nurses can work in a variety of settings across various medical fields. In developing a specialist role, they start to narrow their field of interest and expertise. Advanced practice is something a little different: it is as if nurses have moved through a specialist stage and have now emerged as generalists again, but with more knowledge and skill in nursing, and able to apply their expertise over several areas without losing sight of holistic principles.

Specialization in nursing must not be allowed to follow medical specialization. Nursing is different from medicine and covers wider holistic principles in its application. A nurse who becomes too specialized is in danger of losing this holistic nurturing perspective and may end up in a nursing cul-de-sac. Unfortunately, the 'physician's assistant' movement or 'junior doctors' hours' initiatives have led some nurses in this direction in the UK.

There is no doubt that we are now at a very exciting stage in our nursing development in this country. The UKCC might have fudged the issue over advanced nursing practice, but what it has enabled is an interesting discussion of possibilities and developments. In Birmingham, we are experimenting with various clinical masters programmes for advanced practice, and I believe that, over the next few years, all these and other developments in the UK will give us a better insight into not only what is advanced nursing, but what is the very nature of our profession.

There are many definitions of advanced nursing practice and ANPs in countries outside the UK. This is especially so in North America, where there is a move to merge the clinical nurse specialist title with that of the nurse practitioner, and it is argued by Jones (1994) that the creation of yet another title may cause confusion and threat to existing well-recognized roles. For simplicity, I will not explore any other definitions and titles used in countries such as North America, but restrict myself to describing what I feel should be the criteria, roles and functions of the ANP in this country.

1. ANPs should demonstrate *autonomy*. They should be resourceful enough to work on their own, contributing to either one or more multidisciplinary health care teams, perhaps linking institutional care with community and home based care.
2. ANPs should be *experienced and knowledgeable*. They should be experts in a particular field of nursing, which may be linked closely to a specialist area of medicine or other related subject. They should have at least eight years' postregistration experience, and may have worked as a specialist nursing practitioner. They should have a sound theoretical and practical knowledge base about nursing and the medical and/or other area of practice to which they relate. This knowledge should be at masters degree level and be related to their work.
3. ANPs should be *researchers and evaluators of care*. One of the key areas for ANPs is to be able to conduct research and evaluation into various areas of their work. They should be able to utilize nursing theory and research to analyse problems. A good under-standing of quality assurance and audit is important.
4. ANPs should be able to *conduct a comprehensive health and nursing*

assessment. When working with patients, they should be particularly skilled in the holistic aspects of patient assessment, and at the same time be able to narrow down their focus to the patient's particular medical and/or health concern, identifying the differences between nursing and medical approaches to health assessment.

5. The emphasis of nurse practitioners' roles should be on *case management* and treatment of complex problems/concerns that are within their domain and responsibility. The focus of ANPs should be on *the effects of disease or disability* on the patient and/or the family. Furthermore, they should be working with the patient and/or family to enable the achievement of a productive lifestyle or a peaceful death.

6. ANPs should act as *consultants and educators* in all matters relating to their particular chosen field and role. For this reason, ANPs should be good communicators, change agents and leaders of nursing. There will be times when they will not only teach patients and their families but also teach nurses, doctors and other relevant members of the health care service.

7. ANPs should be *respected and recognized* by their colleagues as an authority in their particular field. Such recognition only comes with time and publication of their work.

Advanced clinical nursing practice and expanded role function should be guided by a nursing model or emphasis. It should not be directed or dictated by physicians or a medical model. The educational preparation of the ANP of the future should be a clinically based masters degree that builds upon the criteria outlined in this chapter. Nursing's scope of practice must be fluid and evolutionary. Many nurses fear that a medical orientation will impact on the ANP role, particularly due to recent changes in junior doctors' hours. We must be careful that such pressure does not compromise its development and implementation within a nursing framework.

In summary, although ANPs are very experienced in nursing practice, are educated to at least masters level, and are often working in technically advanced and clinically demanding areas, they do not have a monopoly on innovation and leading nursing forward. Any nurse may become an innovator, or make a discovery through observation or research that advances nursing practice. However, these nurses do not by virtue of their discovery become ANPs. Advanced nursing practice remains a distinct sphere of nursing in its own right.

References

Castledine, G. (1982). *The role and function of clinical nurse specialists in England and Wales* [thesis]. Manchester: University of Manchester.

Jones, D. A. (1994). Advanced practice: merging the roles of the nurse practitioner and clinical specialist. In *Nursing Issues in the 1990s*. (O. L. Strickland and D. J. Fishman eds.). New York: Delmar.

McGee, P., Castledine, G. and Brown, R. (1996). A survey of specialist and advanced nursing practice in England. *Br. J. Nurs.*, **5**, 682–686.

Ministry of Health and Scottish Home and Health Department. (Salmon Report, 1966). *Report of the Committee on Senior Nursing Staff Structure*. London: HMSO.

United Kingdom Central Council for Nursing, Midwifery and Health Visiting. (1994). *The future of professional practice, the Council's standards for education and practice following registration*. London: UKCC.

Part 1

Understanding advanced practice: the theoretical perspective

1

Advanced nursing practice: an historical perspective

John Albarran and Paul Fulbrook

The nature of advanced practice is unclear. Furthermore, the role of the advanced practitioner, that is, the exponent of advanced practice, has yet to be made explicit in the literature. 'The profession is uncertain about what the advanced practitioner really is' (Castledine, 1991b). It is not only in the UK where there is uncertainty:

> The synonymous use of terms such as expert, specialist and advanced practitioner in the North American literature has led to confusion, since advanced nursing practice may differ from other forms of nursing practice, such as specialist or expert practice (Sutton and Smith, 1995).

> The meaning of advanced practice in the current literature is defined by broad generalizations... however, the common thread which links these roles and explains their common goal has not been made explicit (Patterson and Haddad, 1992).

In the current climate of professional development in nursing, the concepts of 'advanced practice' and 'advanced practitioner' require clarification. Tracing their historical development will help to shape current understanding, and the purpose of this chapter is to place advanced practice within the context of contemporary nursing.

Overview

The concept of the advanced practitioner has long been established in the USA, although it is normally associated with the role of clinical nurse specialist (CNS). The American model of advanced practice is based on the key concepts of clinical judgement and leadership (Spross and Baggerley, 1989) and has been recognized there for many years, having developed from the notion of the nurse clinician, which was first advanced by Reiter in the 1940s (Hamric, 1989), and later written up by her (Reiter, 1966). In 1970, the *American Journal of Nursing* published a collection of papers relating to the CNS (Lewis, 1970). Thus, it was not until the 1970s, and following explication by Georgopoulos and Christman (1970, 1973), that the role was effectively introduced and recognized in the clinical practice setting (Hamric, 1989).

In the UK, the concept of advanced practice (in the guise of a clinical specialist/consultant nurse) was first considered by the Royal College of Nursing (RCN) in the early 1970s in response to the Briggs Report (Department of Health and Social Security (DHSS), 1972). Later, the RCN's *New Horizons in Clinical Nursing* put forward the case for an advanced clinical role and proposed the development of a clinical nurse consultant (Royal College of Nursing (RCN), 1975). However, possibly because it was suggested in the wake of the Salmon report (Ministry of Health and Scottish Home and Health Department, 1966), and the subsequent introduction of a clinical nursing structure with what was arguably an overemphasis on management, the role failed to gain acceptance. An additional obstruction to its development may have been the assertion that the role of clinical nurse consultant 'should attract salary recognition consistent with the level of responsibility and the high degree of expertise' (RCN, 1975). Ironically, the role was also seen as a potential threat to senior clinical nurses (Duberley, 1976; Barrie-Shevlin, 1985).

The literature reviewed in this chapter reveals only limited development of advanced practice in terms of an advanced practitioner role in the UK over the last 20 years or so. However, several advanced roles have been developed, the most notable of which are the consultant nurse (e.g. Wright, 1991) and the lecturer–practitioner (e.g. Lloyd-Jones, 1993). Although these roles are focused on nursing practice, and do include a clinical practice component, the former may be led more by the management structure, whereas the latter appears more educationally based. Logically, the term 'advanced practitioner' suggests that the role should be driven by clinical practice. There are also many examples of CNS roles in the UK (Castledine, 1992), and while most of these roles tend to have a fairly narrow specialist focus, it may be argued by some that advanced practice is implicit within them.

Following the 1983 health service reorganization, many hospitals employed CNSs (Sargeant, 1985), but there was still little evidence mentioned in the literature of advanced practice. In the UK, the role of the CNS appeared to develop on a somewhat individual basis, driven by local service demands, rather than according to a professional framework such as that described by Hamric and Spross (1989). One example of this new CNS role (in the UK) was described by Sargeant (1983), who considered the subroles to be clinical nurse advisor, practitioner, counsellor, educator, manager and administrator. The role, however, seemed to be biased towards a management agenda rather than clinical practice per se.

Thompson and Webster (1986) appraised the role of the CNS in relation to critical care nursing, but were unable to identify clearly its components. They felt that there were many grey areas, that the issues were 'dogged by confusion and lack of uniformity', and that the lack of a clearly defined structure for the role had inhibited its development. They supported their posit by citing McFarlane (1980), who suggested that the bureaucratic nursing structure of the National Health Service (NHS) was not responsive to such changes and did not easily accommodate innovatory development.

In 1988, the career structure of nursing was radically altered with the introduction of clinical grading (Nursing and Midwifery Staff's Negotiating Council, 1988). Although it was intended to reward nurses for clinical advancement, it is arguable that it has failed to do so adequately, since one result of implementing this structure has been that the clinical career ladder of nursing has effectively been cut off at sister level. Kersley (1992) makes the important point that the lack of recognition and financial reward for clinical expertise runs the risk of losing such staff to education and management, leaving the clinical area 'bereft of leaders and lacking direction'. This may be one of several factors that have restricted the growth and development of advanced practitioners.

In order for the role of advanced practitioner to be professionally recognized, it would seem prudent to determine clear guidelines for the role within a defined career structure. The need for a clinical career structure for nursing has been emphasized in the past by the RCN in two publications: *Towards Standards* (RCN, 1981) and *Towards a New Professional Structure for Nursing* (RCN, 1983). The latter publication, whilst proffering a new career structure failed to describe an advanced practitioner role as such. This is somewhat disappointing, since it had been developed from an RCN seminar on advanced clinical roles published only a year earlier (RCN, 1982).

If a career structure was developed that incorporated the advanced practitioner, it would require the distinction to be made between advanced practitioner, clinical specialist, CNS, and in particular, the current nurse practitioner (NP) role which has been widely implemented in recent years.

A decade ago, an RCN working party proposed the concept of a nurse specialist, who they described as an expert 'in a particular aspect of nursing care' who 'demonstrates refined clinical practice, either as a result of significant experience or advanced expertise, or knowledge in a branch or specialty' (RCN, 1988). They went on to state that it is because 'there is no formally recognised position ... within the present structure ... that it is difficult to recognise who is functioning in this role' (RCN, 1988). A number of other professional titles compound the problem, for example, clinical expert, clinical nurse manager, nurse consultant, and senior clinical nurse. It is possible that although there are many different roles, they may all, in fact, be advanced practitioners. It is also possible that there are many practitioners who have a title that suggests they are advanced, when in fact they are not. Much of the confusion regarding advanced nursing practice seems to stem from different terms used to describe the person. This source of confusion may be compounded as these titles are often used interchangeably. Thus, nurses can never be sure they are discussing the same concepts. This can only add uncertainty about the broad nature of advanced nursing practice (Albarran and Whittle, 1997).

The concept of advanced nursing practice has been evident in the UK for the last 20 years or so (Ashworth, 1975; Castledine, 1983; RCN, 1975). In 1990, in its Post-Registration Education and Practice (PREP) Project document, the United Kingdom Central Council for Nursing, Midwifery and Health Visiting (UKCC) stated: 'The standard, kind and content for advanced practice will be specified by the Council. Advanced practitioners must have an appropriate Council-approved qualification recorded on the register' (UKCC, 1990).

Castledine, an advocate of advanced practice since the early 1980s, suggests that this was the first time that an official announcement had ever been made in the UK regarding the development of an advanced practitioner. He bemoaned the fact that the 'political and professional road to identification of advanced practice has been a continual uphill struggle' (Castledine, 1992). Indeed, this was underlined by the extremely slow progress made following the publication of PREP (UKCC, 1990). Despite wide consultation and debate, consensus about the nature, scope and criteria of advanced practice has not been reached (UKCC, 1996).

The current professional view, which is accepted by many, is that individuals who are at an advanced level should be engaged in developing and advancing clinical practice, research, and education, stretching professional boundaries in the delivery of patient care, and pioneering new roles that reflect changing needs, as well as influencing local and national health care policies (UKCC, 1994, 1997).

To give context to the present situation, it is necessary to trace and examine the major forces that have shaped the evolution of a clinical career structure that currently revolves around the professional, specialist and advanced levels of clinical practice (UKCC, 1994). Movement has been influenced by a number of factors, including professional developments, educational and health service reforms, a desire to retain clinical experts at the bedside, and a drive to advance excellence in the delivery of nursing services and strengthen the profile of clinical practice (Ashworth, 1975; Castledine, 1983; Pearson, 1983; Wright, 1986). However, this path has been neither coherent nor based on a systematic approach.

In the light of the above, the aim of this chapter is to discuss the historical development of advanced nursing practice and to identify how various milestones have influenced its passage.

The American influence

Concepts of advanced nursing practice have long been recognized in the USA, where they have traditionally been associated with the characteristics of the CNS. However, most commentators credit Reiter (1966) as a key protagonist of advanced practice, whose ideas on the nurse clinician (a term that she first coined in 1943) later evolved to become central to the CNS role. For Reiter (1966) a nurse clinician was 'a master practitioner throughout all the dimensions of nursing practice'. Additionally, other responsibilities entailed being able to demonstrate advanced knowledge, high levels of clinical judgement, and competence in a particular field of nursing. Moreover, the sole purpose of introducing nurse clinicians with a high level of skill and theoretical insight was to improve patient care, which Reiter (1966) conceived to be in jeopardy. With subsequent publications (Lewis, 1970) and further research, the role of the CNS began to be widely adopted and accepted in the USA. Statutory bodies also supported this clinical enterprise and mandated the level of education for such positions as graduate preparation (Amos-Taylor and Elberson, 1989). It was, presumably, reasoned that the grounding of nurses to the level of CNS would equip them with the leadership to enhance quality of care by advancing clinical theory and practice. However, these expectations were based on anecdote, assumption, speculation and belief, rather than on empirical evidence. There was also a lack of agreement on the attributes required to define the role of the CNS, and the position such an individual should hold in existing nursing hierarchies.

It was a small experimental study lasting 13 months, however, which suggested that nurses who were prepared for CNS roles were able to deliver sophisticated individualized nursing care based on careful systematic planning, scientific knowledge in patient care, and innovation (Georgopoulos and Christman, 1970). The CNSs in the study exercised discretionary judgements and acted as expert role models and as a resource for members of the health care team. In contrast, it was observed that the work of the non-CNSs in the control group tended to be dominated by crisis management and administrative tasks, with care organized around rituals and based on a physician-led model of practice. Thus, for Georgopoulos and Christman (1970), a CNS was a registered nurse in possession of postgraduate preparation relating to a specialist area of nursing practice, who was able to provide a comprehensive and competent level of care as well as an informed expertise about patient needs. They suggested that the contribution of such roles was encouraging, and long-term benefits would result if the appropriate organizational supportive measures were instituted.

Concurrent with the above project, another study set out to investigate the influence of CNS behaviour, as determined by 'Kardex' entries (nursing notes), when compared with a non-CNS control group (Georgopoulos and Jackson, 1970). Although all subjects demonstrated improvement in key categories of documentation, the experimental group tended to be more patient focused, with greater detail and coverage of nursing activity. As such, it was concluded that nursing practice was superior in those units led by a CNS.

As empirical evidence accumulated on the impact of advanced practitioners based on the positive effects on patient outcomes (Sparacino, 1986; Amos-Taylor and Elberson, 1989), the CNS role was endorsed by the American Nurses Association (American Nurses Association (ANA), 1976). Later, in a social policy statement (ANA, 1980), they proposed that a CNS should be a qualified nurse who, through study and supervised practice at graduate level (master's or doctorate), has become an expert in a selected sphere of nursing. Additionally, the earlier document (ANA, 1976) emphasized that the CNS must provide leadership for staff development, education, consultation and research, and for directing patient care. These reports alluded to core values that have since been aligned under the umbrella of advanced nursing practice, although role components within models of advanced practice varied (Spross and Baggerly, 1989; Sparacino et al., 1990; Heffline, 1991).

Sparacino (1986) argued that persistent disagreement regarding the functional division of CNS roles had led to slow maturity and sanctioning of this level of nursing practice by the profession, as well as explaining why these roles have been often either underutilized or misunderstood.

Georgopoulos and Christman's (1970) work drew much interest in the UK, and, since their work was based on ward sisters, Duberly (1976) thus reasoned that these individuals were the natural CNSs, and, as experts in their own field, were most appropriately suited to improve perceived falling standards. For Duberly (1976), a separate CNS role was unnecessary, and, if implemented, would 'only result in disillusionment and frustration'. However, it was in response to other contemporary nursing initiatives, including the introduction of nationally validated clinical courses in a range of specialty settings, practice and academic developments, and the impact of NHS reorganizations, which began slowly to materialize into a trajectory that placed advanced nursing practice on the professional stage. Castledine (1991a) charted how various events in nursing history have converged into the concept of advanced nursing practice. These events will now be discussed in greater detail.

The specialization of clinical practice

Many nurse theorists have credited recognition of the importance of delivering specialized and advanced patient care to Florence Nightingale, who recruited and taught her nurses how to care and treat wounded and injured soldiers during the Crimean War (Amos-Taylor and Elberson, 1989). A landmark publication was Nightingale's *Notes on Nursing* (1859), which was specifically aimed at professionally trained nurses, and the establishment of the Nightingale School of Nursing in 1860. In addition, Nightingale was responsible for seeking to emphasize the relationship between nursing as a profession and as a specialization, and did so by highlighting the difference between hired untrained workers and practitioners who had been prepared at St Thomas' Hospital in London (Castledine, 1994). Nightingale (1859) also observed that it was 'not uncommon, in small country hospitals to have a recess or a small room leading from the operating theatre; in which patients remain until they have recovered from the immediate effects of the operation'. Implicit in this was the recognition that patients needed to be cared for by nurses who were prepared with a distinct set of skills for closer observation. Moreover, as surgical techniques and interventions evolved, hospitals began to design recovery rooms, special care units, and cubicles to contain infectious patients. Thus the term 'specialist' began to be applied to nurses who had experience of these fields (Amos-Taylor and Elberson, 1989).

Like medicine, specialization within nursing began to grow during Nightingale's era. Subsequent world conflicts resulting in other developments in, for example, resuscitation, triage, and surgical and anaesthetic techniques, demanded that nurses should acquire additional clinical expertise to care for the victims of war (Menard, 1987). It was, however, the Nurses' Registration Act of 1919 that first formally divided nursing into four specialties, namely: sick children, mental nursing, care of the mentally handicapped, and fever nursing, although specialty in this sense related to the skills and knowledge associated with a particular medical disorder or disease process (Castledine, 1994).

The ensuing provision of different training courses that were open to recruits entering the profession can in itself be viewed as an acknowledgement that meeting the demands of a changing population required nurses who were prepared according to specialist educational programmes.

Indeed, qualification and appointment to staff nurse, on whatever part of the register, meant, in the view of Kratz (1976), being on the road to specialization. Kratz did, however, make the distinction that a specialist working in a particular field of medicine did not equate with the range of responsibilities, knowledge, expertise and authority associated with a CNS role.

The title of CNS, while originally American, had been introduced and adopted by the RCN (1975). However, notions of advanced nursing practice remained implicit in the role (Castledine, 1992). The growth of specialization and clinical expertise was equally due to progress in health care technology, and as a result of patient treatments becoming more sophisticated and elaborate, which, in turn, led to the division of medicine into specialties (Castledine, 1982; Menard, 1987). This was rapidly followed by the creation of specialist wards or care units. As a consequence of nurses practising in such areas, their skills and knowledge were enhanced and their perspectives on patient care more focused. In response to these develop- ments, demands for nursing expertise increased, as did the recognition of the content embedded in clinical nursing (Castledine, 1982). Stemming from these changes, nurses' traditional roles began to extend and expand into new spheres, although, in many instances, these were discarded technical skills and/or responsibilities that were traditionally exclusive to medicine. Measuring blood pressure was the earliest example, although a more significant development, perhaps, was when nurses undertook intravenous drug administration. More recent examples include such skills as venous cannulation, defibrillation, electrocardiography and urethral catheteriza- tion.

Weston (1975) points out that in the USA, with regard to the community services, roles such as paediatric NPs and physician assistants emerged as a result of new medical graduates pursuing a hospital based career rather than entering general practice, which, in turn, left the family health care services without the necessary medical resources. Subsequently, concern was expressed about the possible loss of nursing core values, as it was uncertain that nursing care was consistently incorporated into such roles, since nurses were being trained according to a medical model of treatment. Weston (1975) questioned whether these developments were legitimate areas for the profession, as it seemed that nurses in these roles were being utilized as a means of cost containment and to ameliorate service deficiencies. It is interesting to note that support for these roles, and that of the CNS, was forthcoming by some physicians who viewed such innovations as complementary to medicine and a further opportunity to collaborate and improve patient care (Bates, 1970). More recently, with the projected shortage of physicians entering medicine, the American College of Physicians (1994) has also reiterated its commitment to supporting the need for collaboration and for the regulated expansion of NPs and physician assistants.

With regard to the UK, the development of specialist nursing practice can be in part ascribed to the innovations of some key centres. The Royal Marsden Hospital, for example, was one of the earliest institutions to appreciate the need for specialization, and thus began to educate the nurses working there with the relevant skills and knowledge to enable them directly to meet the increasingly complex needs of patients and instigate innovations to improve the provision of care (Tiffany, 1984; Markham, 1988). Moreover, there was an emphasis on continuing education, which was viewed not as 'a luxury for the privileged few, but rather a necessity for advanced nursing practice' (Tiffany, 1984). These CNSs were also expected to incorporate research and educational functions, as well as provide advice when consulted. The specific areas where such roles were developed included intravenous therapy, nutritional support, stoma care, community liaison, infection control and care of the terminally ill (Tiffany, 1984; Wilson-Barnett, 1985).

Throughout the UK, nurse specialism spread across many settings. In most cases, however, nurses were only providing technical competence with prescribed procedures or tasks, rarely with an opportunity for forging new directions in clinical nursing. In reality, as nurse specialists, they were either relieving the work of doctors or had chosen to specialize in certain aspects of nursing rather than within the clinical setting (Thompson and Webster, 1986).

Other pioneering roles evolved from the Bethlem and Maudsley Hospitals, where the nurse therapist became established in answer to progress made in behavioural psychotherapy (Castledine, 1991a). Community psychiatric nurses also began to broaden their expertise and increase their contribution to patient care. At Guy's Hospital, the liaison psychiatric nurse was one role that was introduced in response to a recognition that specialist care was required for patients who became confused, or suffered psychosis or depression after a surgical operation or illness. The postholder was regarded as an expert who was available for consultation and for advice to general nurses. While this particular innovation did not receive the wide publicity (Wilson-Barnett, 1985) of those cited by Tiffany (1984), they were nevertheless all perceived as examples of advanced practice, as each was effectively breaking new ground in nursing.

Head (1988) described one of the forerunning specialist roles in the accident and emergency department in the guise of a NP whose purpose was to assess, treat and refer patients, utilizing individual nursing knowledge and skills to enhance the quality of services. However, this role arose to a great degree from the external pressures of deficiencies in service provision and a need to ensure the effective use of manpower resources.

In the opinion of Wilson-Barnett (1985), advanced nursing roles were about improving the well-being of patients and meeting any inadequacies within health care. Thus, the 1970s and 1980s witnessed the proliferation of clinical specialization in the health service. This, in turn, appeared to mandate that nurses working in specialist units/departments should be equipped with a combination of attributes that involved clinical expertise and additional education in order to deliver sophisticated and advanced care, as well as improve standards of practice. By implication, this seemed to denote a distinct level of practitioner.

In spite of the above, the adoption of a specialist ideology within nursing has not been smooth. In the past, many in the profession have felt threatened or have sought to control the growth of specialisms and professional education by adhering to a generalist view of nursing as a practical occupation (Dulfer, 1981; White, 1985). Others, for example

Chapman (1983), have argued that the specialization of nurses would potentially fragment the care of patients rather than augment the holistic concept. For Thompson and Webster (1986), there was an equal risk that future clinical nurse specialisms may arise from 'medically derived or politically instigated need' as opposed to a nursing core. Additionally, some claimed that specialists resented sharing their knowledge, jealously guarding it and using it principally as a source of power and status (Chapman, 1983). Similarly, Georgopoulos and Christman (1970) had earlier warned that the manner in which the role developed should not relate to the degree of specialist knowledge, but to the abilities and personality of each individual in motivating and collaborating in their commitment to innovation. Yet, as White (1985) notes, the generalist view of nursing opposed the acquisition of additional education as well as the development of professional accountability, preferring practitioners to have a broad knowledge base. This contrasted with the interests of the specialist lobby, who, through academic study, sought to develop beyond first level registration, increase their clinical competence, and deepen their knowledge within their chosen field, as well as achieve professional autonomy and accountability for their practice (White, 1985).

Apart from internal mechanisms, specialties in nursing have also arisen in response to a number of other factors. Economic constraints, cultural diversity, changing patterns in health care needs (HIV, for example), and the increased age of many within the population, have collectively affected the provision and delivery of health services. Similarly, national priorities such as *The Health of the Nation* (Department of Health (DoH), 1992) have led to specialty roles being forged in order to meet the needs of patients with heart disease or strokes, or those affected by cancer. Such roles now include rehabilitation and palliative nursing. In more technical areas, perhaps as a result of financial and efficiency drives, nurses are now able surgically to remove veins in preparation for coronary artery bypass grafting (Holmes, 1994) as well as insert central venous lines (Hamilton et. al., 1995). However, as will be seen later, these developments only cloud the issue further when attempting to unravel the essence of advanced nursing practice.

Academic and clinical initiatives

Running parallel with global specialization (Handy, 1985), British nursing also witnessed a number of clinical and academic initiatives that were inspired by Manchester University and the Manchester Royal Infirmary (MRI). This impetus was directed by a growing awareness that, with clinical promotion, expert nurses either lost contact or were rarely able to participate in direct patient care (Castledine, 1982; Pearson, 1983). The work of Biddulph (1976) was an important clinical landmark. In this project, three experienced sisters based at the MRI were supported in advancing their existing roles as clinical specialists in the areas of orthopaedics, psychiatric liaison and neurosurgical nursing. Concurrently, the department of nursing at Manchester was actively pursuing the development of practice through the introduction of the nursing process, nursing models, nursing curriculum and master's degree courses in clinical nursing (Castledine, 1991a, 1994).

Prior to this, clinical practice and educational programmes had been dominated by the achievement of tasks, traditions, administration and a medicalized framework of care based on disease management. With the implementation of the nursing process and models of care, the visibility of clinical nursing began to increase (for example, McFarlane and Castledine, 1982; Webb, 1986). Nurses began to adopt ward philosophies in order to make explicit their perceptions about nursing and their role, the nature of their patients, and health-related needs that underpinned their approach to nursing care (Wright, 1986). Coupled with this, an emphasis on collaborative partnerships with patients and the need for individualized care became a professional priority. As a result of the close links between the MRI and Manchester University, joint appointments were established in 1980, an idea that was later taken up in other centres (Tiffany, 1984; Wright, 1986).

As the demand for CNSs escalated, Castledine (1982) set out to examine their role in the UK. In his research, CNSs were questioned by means of a Delphi technique, with some additional more detailed data being generated from a subset of respondents by interview. The data analysis generated 11 factors that were considered necessary to the role of the CNS (Table 1.1), although it is interesting to note that only a few of the respondents in the study fulfilled all the criteria.

Table 1.1. Criteria for the CNS role (after Castledine, 1982)

1. Continued involvement in direct patient care
2. Directly responsible and accountable for nursing actions
3. Ideally should be clinically educated above registration level and possess a bachelor of nursing degree, but preferably a masters degree
4. Involved with clinical nursing research
5. Involved in education programmes and have teaching responsibilities that may include patients, relatives and any member of the health care team
6. Able to co-ordinate care with other health care professionals, or lead the organization of a patient's total health care
7. Should be expert in the nursing process approach to nursing care
8. Viewed as an expert by peers and thus able to act in a consultant capacity
9. Has freedom and flexibility within the role
10. Is actively engaged in and concerned with the dissemination of practice through publication and conferences
11. Act in a liaison capacity between hospital and community

What was evident from this investigation was the recognition that there were no national guidelines on professional preparation for such posts, nor was there a system for rewarding higher levels of clinical practice; indeed, some CNSs held low-paid positions. With regard to the suggested educational preparation, only a few facilities offered a masters programme with a clinical option, thus a postbasic course and a diploma in nursing were viewed as more realistic achievements. This position had been previously reached by the RCN (1975).

In other spheres, Pearson (1983) and Wright (1986), also from Manchester, pioneered innovations in practice. The Burford Clinical

Nursing Unit was successfully established by Pearson with the aim of providing a holistic approach to nursing care, led and managed by nurses. This was also realized by the implementation of primary nursing, which was viewed as a means of enhancing the quality of care, and considered well-suited to enabling nurses to build closer therapeutic relationships with patients. It was also an approach that allowed the devolvement of autonomy and accountability to those making decisions for the patient's well-being. Pearson's view of advanced clinical roles was linked with the growing professionalism taking place within nursing, as well as with increasing opportunities for independent practice and for decision making (Pearson, 1983). However, for him, the vision of the clinical nurse consultant was more appealing, and was differentiated from the CNS by virtue that the former worked independently as a specialist in nursing, whereas the latter worked in collaboration, concerned with the care of patients under medical treatment.

Pearson (1983) also supported the introduction of a clinical nursing structure, which was conceived as a means of preserving the expertise of senior nurses at ward level, enabling the contribution of these individuals to the quality of patient care to be formally recognized and celebrated in terms of status and financial remuneration. In summary, Pearson speculated that advanced practitioners, in the role of clinical nurse consultants, should be: engaged in teaching and supervision; concerned with the forward movement of nursing practice; improving techniques for solving patient problems; and providing professional advice as requested. It was, however, the expansion of nursing horizons that would ensure that nurses could work towards independent practice.

Meanwhile, Wright (1986) was working with similar concepts at the Tameside Development Unit, where he pursued the ideal of the consultant nurse as an advanced practice role. He suggested a registered nurse, qualified as a teacher with higher academic profile, who would be a provider of clinical excellence and expertise similar to the professional responsibilities identified by Castledine (1983) and Pearson (1983). Wright (1986) equally stressed the roles of change agent and educationalist as essential for advancing nursing practice. In addition, he promoted personalized care by redefining the bureaucratic model of care into a professional one in which clinical practice was central, and where nursing care was planned systematically in partnership with the patient and the nurse, who would assume accountability for all decisions. Such innovations in practice were key milestones in the development of advanced nursing practice, and were described as 'new nursing' (Salvage, 1990), as they had begun to challenge the accepted orthodoxy of nursing care provision.

It is worth noting that during this period, the drive that was leading these nursing initiatives was a philosophy that was embedded in the practice of nursing. Another feature of 'new nursing', spearheaded solely by practitioners, was that some clinical developments had impacted on the political agenda. Most notable of these were the adoption of primary nursing (DoH, 1989) and the named nurse concept (Wright, 1992). Additionally, the impact of the dynamic standards project (RCN, 1990), nursing development units, and the integration of a culture that fostered individualism, collaboration and sensitive nursing, contributed to transform the delivery of nursing care. Perhaps more importantly, the 1980s accentuated the growing strength and scope of clinical practice and nurtured a vision of wider possibilities for practitioners. It was an era that reclaimed and exhorted the values of clinical excellence, creative nursing care and patient centred approaches.

More recently, at the University of Central England (formerly the Birmingham School), ongoing evaluation of their masters programme in advanced nursing practice (Brown, 1995), and of national trends, continues (McGee et al., 1997), an association of Specialist Nurses and Advanced Nursing Practitioners has been established, and a new clinical career structure in nursing, which would enable practitioners to progress to the level of advanced nurse practitioner, has been proposed (Castledine, 1997).

Royal College of Nursing

The RCN has been a key forerunner in promoting the case for advanced nursing practice and for a clinical nursing structure. It was in 1971 that the RCN (RCN, 1975) first put forward submissions to the Committee on Nursing (DHSS, 1972) that roles such as the clinical nurse consultant should be introduced to exploit the wide contribution of nurses to the profession, and to enhance further the quality of care in an era of change and specialization. In addition, the proposals made reference to the need to provide a promotion ladder for clinical staff and the type of preparation required. However, the committee made no specific recommendations regarding the nurse consultant role; instead, it acknowledged the diverse contribution and increasing responsibilities of ward sisters, suggesting that they should be accorded increased status and reward.

Much of the opposition to nurse consultants was based on the misconceptions of nurse managers, educationalists and some practitioners. As a result, the RCN set up a working party to investigate the usefulness of these roles. The working party accepted its terms of reference with minor alterations, which included changing the title of 'clinical nurse consultant' to 'clinical nurse specialist', and, with evidence gathered from a seminar held at Leeds Castle in Kent, produced a short document entitled New Horizons in Clinical Nursing (RCN, 1975). Contained within were discussions about why the profession was in need of bedside experts, and it pointed to the failure of the Salmon management structure (Ministry of Health and Scottish Home and Health Department, 1966) to implement a framework that would promote the value of clinical roles. Indeed, the introduction of the nursing officer grade only served to distance the postholders away from patient care by an overemphasis on the management role at the expense of clinical activity. The additional confusion regarding the responsibilities relating to the role of a nursing officer led to dissatisfaction amongst many at a time when standards of patient care were deteriorating; thus, the need for a senior clinical leader was viewed as mandatory (Ashworth, 1975).

Following study of existing senior grades of nurses, Kerrane (1975) concluded that only the clinical teacher had the potential of becoming a CNS, although even this was uncertain. However, in the role of CNS, an individual would be required to improve/maintain high standards of patient care by direct participation, liaison and consultation. To convert this ideal into reality, it was duly articulated that for CNSs to succeed, it was imperative that they should be suitably qualified and carefully appointed. Additionally, they should have the freedom, flexibility and necessary support in pursuit of their objectives (Ashworth, 1975). In terms of the desirable qualities for the role, substantial clinical expertise, a nationally validated certificate from the Joint Board of Clinical Studies (established in 1972) relating to the nurse's particular field of practice, and a diploma in nursing, were regarded as necessary. Once in post, it was speculated that the CNS would promote the understanding of core nursing values (which were to some extent perceived to be under threat) among other health care professionals. The findings of the seminar were presented to the Department of Health and Social Security, with the recommendation that more work needed to be undertaken.

Later, in their expression over safeguarding standards of care, an RCN (1980) discussion paper continued to endorse clinical specialists. For the RCN (1980), in order to improve the quality of service provision, it was desirable that nurses should be armed with the skills of assessing, planning, implementation and evaluation. While the ward sister was recognized as the lynch pin, and most able to set, implement and monitor standards of care, the recommendations of the working party suggested that avenues should be considered for enhancing and expanding this role in terms of a clinical career structure that could facilitate the establishment of posts such as clinical nurse consultant. Thus, in summary, the RCN (1980) was reflecting views that had been expressed earlier (RCN, 1975). In a follow-up paper, Towards a New Professional Structure for Nursing (RCN, 1983), it was emphasized that a greater need for knowledge was necessary in nursing, as this would enable practitioners to become systematic and analytical in their practice and thus contribute to the quality of patient care. However, as Fulbrook (1996) notes, while the document proffered a new vision of a clinical career structure, it was notable that descriptions of advanced nursing practice were absent. This was disappointing, as only a year earlier the College had published a proposal for advanced clinical roles (RCN, 1982).

Amid the continued proliferation of specialist roles and concerns about the misuse of titles, the RCN responded by convening a group charged with investigating the development of specialties in nursing, as well as providing criteria that would distinguish the nurse specialist from other roles (RCN, 1988). The arguments put forward for having nurse specialists were linked to the increased and diverse knowledge base of nursing and the need to integrate further a broader theoretical basis into practice. It is interesting to note that no reference was made to previous work, or to the roles of a clinical nurse consultant or a CNS. The document stated:

> Nurse specialists are experts in a particular aspect of nursing care...they demonstrate refined clinical practice, either as a result of significant experience or advanced expertise, or knowledge in a branch or specialty...Specialist practice involves a clinical and consultative role, teaching, management, research and the application of relevant nursing research. Only if a nurse is involved in all of these is [he or] she a specialist (RCN, 1988).

It was reasoned that nurse specialists would bring about significant changes and co-ordinate clinical practice, and that their authority would stem from clinical credibility and managerial expertise, as well as from their position within the team. Moreover, in order to demonstrate advanced clinical practice, continuing education relating to the role was considered to be vital. However, it was also concluded that due to a lack of a 'formally recognised position for the nurse specialist within the present structure... it is difficult to recognise who is functioning in this role' (RCN, 1988). Wide professional discussion followed publication of the document. However, a small study conducted in the late 1980s reported continuing misconceptions regarding specialist nurse functions from both managers and practitioners: 'Many of the job descriptions were compiled by rather unknowledgeable managers who described the role as they would like to see it without consulting a CNS first' (Stafford, 1991).

Political and professional influences

According to Castledine (1991a, 1994), various government reforms endorsed the role of clinical nurses, whereas the Department of Health sought possibilities to enable specialist nurses to be recognized. The Royal Commission on the NHS (DHSS, 1979) pressed for an improved career structure and suggested that there should be greater rewards available in clinical nursing and that these should be accorded on the basis of developing expertise and increased responsibility for decision making.

Within the community, Stilwell (1982) promoted the alternative, yet complementary, role of the NP as a means of assisting general practitioners in meeting the primary health care needs of patients. In this role, patients were able to seek consultations with NPs, who performed some physical examinations and provided health education on a range of conditions. They were also able to offer some treatments according to written guidelines. Stilwell (1982) acknowledged that this new independent role was challenging the traditional boundaries of nursing and medicine. Similarly, Andrews (1988) emphasized that district nurses were providing a specialist service in terms of giving direct care, co-ordinating service provision, demonstrating consultancy skills and prescribing treatment. Amongst the examples of autonomous practice achieved by highly experienced and educated nurses, Andrews (1988) lists initiating well-woman/man clinics, instigating treatments, conducting pelvic and breast examinations, and obtaining cervical smears, all of which combined relevant aspects of health education and promotion.

The drive for advanced practice roles within the community setting reflected the aspirations of the Cumberlege Report (DoH, 1986), which had given firm support for the growth of a limited number of autonomous nurse practitioners, who, with the appropriate advanced skills of health promotion, diagnosis and treatment of disease, would be able to provide a comprehensive range of, and access to, health care services. The impetus for this and other similar roles was a deficiency in the service, changing health care trends, and a lack of appropriately qualified doctors (Trnobranski, 1994). However, nurses who had attained this calibre of practice were both well-placed to serve the community and those who were most disadvantaged regarding access to health care, and able to assist in the implementation of national and international priorities for health promotion (Trnobranski, 1994).

With the disciplines of district nursing, health visiting, school nursing and community midwifery becoming part of the health service in the mid-1970s, interprofessional divisions became less evident, and are now, with other established branches, part of community health care nursing (UKCC, 1994). Prior to this, Butterworth (1988) had reasoned that an integrated team approach bringing all eight community-based specialties together would allow community practice to develop and stimulate innovation in all areas. This would require the provision of a career structure to retain clinically based experts who could then encourage excellence in practice (Butterworth, 1988).

The Heathrow Debate (DoH, 1994) indicated that, as primary health care widens in scope, opportunities for nurses with the appropriate blend of skills and expertise will be recognized and demanded by a number of health care workers. This document indicated that the number of specialist nurses in the community should be balanced with generalist teams, but that it was important that nurses should be able to prepare themselves for a constantly changing environment. A more recent government initiative suggests that there should be greater scope for professional and personal achievement, as well as career opportunities for those based in primary settings (DoH, 1997). Presumably, this is in recognition that nurses are now better qualified and better able to exercise appropriate discretionary judgements and autonomy (Morrall, 1997) when entering into areas traditionally within the domain of medicine, such as nurse-led minor injury and rehabilitation clinics, nurse-led specialist services, for example, in respiratory care and dermatology, and nurse prescribing.

The implementation of community based roles has also seen the provision of a range of other specialist services that benefit patients and other professionals (Layzell and McCarthy, 1993; Briggs, 1997). Inevitably, the Government has been keen to support nurses in the expansion of their roles, since, in doing so, the quality and the effectiveness of community services should be enhanced. However, it has been assumed that new education programmes of preparation will embrace the expanded roles so that nurses can play a wider role and function as specialists in community health (DoH, 1997).

Government affirmation for clinical role development and structures that would enhance 'care provision and realise the potential for clinical practice' (DoH, 1989) was stated towards the end of the decade in the wake of Project 2000 (UKCC, 1986). A *Strategy for Nursing* went a little further by recommending that the 'contribution of specialist practitioners should be explored and developed' (DoH, 1989). It was also assumed that each of the nursing disciplines would have its own advanced practitioners, who would be engaged in the care of patients, available for advice, and actively contributing to education, training and research activities. This was a major step forward, particularly following the publication of the *NHS Management Inquiry* (DHSS, 1983), which had effectively resulted in the voice of nursing being diluted at executive level, with hierarchies undergoing reorganization, and an era of imposed general management, which lasted most of the decade. This is nowhere more evident than in the words of Sargeant (1985), whose CNS role arose following the 1983 health service reorganization: 'My responsibilities give me few chances to nurse patients myself.' Management and administrative duties appeared to limit her clinical remit, and, for Fulbrook (1996), this role had a bias towards management rather than direct patient care, possibly reflecting the dominant ideology at that time.

Perhaps the most disappointing government publication was *A Vision for the Future* (DoH, 1993a), which, apart from suggesting that all nurses progress professionally, adds that some clinicians may develop roles as independent practitioners, providing services through private care. Clearly, the emphasis in this report was on health service policy initiatives and their achievement, though it may be reasoned that the fulfilment of these and other national health targets may be realistically and effectively expedited by the presence and contribution of advanced nurse practitioners.

In contrast, since the UKCC became established, it has, through various professional documents, recognized the expertise of practitioners. Castledine (1991a) acknowledges the progress made in stating that the Council 'has opened the door to further expansion and development in clinical practice'. Other policies and documents, such as the *Code of Professional Conduct* (UKCC, 1984) and the *Scope of Professional Practice* (UKCC, 1992) have stressed the increased responsibility and accountability of each registered nurse in assuring excellence in the delivery of care. Implicit within the latter, the Council empowered nurses to broaden and adjust the boundaries of professional practice with the proviso that any such expansion of their role was in response and relevant to patients' needs.

Coupled with the earlier professional educational reforms (UKCC, 1986) and later initiatives in practice development (Wright, 1992), the research of Benner (1984) drew attention to the fact that nursing expertise in the management of patient care was variable, and that nurses were not interchangeable. Indeed, the education, clinical experience and skills of practitioners meant that individuals practised at distinct levels of competency that were characterized by mastery in discerning accurately the priorities of a situation, making professional judgements, and decision making. On the strength of mounting evidence and recognition that patients with unique needs require nurses with specialist skills, the PREP report (UKCC, 1990) proposed a model of professional practice that added weight to the conviction that clinical expertise varied according to an individual's state of professional development, and officially acknowledged that advanced nursing practice was a legitimate sphere of practice.

Initially, the proposals advocated a career structure comprising three distinct areas of practice, thus enabling a newly qualified nurse at primary level to proceed to advanced practice and finally (for an elite few) to consultant level. This would be on the basis of clinical expertise and academic achievements (UKCC, 1990). The rationale for this approach was the desire to offer nurses a practice based, but academically credible, pathway for future progression, which would add coherence to postregistration educational provision. Past models of professional education had encouraged the duplication of studies, which were often unrecognized or not credited by other professionals. The project report indicated that there would not be a registrable qualification linked with the consultant level of practice, and, although the vision was there, the terms of reference for the consultant nurse were rather vague. Possibly because it was such a new, unorthodox role, the professional body itself was uncertain what educational characteristics or clinical experience were required for this level of practice. The recommendations contained in the PREP report were widely discussed (Cole, 1991) and contested, but were finally approved with the publication of *The Future of Professional Practice* (UKCC, 1994).

The newly demarcated areas of clinical nursing included professional and specialist levels, as well as the sphere of advanced nursing practice, which:

is not an additional layer of practice to be superimposed on specialist nursing practice. It is, rather, a description of an important sphere of professional practice which is concerned with the continuing development of the professions in the interest of patients, clients and health services (UKCC, 1994).

General descriptions of the expectations associated with each level were provided, including the level of education required to progress. With regard to advanced nursing practice, it was stressed that individuals should be concerned with adjusting the boundaries of future practice, pioneering and developing new roles that were responsive to the changing health needs of the population, as well as exploring new avenues for clinical practice, research and education that would enhance professional practice. Although the domain of advanced nursing practice was not to be accorded registration, it was proposed that the level of educational preparation should equate with a masters degree.

The UKCC (1994) clearly recognized that the advanced practitioner role was critical in order to further clinical practice developments, not only as a means of establishing new horizons in clinical practice but also to serve the public and the health service in a more effective manner. In many ways, the profession was responding to increased pressures, which expected nursing practice to be comprehensive, systematic and value for money (Casey, 1991; Boylan, 1992). However, there was no blueprint to support the realization of the advanced practitioner role, and there was neither a professional nor a clinical framework for its development. It seemed that by avoiding being prescriptive, the Council appeared to many as being uncertain about how to progress.

Fulbrook (1994) was one of the few whose research sought to tackle various questions and related issues about the nature and scope of advanced nursing practice from the perspective of the practitioners themselves, concluding that advanced practice was 'a complex composite of knowledge and experience applied in a unique way according to each situation through the medium of the self...the advanced practitioner'. Two years later, Holyoake (1996) argued that advanced nursing practice should not be about seeking to shift the boundaries of practice, but rather that it should strive to push beyond them with the key aim of legitimizing nursing as a profession in its own right. On a more practical level, Sparacino (1992) suggested that the skills of the advanced nurse would include conducting comprehensive assessments and diagnoses, formulating strategies, and implementing treatment for a wide range of conditions or situations. Furthermore, these nurses would be differentiated from others by their ability to discern priorities rapidly. They would combine their knowledge of the range of social, biological and psychological variables related to the patient to inform their professional judgement.

Other nurse theorists from a range of settings have proposed models that have variously attempted to analyse and illuminate the nature and competencies congruent with advanced nursing practice, and endeavoured to identify the conditions that may facilitate the integration of advanced roles into clinical practice (Jukes, 1996; Albarran and Whittle, 1997; Manley, 1997). Central to these examples has been cognizance of the nursing perspective, which must embrace every feature of patient treatment or care. This belief is that, unlike in many new clinical posts whose expansion has been through the medicalization of nursing practice, the essence of advanced nursing practice is in the *nursing* role (Smith, 1995; Manley, 1996).

The current situation has been confounded by the promotion of medical models of advanced practice. This thrust has been attributed in part to the reduction in junior doctors' hours (DoH, 1993b) and in part to a need to control escalating costs, to such an extent that nurses have been trained to develop the skills to assume the on-call rota job of junior doctors (McDougall, 1994). The development of such roles has been supported by government task force funds, and has most frequently been associated with nurse practitioner posts. This momentum has portrayed a false impression about the competencies and ideals linked with advanced nursing practice. What is equally relevant is that this trend has been seen as stifling opportunities for practice and displacing the unique vision of nursing (English and Lindsay, 1993; Holyoake, 1996). However, a recent study has highlighted the legal ramifications and raised questions of the professional accountability of nurses in assuming these quasi-medical posts (Dowling et al., 1996). Not only is it argued that values at the heart of nursing are being compromised, but there are warnings that:

> while the traditional margins between health care disciplines begin to disappear, nurses must not lose sight of the fact that skilled specialist and advanced nursing is not about performing technical tasks but about delivering holistic patient care, a challenge that is far more demanding to fulfil . . . it is the benefit of intelligently planned nursing intervention rather than the performance of certain handed down technical skills that create a more lasting impression for the patient and their families (Albarran, 1996).

Conclusion

Historically, a point has been reached in which the sum and substance of advanced nursing practice has to be made explicit, otherwise there is a risk that political forces or medico-economic agendas will either hijack or redirect the concept away from a nursing paradigm. Clearly, without the input of all health care professionals, it is likely that neither will the role of the advanced nurse practitioner gain the recognition it rightly warrants nor will the nature of advanced nursing practice encompass the broad philosophical values embodied within nursing. The visionary ideal of advanced practice, achieved through educational and experiential preparation, may be lost. Shaping the destiny of advanced nursing practice should be viewed as an urgent priority as the profession enters the next millennium, since the decisions of today will determine the clinical practice of tomorrow.

The struggle for advanced nursing practice has been neither coherent nor deliberate, with progress being influenced by a number of internal and external forces, some of which have hampered recognition, whilst others have promoted the motives and wide benefits of advanced nursing practice. The positive drive has been propelled by a need to acknowledge and celebrate the impact that clinical nursing initiatives have on the development of high quality patient care, which goes hand in hand with meeting NHS objectives.

It has recently been suggested that advanced nursing practice may be 'the engine room for moving nursing into the 21st century' (Holyoake, 1996). However, a failure by the nursing profession to take control and to capitalize on accumulated professional strengths will openly invite others to assume the driving seat, and thus the collective efforts of the past will not have been served well.

From the history outlined above, it is clear that there is still little real understanding about the nature of advanced practice and the role of the advanced practitioner, not just in the UK, but throughout the developed world. Nursing has yet to answer two fundamental questions: 'What is advanced practice?', and 'What is an advanced practitioner?' We hope that the following chapters will go some way towards providing the answers.

References

Albarran, J. W. (1996). Exploring the nature of informed consent in coronary care practice. *Nurs. Crit. Care*, 1, 127–132.

Albarran, J. W. and Whittle, C. (1997). An analysis of professional, specialist and advanced nursing practice in critical care. *Nurse Educ. Today*, 17, 72–79.

American College of Physicians. (1994). Physician assistants and nurse practitioners. *Ann. Int. Med.*, 12, 714–716.

American Nurses Association. (1976). *The Scope of Nursing Practice*. Cited in Briody, M. E. (1996). The future of the clinical nurse specialist in the USA. *Int. Nurs. Rev.*, 43(1), 17–20, 31–32.

American Nurses Association. (1980). *Congress for Nursing Practice: a Social Policy Statement*. Kansas City, MO: ANA.

Amos-Taylor, R. P. and Elberson, K. (1989). Quality care: the emerging role of the CNS. *Crit. Care Nurse*, 9(4), 28–37.

Andrews, S. (1988). An expert in practice. *Nurs. Times*, 84, 31–32.

Ashworth, P. (1975). The clinical nurse consultant. *Nurs. Times*, 71(15), 574–577.

Barrie-Shevlin, P. (1985). Creativity, enthusiasm, diplomacy. *Nurs. Mirror*, 160(20), 46–47.

Bates, B. (1970). Doctor and nurse: changing roles and relations. *N. Engl. J. Med.*, 383, 129–134.

Benner, P. (1984). *From novice to expert: excellence and power in clinical nursing practice*. Menlo Park, CA: Addison-Wesley.

Biddulph, C. (1976). The clinical specialist. In *Nurses and Health Care*. (E. Lucas, ed.) London: King Edward's Hospital Fund.

Boylan, A. (1992). Prove your worth. *Nurs. Times*, 88(1), 28–29.

Briggs, M. (1997). Developing nursing roles. *Nurs. Stand.*, 11(36), 49–55.

Brown, R. (1995). Education for specialist and advanced practice. *Br. J. Nurs.*, **4**, 266–268.

Butterworth, T. (1988). Breaking the boundaries. *Nurs. Times*, **84**(47), 36–39.

Casey, N. (1992). A vexed question of value. *Nurs. Stand.*, **6**(37), 3.

Castledine, G. (1982). *The Role and Function of Clinical Nurse Specialists in England and Wales* [thesis]. Manchester: University of Manchester.

Castledine, G. (1983). The nurse for the job. *Nurs. Mirror*, **156**(3), 63.

Castledine, G. (1991a). The advanced nurse practitioner, part 1. *Nurs. Stand.*, **5**(43), 34–36.

Castledine, G. (1991b). The advanced nurse practitioner, part 2. *Nurs. Stand.*, **5**(44), 33–35.

Castledine, G. (1992). The advanced practitioner. *Nursing*, **5**(7), 14–15.

Castledine, G. (1994). Specialist and advanced nursing and the scope of practice. In *Expanding the Role of the Nurse: the Scope of Professional Practice*. (G. Hunt and P. Wainwright, eds.) pp. 101–113 London: Blackwell Scientific.

Castledine, G. (1997). Framework for a clinical career structure in nursing. *Br. J. Nurs.*, **6**, 264–271.

Chapman, C. (1983). The paradox of nursing. *J. Adv. Nurs.*, **8**, 269–272.

Cole, A. (1991). Advance to go? *Nurs. Times*, **87**(7), 48–49.

Department of Health. (Cumberlege Report, 1986). *Neighbourhood Nursing – A focus for Care*. (Report of the Community Nursing Review.) London: HMSO.

Department of Health. (1989). *A Strategy for Nursing*. London: HMSO.

Department of Health. (1992). *The Health of the Nation: a Strategy for Health in England*. London: HMSO.

Department of Health. (1993a). *A Vision for the Future*. London: National Health Service Management Executive.

Department of Health. (1993b). *Hospital doctors: Training for the Future*. (Report of the Working Group on Specialist Medical Training.) London: HMSO.

Department of Health. (1994). *The Challenges for Nursing and Midwifery in the 21st Century – The Heathrow Debate*. London: HMSO.

Department of Health. (1997). *Primary Care: Delivering the Future*. London: HMSO.

Department of Health and Social Security. (Briggs Report, 1972). *Report of the Committee on Nursing*. London: HMSO.

Department of Health and Social Security. (1979). *Report of the Royal Commission on the National Health Service*. London: HMSO.

Department of Health and Social Security. (1983). *NHS Management Inquiry*. London: HMSO.

Dowling, S., Martin, R., Skidmore, P. et al. (1996). Nurses taking on junior doctors' work: a confusion of accountability. *Br. Med. J.*, **312**, 1211–1214.

Duberley, J. (1976). The clinical nurse specialist. *Nurs. Times*, **72**, 1794–1795.

Dulfer, S. (1981). Danger: specialists at work. *J. Community Nurs.*, **5**(1), 2.

English, I. and Lindsay, G. (1993). Task orientated hospital workers threaten the role of nurses. *Br. J. Nurs.*, **2**, 643–645.

Fulbrook, P. (1994). *Advanced Practice and the Advanced Practitioner: an Emic Perspective* [dissertation]. Manchester: Royal College of Nursing/Manchester University.

Fulbrook, P. (1996). Advanced practice: do we know what it is? *Nurs. Crit. Care*, **1**(1), 9–12.

Georgopoulos, B. S. and Christman, L. (1970). The clinical nurse specialist: a role model. *Am. J. Nurs.*, **70**, 1030–1039.

Georgopoulos, B. S. and Christman, L. (1973) The clinical nurse specialist: a role model. In *The Clinical Nurse Specialist: Interpretations*. (J. P. Riehl and J. W. McVay, eds.) New York: Appleton-Century-Crofts.

Georgopoulos, B. S. and Jackson, M. (1970). Nursing Kardex behaviour in an experimental study of patient units with and without clinical nurse specialists. *Nurs. Res.*, **19**, 196–218.

Hamilton, H., O'Byrne, M. and Nicholai, L. (1995). Central lines inserted by clinical specialists. *Nurs. Times*, **91**(17), 38–39.

Hamric, A. B. (1989). *History and overview of the CNS role*. In *The Clinical Nurse Specialist in Theory and Practice*, 2nd ed. (A. B. Hamric and J. A. Spross, eds.) pp. 3–18. London: Saunders.

Hamric, A. B. and Spross, J. A. eds. (1989). *The Clinical Nurse Specialist in Theory and Practice*, 2nd ed. London: Saunders.

Handy, C. (1985). *Understanding Organisations*, 3rd ed. London: Penguin.

Head, S. (1988). Nurse practitioners: the new pioneers. *Nurs. Times*, **84**(26), 26–28.

Heffline, M. S. (1992). Establishing the role of the clinical nurse specialist in post-anesthesia care. *J. Post-Anesth. Nurs.*, **7**, 305–311.

Holmes, S. (1994). Development of the cardiac surgeon assistant. *Br. J. Nurs.*, **3**, 204–210.

Holyoake, D. (1996). Medicine is still big brother. *Nurs. Stand.*, **10**(28), 11.

Jukes, M. (1996). Advanced practice within learning disability nursing. *Br. J. Nurs.*, **5**, 14–27.

Kerrane, T. (1975). *Role relations*. In *New Horizons in Clinical Nursing*. (Royal College of Nursing.) London: RCN.

Kersley, K. (1992). The clinical nurse specialist – a personal perspective. *Intensive Crit. Care Nurs.*, **8**, 71–75.

Kratz, C. (1976). The clinical nurse consultant. *Nurs. Times*, **72**, 1792–1793.

Layzell, S. and McCarthy, M. (1993). Specialist or generic community nursing care for HIV/ AIDS patients? *J. Adv. Nurs.*, **18**, 531–537.

Lewis, E. P. ed. (1970). *The Clinical Nurse Specialist*. New York: American Journal of Nursing Company.

Lloyd-Jones, N. (1993). The lecturer–practitioner role and the development of intensive care nursing practice. *Intensive Crit. Care Nurs.*, **9**, 232–236.

Manley, K. (1996). Advanced practice is not about medicalising nursing roles. *Nurs. Crit. Care*, **1**(2), 56–57.

Manley, K. (1997). A conceptual framework for advanced practice: an action research project operationalizing an advanced practitioner/consultant role. *J. Clin. Nurs.*, **6**, 179–190.

Markham, G. (1988). Special cases. *Nurs. Times*, **84**(26), 29–30.

McDougall, J. M. (1994). The role of the neonatal practitioner. *Care Crit. Ill*, **10**, 207–209.

McFarlane, J. (1980). *Essays on Nursing*. London: King Edward's Hospital Fund.

McFarlane, J. K. and Castledine, G. (1982). *The Practice of Nursing using the Nursing Process*. London: Mosby.

McGee, P., Castledine, G. and Brown, R. (1997). A survey of specialist and advanced nursing practice in England. *Br. J. Nurs.*, **5**, 682–686.

Menard, S. (1987). *The Clinical Nurse Specialist: Perspectives on Practice*. New York: Delmar.

Ministry of Health and Scottish Home and Health Department. (Salmon Report, 1966). *Report of the Committee on Senior Nursing Staff Structure*. London: HMSO.

Morrall, P. A. (1997). Professionalism and community psychiatric nursing: a case study of four mental health teams. *J. Adv. Nurs.*, **25**, 1133–1137.

Nightingale, F. (1859). *Notes on Nursing*. London: Harrison.

Nursing and Midwifery Staff's Negotiating Council. (1988). *A Guide to the Clinical Grading Structure*. London: Macdermott and Chant.

Patterson, C. and Haddad, B. (1992). The advanced nurse practitioner: common attributes. *Can. J. Nurs. Admin.*, **5**(4), 18–22.

Pearson, A. (1983). *The Clinical Nursing Unit*. London: Heinemann.

Reiter, F. (1966). The nurse-clinician. *Am. J. Nurs.*, **66**, 274–280.

Royal College of Nursing. (1975). *New Horizons in Clinical Nursing*. London: RCN.

Royal College of Nursing. (1980). *Standards of Nursing Care: A Discussion Document*. London: RCN.

Royal College of Nursing. (1981). *Towards Standards*. London: RCN.

Royal College of Nursing. (1982). *Report of the Seminar on Advanced Clinical Roles*. London: RCN.

Royal College of Nursing. (1983). *Towards a New Professional Structure for Nursing*. London: RCN.

Royal College of Nursing. (1988). *A Report of the Working Party Investigating the Development of Specialties within the Nursing Profession*. London: RCN.

Royal College of Nursing. (1990). *Quality of Patient Care: The Dynamic Standard Setting System*. London: RCN.

Salvage, J. (1990). The theory and practice of the 'New Nursing'. *Nurs. Times*, **86**(1), 42–45.
Sargeant, L. (1985). Intensive care nursing: clinical nurse specialist, part 1. *Nurs. Mirror*, **160**(9), 24–25.
Smith, M. C. (1995). The core of advanced practice nursing. *Nurs. Sci. Q.*, **8**, 2–3.
Sparacino, P. (1986). The clinical nurse specialist. *Nurs. Pract.*, **1**, 215–228.
Sparacino, P. (1992). Advanced practice: the clinical nurse specialist. *Nurs. Pract.*, **5**(4), 2–4.
Sparacino, P., Cooper, D. and Minarik, P. (1990). *The Clinical Nurse Specialist: Implementation and Impact*. Norwalk, CT: Appleton and Lange.
Spross, J. A. and Baggerley, J. (1989). Models of advanced nursing practice. In *The Clinical Nurse Specialist in Theory and Practice*, 2nd ed. (A. B. Hamric and J. A. Spross eds.), pp. 19–40. London: Saunders.
Stafford, R. (1991). The evolution of the specialist. *Nurs. Times*, **87**(16), 39–40.
Stilwell, B. (1982). The nurse practitioner at work. *Nurs. Times*, **78**, 1799–1803.
Sutton, F. and Smith, C. (1995). Advanced nursing practice: new ideas and new perspectives. *J. Adv. Nurs.*, **21**, 1037–1043.
Thompson, D. R. and Webster, R. A. (1986). The clinical nurse specialist in critical care. *Nurs. Pract.*, **1**, 236–241.
Tiffany, R. (1984). The Marsden experience. *Nurs. Mirror*, **159**(21), 28–30.
Trnobranski, P. (1994). Nurse practitioner: redefining the role of the community nurse? *J. Adv. Nurs.*, **19**, 134–139.
United Kingdom Central Council for Nursing, Midwifery and Health Visiting. (1984). *Code of Professional Conduct*. London: UKCC.
United Kingdom Central Council for Nursing, Midwifery and Health Visiting. (1986). *Project 2000: A New Preparation for Practice*. London: UKCC.
United Kingdom Central Council for Nursing, Midwifery and Health Visiting. (1990). *Post-registration Education and Practice Project*. London: UKCC.
United Kingdom Central Council for Nursing, Midwifery and Health Visiting. (1992). *The Scope of Professional Practice*. London: UKCC.
United Kingdom Central Council for Nursing, Midwifery and Health Visiting. (1994). *The Future of Professional Practice – the Council's Standards for Education and Practice Following Registration*. London: UKCC.
United Kingdom Central Council for Nursing, Midwifery and Health Visiting. (1996). *PREP – The Nature of Advanced Practice – An Interim Report*. London: UKCC.
United Kingdom Central Council for Nursing, Midwifery and Health Visiting. (1997). *UKCC Position on Advanced Practice*. (Press Statement 8/1997.) London: UKCC.
Webb, C. (1986). *Women's Health: Midwifery and Gynaecological Nursing*. London: Hodder and Stoughton.
Weston, J. (1975). Whither the 'nurse' in nurse practitioner? *Nurs. Outlook*, **23**, 148–152.
White, R. (1985). Political regulators in British nursing. In *Political Issues in Nursing: Past, Present and Future*. (R. White, ed.) pp. 19–43. Chichester: Wiley.
Wilson-Barnett, J. (1985). Learning from specialists. *Nurs. Mirror*, **160**(2), 20–21.
Wright, S. (1986). *Building and Using a Model*. London: Edward Arnold.
Wright, S. (1991). The nurse as a consultant. *Nurs. Stand.*, **5**(20), 31–34.
Wright, S. (1992). Advances in clinical practice. *Br. J. Nurs.*, **1**, 192–194.

2

Perspectives on advanced practice: an educationalist's view

Sue Frost

One of the major challenges in taking forward nursing practice is to identify whether and if the profession should establish any parameters or boundaries to determine the nature of nursing. In particular, the debate about 'advanced' nursing practice has become so vexed that those who are responsible for organizing professional courses are discouraged from using the term 'advanced' in course titles, for fear of confusing participants and their funding source. It could be argued that nursing has reached a crossroads and must make a decision about how to move forward. Should nursing protect its core skills and retain the role conventionally and traditionally assigned to it, or should it develop into new arenas, assuming new and less traditional roles? Benjamin Disraeli captured the essence of the challenge: 'Next to knowing when to seize an opportunity, the most important thing in life is knowing when to forego an advantage.' In this chapter, I do not wish to contribute to the lack of coherence on this subject but to share an overview from the perspective of education.

In 1995, the English National Board for Nursing, Midwifery and Health Visiting (ENB) approved two new educational programmes: 'The nurse as first assistant to the surgeon' and 'Upper gastro-intestinal endoscopy; nurse practitioner programme'. The approval of these programmes caused the ENB to receive considerable correspondence. Approximately half of the many letters received expressed outrage and concern that such programmes should be approved. The essence of the comments in these letters expressed concern that nursing would be greatly harmed by moving into areas of medical practice. Nursing, it was suggested, would lose its focus on caring and supporting patients in a search for a professional identity that was better located within medical practice. The other half of this correspondence extended congratulations. The view here was that nursing was, at last, being permitted to develop new and complex skills, to take new responsibilities, and develop practice in different and innovative ways.

To understand why there should be such a disparate view, it is necessary to take a step back and consider what defines nursing practice and how it is taken forward. In this chapter, I want to explore some of these issues and examine the contributions of some of the stakeholders, including individual practitioners and their employers, as well as the statutory and professional bodies. I will share some personal thoughts on ways of taking the debate forward; indeed, I would suggest that the fact that nursing is engaged in such a debate demonstrates the increasing maturity of the profession as it wrestles with complex issues about role, function and practice.

Taking practice forwards: the drivers

Nurses, midwives and health visitors have always sought to redefine and develop the roles that they undertake. If this was not the case, then nurses would not be taking patients' blood pressure readings, and health visitors would still be functioning as the Salford Lady Sanitary Inspectors. The drivers for change have come from outside as well as from within the professions. In the 1990s, many of the reports reflecting the government agenda have been influential:

- The National Health Service and Community Care Act (Department of Health, 1990a)
- The GP contract (Scott and Maynard, 1991)
- The new deal on junior hospital doctors' hours (Department of Health, 1990b)
- *New World, New Opportunities* (Department of Health/National Health Service Management Executive, 1993)
- *A Service with Ambitions* (Department of Health, 1996)

These reports reflect the context of the government's health and social care agenda. Within the profession, one of the initiatives for change was to give practitioners responsibility for their own scope of practice and for the roles that they undertook. The United Kingdom Central Council for Nursing, Midwifery and Health Visiting (UKCC) *Scope of Professional Practice* (1992) was one of the most important factors in enabling nurses to develop and lead practice in response to the changing world of health care. The UKCC gave recognition to roles with more complexity and higher order skills through the development of new qualifications presented in *Standards for Education and Practice following Registration* (UKCC, 1994).

Traditional roles are changing and disappearing, new roles are emerging, and the expectations from the £1 billion investment in professional education have changed. Nurses, midwives and health visitors are expected to operate effectively in a health service environment where the following issues are important:

- Patient focused care;
- Vertically integrated services with managed care pathways;
- Service re-engineering;
- Multiprofessional/disciplinary/agency delivery of care;
- Evidence based practice;
- Clinical effectiveness and efficiency;
- Clinical governance;
- Clinical guidelines and protocols.

In this context, nursing needs to reflect on how decisions are made about changing roles. More importantly, nursing needs to examine who makes such decisions and what are the consequences for nursing practice, nursing education and the nursing profession.

How are roles evolving?

In 1995, the ENB undertook a review of nurse practitioner developments in England. Lovett and Norwood (ENB Officers) prepared a report for the Board, and drew the following conclusions:

- There is no national standard for role definition or role preparation following registration.
- There is not a coherent view about the definition of roles and educational opportunities between the interested people, including statutory bodies, employers, professional organizations, educational institutions and individual practitioners.
- There are fundamental differences in the development of nurse practitioners within primary health care settings and institutional health services.
- Primary health care services have made considerable use of research and evaluative methodologies to explore the development and value of nurse practitioners.
- The relationship between advanced practice, specialist practice and nursing practice is unclear and confused.

In presenting his work to the Board, Peter Lovett commented:

Role boundaries are arbitrary and changing. At a time of workforce scrutiny, activity analysis and cost effectiveness, we should not be surprised that policy makers and health care providers look to nursing to contribute to improving health care and health gain. It is not surprising, therefore, that role enhancement is seen as the natural opportunity (Lovett and Norwood, 1995).

Nurses, arguably, have always expressed some confusion about what they can and cannot do; the problem is that the speed and scale of change have increased the urgency for a coherent view. The evolution of roles results in either the enhancement of nursing or the extension of nursing into new roles.

Much of the literature about role development refers to role expansion or role extension. Role *expansion* tends to refer to skill and knowledge development within the concept of nursing as a separate therapeutic activity, and may be seen as a development that results from professional autonomy and self-determinism. Enhanced roles are thus developed from activities and skills that are conventionally within nursing, midwifery or health visiting.

The *extension* of nursing roles has been recognized and supported since the days when the former Joint Board of Clinical Nursing Studies published papers on 'The extended role of the nurse'. Extension of role generally refers to development that goes beyond conventional nursing boundaries. Preparation for extended roles is not always predicated upon a nursing qualification, and may lead to roles well outside of the conventional sphere of nursing practice. The model of expansion and extension of roles described by Lovett and Norwood in the ENB report is best summarized as follows:

- *Role expansion* Core of nursing is primary practice with a range of postqualifying specialist developments. Expansion takes the boundary of specialist development further to embrace new dimensions within the broadest concept of nursing.
- *Role extension* Extending a nursing role tends to focus on one area of practice or skill. The boundary of this area is then extended outside of nursing into another professional domain.
- *Nursing role development* Most role development in nursing embraces both expansion and extension of conventional roles. The consequence is that the boundary of nursing is shifted and the fundamental nature of nursing is gradually changed.

Nursing roles are extending in many different ways. Within adult nursing, the move to undertake medical roles has resulted in considerable change in practice. A research project undertaken for South West Thames Regional Health Authority (Touche Ross et al., 1994) examined a number of new practitioner roles that were undertaken by nurses. Eighteen roles were examined and assessed against a number of measures, including patient safety, patient and nurse satisfaction, cost efficiency and cost effectiveness. The findings of the study indicated that the development of the roles examined in the study did not reduce the safety of care to patients or clients. The study found that some roles may be less cost effective when undertaken by nurses, whereas other roles resulted in a greatly improved service to patients/clients. The study supported the development of new nursing roles, but concluded that it is not always a cost effective option to move medical roles to nurses. This study also concluded that where nurses develop roles traditionally undertaken by other professions, it should not be assumed that only the lower-skilled tasks should be assigned to nurses. The study found that it is appropriate and cost effective for nurses to develop new roles that require highly complex skills. Developing new roles requires support and skill development.

Redshaw and Harris (1995) undertook an exploratory study of the role of the advanced neonatal nurse practitioner (ANNP) and the requirements for educational preparation. The main findings of the study indicated that the development of new nursing roles requires greater thought and support than was given to the subjects in the ANNP cohorts. The main findings of the study have important implications for the development of new nursing roles:

- Advanced neonatal practice development appears to be qualitatively different from the specialist neonatal postregistration programme.
- The role of the ANNP encompasses clinical practice development, teaching, consultation and research.
- Experienced nurses are capable of undertaking an advanced training programme with other professional colleagues and of functioning as advanced practitioners in their own right.
- A number of issues have to be addressed more effectively if developments such as ANNP are to continue. These include accountability, nurse prescribing, role definitions and transfer of skills.

Redshaw and Harris (1995) concluded that 'a significant and qualitatively different development of this kind needs recognition, some central degree of support and continued monitoring'. Their study demonstrated the vulnerability of these practitioners and highlighted an urgent need to address the nature of advanced and specialist practice and their requisite preparation.

The development of extended and expanded roles is not solely the domain of adult nursing. Within other branches, there has been considerable role development. A senior nurse within children's nursing recently expressed the view that intravenous cannulation is now a core skill of all children's nurses and should be taught in preregistration programmes. In learning disability nursing, role development has included the acquisition of behavioural programming skills, behaviour modification, and complex management of people with challenging and difficult behaviours. In mental health nursing, the development of managed care pathways has enabled nurses to enhance their roles across a range of activities, including family therapy, behaviour therapy, and the management of people with dementia. Indeed, nursing development often focuses on areas of practice where there is little input from other professions, such as offering health care to homeless vagrants in large cities, refugee support in war zones, and other vulnerable groups.

Who decides on new roles for nurses?

That nursing is undergoing change is self-evident. The question of who should decide on such developments is less clear. The consequences of these changes are also in need of greater consideration. Nursing is a self-regulated profession; decisions about new roles are derived from a creative tension between the regulating bodies, employers, and practitioners and their professional organizations.

Employers have a major role in deciding what roles nurses may assume. Nurses may be employed in a wide range of roles, providing they do not use titles that suggest they have a qualification to which they are not entitled. This means that nurses may be employed to undertake duties that extend their role, providing they do not claim to be medical practitioners, psychologists, physiotherapists, and so on (unless they happen to have these qualifications). Employers have a responsibility to ensure that the people employed are prepared and equipped to undertake the responsibilities of their job. Employers may well have the view that the extension and enhancement of nursing roles is an employment issue.

The regulatory bodies have a statutory responsibility to ensure that the public is protected from inappropriate practice. The UKCC *Scope of Professional Practice* (1992) empowers nurses, midwives and health visitors to extend and expand their sphere of practice, but the responsibility for safe and effective practice remains with the individual through professional accountability. This means that nurses are able to work outside their area of specialism if they have undertaken appropriate education that assesses and assures their competence. The consequence is that, until very recently, statutory bodies (UKCC and National Boards) have seen the issue of advanced practice as a matter of effective education to protect the public from unsafe practice.

The individual practitioner has professional responsibility. Nurses undoubtedly want to develop and expand their roles, although there is evidence that many practitioners underestimate their responsibilities within *The Scope of Professional Practice,* and undertake certain roles simply because their employer expects that they will do so. The majority of nurses who are developing new roles, however, understand the need to explore and try out new ways of providing effective nursing within a multidisciplinary team. In this way, new and interesting roles are developed that benefit nursing and the patient/client. Practitioners are developing roles that combine a range of professional skills, to provide a comprehensive service to patients across social and health care boundaries.

The Royal Colleges and other professional bodies are also interested in the development of nursing roles, and are entering into discussion with a wide range of people to offer appropriate support to nurses within rapidly changing areas of practice. The professional bodies offer a different and important perspective on the expansion and extension of roles.

Amongst nurses and their professional and statutory bodies, there are many concerns about what extension of roles 'does to nursing'. Undoubtedly, there has to be a paradigm shift if nurses are to continue to operate within modern, reconfigured health services. The major challenge is to understand the extent to which the substitution of medical roles by nurses changes the essence and core function of nursing. A number of questions should be explored and debated to support nurses and their employers who are operating within the difficult area of advancing practice:

- Who should deliver the essential care required by people who are dependent on nurses?
- Will an extended role model for nursing be reductionist and move nurses to a technician or medical support role?
- Are these new roles the most appropriate use of highly skilled nurses?
- Should the new extended roles that are emerging be considered as advancing nursing practice?

Taking the debate forward

As nursing roles change, it is inevitable that there will be a time of confusion and a lack of coherence. The first stage is probably to examine whether these new developments cause a problem for any of the people concerned.

The problems for the individuals and their employers are resolved if appropriate educational preparation is undertaken, with practice supported by clinical supervision, practice protocols and agreements between professional colleagues. This reduces the risk to patients and the liability of health service employers. Clearly, there is a need to agree what constitutes appropriate education, supervision and protocol, but within this context the boundaries become limited by the professional account-ability of the nurse, and the employer's responsibility of the health service.

The challenge for the statutory bodies is to be clear about their contribution, and to decide to what extent they should manage these professional boundaries and regulate through their standards frameworks.

The issues for the nursing profession are perhaps more complex in terms of where nursing positions itself within the delivery of health care. Nursing is respected as one of the seven self-regulated professions, and there is a need for the profession to debate the extent to which a shift in the fundamental nature of nursing would undermine the ability of the profession to determine its boundaries, roles and responsibilities. The more cynical would indeed see the issue of role extension as part of an overt move to undermine professional autonomy and control.

The profession has had some opportunity for debate to identify the scale and extent of the problem. The UKCC has undertaken wide discussion and consultation to secure views on the development of advanced practice, but this debate needs to be taken further to examine ways of identifying and valuing the essential and core functions of nursing. Evidence from the field indicates an increasing disquiet about the quality of health care received by many patients. This is particularly interesting in the light of new and exciting developments within the NHS, including considerable commitment to improving the quality of care offered to patients and clients. Nursing will only move forward if the debate about roles and responsibilities embraces the real experience of patients and their families.

In a recent discussion with the Chief Executive of an NHS trust, he pointed out that his small-to-medium sized trust had no need of developing specialist or advanced practice for nursing. He went on to explain that this was because his NHS trust had no intensive or 'high tech' service. This popular view, echoed by this Chief Executive, assumes that advancing practice is about the acquisition of an increasingly narrow skill set, albeit at a highly complex level. It is my view that advancing practice is about developing the way in which nurses understand how they make decisions, analyse the consequences of what they do, and adapt nursing to improve the health outcomes for the people they serve. Advanced practice is concerned with leadership through knowledge and skill, and the advanced practitioner, in my view, is not someone who solely undertakes the most technical tasks, but who manages the delivery of nursing in ways that exploit all of the nurse's skills to collaborate with patients/clients and other members of the health team to achieve the best outcomes. I believe that was what was intended by the UKCC in establishing the 'specialist practitioner' specification.

Developing skills in one area to expand roles is not a threat to the core of nursing unless this replaces that core. I would argue that it is important, however, not to see this debate in its narrowest sense. It is possible to envisage nursing in a multiplicity of role definitions that embrace the ability of nursing to expand and to extend across professional boundaries. This has to be considered in the context of how such new roles would then be effectively regulated. Regulation is not simply about power and control, it is about ensuring public safety and confidence in nursing, and there are clearly issues about how roles that extend into other professional domains are supported and regulated.

Another challenge is to build a common vocabulary. People are confused about titles that imply expertise but which are used inconsistently; there is a plethora of terminology that makes it difficult for practitioners and their employers to interpret clearly. This might be partly as a result of underestimating the value of core nursing roles. The UKCC 'specialist practitioner' might have a clear meaning within the statutory bodies, but its relationship to clinical expertise is far from universal. A number of titles are used interchangeably:

- Nurse practitioner
- Clinical nurse specialist
- Specialist practitioner
- Advanced practitioner
- Nurse specialist
- Nurse therapist

It may, of course, not matter whether different titles are used, but I would argue that there is a need to establish a framework of language that is clear about the roles and competence that can be expected. In particular, there is a need to be clear about the relationship between specialist practice and advanced practice. The UKCC concluded in 1996 that it would not provide standards for advanced practice (Murray and Thomas, 1997). The problem is that defining advanced practice is a bit like trying to secure jelly with drawing pins. Every time you get near to succeeding, it slips away. The only way to arrive at a definition would be to be so prescriptive and narrow that *The Scope of Professional Practice* (UKCC, 1992) is undermined. The current framework does enable nurses to take practice forward in many ways, and nursing education can contribute by ensuring that nurses develop the analytical thinking skills that enable practitioners to make decisions about the nature of their practice. In this way, the UKCC *Scope of Professional Practice* can give meaning and coherence to role development in ways that support rather than constrain initiative.

The approval of new programmes of education is not a threat to nursing, but signals change in assumptions about conventional practice and nursing roles, and the statutory bodies should support and embrace such development. Nursing should celebrate the opportunity to discuss ways of advancing practice, and it is important not to reject new roles or developments simply because they do not easily fit into our 'map of the world'. It is important, however, to become active in considering the consequences and implications of new roles, whether it is the 'nurse anaesthetist' or 'nurse counsellor'. Educators have to be aware that they are part of shaping these developments; they have to ensure that understanding and analysing issues around role development is an explicit part of the skills developed by students of nursing.

The prevailing ethos in nursing has been about safety: I would certainly like the nurse who is giving me my next injection to be safe! This ethos, however, can constrain and limit the rich contribution that nurses are able to make. Nurses have to learn about the notion of risk, and gain the skills to evaluate how they develop new ideas within a framework of acceptable risk. The challenge of developing new roles is more likely to be addressed if nurses articulate the risks involved. Nursing roles will be changed and extended regardless of whether any one stakeholder objects, but, unless nurses take some risk, then nothing will change and nursing practice will not move forward.

Whoever said, 'If you're in a hole, stop digging', was quite right. Nursing should stop 'digging a hole' for itself in relation to advanced practice. We have to let go of some of the things that are part of our ritual and practice, and make way for new ideas and new spheres of practice. Nursing can only do this if individual practitioners have the skills to question and analyse what they do and understand the consequences of clinical practice. Employers can only do this if they understand their responsibilities and the advantages of employing qualified nurses. Statutory and professional bodies can only make a contribution if they accept the changing influences on practice and work together to establish a common framework for standards, a common language, and a shared commitment to work with practitioners and their employers.

Educationalists cannot ignore their responsibility for supporting and underpinning new initiatives in practice. Education has a dynamic role in relation to practice, in that education should inform and be informed by good practice. The lead time for developing new programmes is often underestimated by purchasers; education has to prepare nurses for 'what will be' as well as 'what is'.

The preparation and development of teachers of nursing, midwifery and health visiting has to be derived from a deep and enduring understanding of practice. It is not simply a question of obtaining current anecdotes to make nursing theory applicable to practice; education has to root theory within practice. This means an understanding of the relationship between theory and practice in ways that support the student in questioning and challenging concepts and conventional models. Students have to learn about the nature of argument, they must understand the elements of logic and reasoning. The skills of using argument, logic and reason have to be translated into the practice contexts that have meaning to practitioners. This will enable nurses to improve the way in which they make decisions about the roles they undertake.

The value of locating nursing education within higher education institutions will be little more than an expensive experiment unless nursing education supports the development of these higher order skills of thinking and reasoning. The advancement of teachers has to take account of this development and ensure that students are exposed to teachers who are capable of managing the intellectual discourse that should underpin practice. This means that teachers need to draw on contemporary literature and research, and interweave this with knowledge of contemporary practice development. The purpose of professional education should be to ensure that students are given the courage and confidence to face the real dilemmas of practice in ways that improve rather than weaken them as practitioners.

Nurses will and should enhance and extend their roles. The difficulty is that in order to face up to the challenges brought about by such role developments, employers, statutory and professional bodies, and policy makers in a number of professions have to work together in ways that cross conventional boundaries. If this is not orchestrated effectively and efficiently, then the strength and power of self-determinism will be lost as nursing roles are determined and directed by others.

References

Department of Health. (1990a). *National Health Service and Community Care Act 1990*. London: HMSO.

Department of Health. (1990b). *Heads of Agreement: Ministerial Group on Junior Hospital Doctors' Hours*. London: HMSO.

Department of Health. (1996). *The National Health Service, a Service with Ambitions*. London: HMSO.

Department of Health/NHS Management Executive. (1993). *Nursing in Primary Health Care: New World, New Opportunities*. London: HMSO.

Lovett, P. and Norwood, S. (1995). *Nurse Practitioners – Developments in England*. (Paper presented to UKCC and National Boards annual seminar.)

Murray, C. and Thomas, M. (1997). Advanced Nursing Practice: role or concept? *British Journal of Nursing*, **6**(9), 474

National Health Service Management Executive. (1993). *Day Surgery: Report by the Day Surgery Task Force. London: HMSO*.

Redshaw, M. and Harris, A. (1995). *An exploratory study into the role of the advanced neonatal nurse practitioner and the education programme of preparation*. London: ENB.

Scott, A. and Maynard, A. (1991). *Will the new GP Contract Lead to Cost Effective Medical Practice?* (Discussion paper.) York: Centre for Health Economics, University of York.

Touche Rosse, South Thames Regional Health Authority, NHS Executive, South Thames (1994). *Evaluation of Nurse Practitioner Pilot Projects*. London: Touche Ross.

United Kingdon Central Council for Nursing, Midwifery and Health Visiting. (1992). *The Scope of Professional Practice*. London: UKCC.

United Kingdon Central Council for Nursing, Midwifery and Health Visiting. (1994). *Standards for Education and Practice Following Registration*. London: UKCC.

3

The search for meaning in advanced nursing practice

Barbara Stilwell

Introduction

The quest to describe the nature of nursing practice has become something of a professional crusade in nursing, and most surely stems from a persistent wish to clarify the knowledge base for nursing. Recent discussions on nursing policy formation, as well as in the nursing literature, attempt to clarify the differences between specialists, experts and advanced practitioners in nursing, but there appears to be little consensus of views (Brown, 1995; Holyoake, 1995). Health systems, of which nurses are a component, are changing fast, driven by the need for cost-constraint and efficiency in service provision. It is these changes, outside of nursing's control, that demand new skill-mixes and new roles for nurses, which appear to be focused on traditional medical models, and the taking over of traditional medical skills and responsibilities (Richardson and Maynard, 1995).

However, changes in health systems are not happening in isolation; there are profound societal and economic changes too. Family structures, expectations of work, technology, travel and experience of illness and health have all changed and are still changing (Salvage, 1993). Nurses and their patients are part of these larger societal changes, and their encounters must be given meaning in these dynamic contexts. The search for definitions of advanced nursing practice, as well as for specialist and expert practice, reflect this current need for interpretation and meaning in nursing as it faces the challenges of a changing society, as well as demands for new roles in a changing health care system.

Nurses have tried to clarify the nature of nursing practice and the knowledge base required for practice for many years, often through the application of scientific meaning to nursing (Robinson, 1994). Robinson suggests, however, that nursing is not amenable to scientific analysis, it being unscientific in nature itself. She uses work by Becher (1989) to substantiate her argument. Becher studied over 200 academics to elicit the forms of knowledge that they used, and found a spectrum of knowledge that lay between such boundaries as restricted and unrestricted knowledge, hard and soft knowledge, and pure and applied disciplines. At one end of the spectrum stood physics, its academics characterized by 'consensual understanding of profound simplicities... a particular way of approaching problems', while at the other end was geography, with 'unclear boundaries, problems which are broad in scope but loose in definition, a relatively unspecific theoretical structure, a concern with the qualitative and particular, and a reiterative pattern of enquiry'. Robinson (1994) maintains that nursing is far more akin to geography in its place on this spectrum, and its attempts to become more scientific by using the language and classifications of science are therefore inappropriate.

Nursing literature also alludes to the importance of highly unscientific concepts, such as intuition, caring and empathy, in the process and outcomes of nursing care (Carper, 1978; Benner, 1984; Kitson, 1987; Paterson and Zderad, 1988; Lawler, 1991; Sutton and Smith, 1995). These processes, which cannot be classified as nursing science, are often expressed as nursing art, and nursing is seen as a complex activity that encompasses scientific and artistic knowledge for its successful practice (Gendron, 1994; Johnson, 1994). It is expression of the relationship between the science and art of nursing that appears to elude exact description. A parallel analogy can be seen in the performance of music: a pianist, for example, can perform with technical brilliance, but in order to be a truly great performer, technical competence has to be combined with sensitive interpretation and a deep understanding of, and feeling for, the music.

The following description of nursing practice is an attempt to address the issue of the changing context of care for nursing, as well as to express the complexity of nursing practice. It is based on observations of nurse practitioners, mostly, but not solely, in primary health care settings, and involvement with curriculum development for courses to prepare nurse practitioners. It is descriptive rather than interpretive, assuming that meaning in nursing encounters is found by the participants, usually the nurse and the patient. The description accepts the integrity of art and science in nursing, because it seems that, the more nursing is reduced to its component parts, the more it demands to be put together again in order to represent what it really is.

What nurses do

Paterson and Zderad (1988) contend that nursing 'is an experience lived between two human beings', and that nursing interventions are 'directed towards nurturing the well-being... of a person with perceived needs related to the health–illness quality of living'. Because each human being is an individual with unique needs and responses, no two nursing encounters can ever be the same, and, to practise successfully, nurses must be highly self-aware, as well as open to the singularity of each person. Paterson and Zderad suggest that successful nursing is founded on an existential awareness of self and others (by the nurse), and it is this awareness that leads the nurse to help patients to identify and achieve their personal health goals, rather than those of nursing or the health system.

This existentialist approach to nursing practice has inherent risks: if each encounter with a patient is different, then protocols of care cannot account for every situation. Nurses are set free from routinized and impersonal care, but at the same time lose all the supposed security offered by predictable assessments, treatments and outcomes. In the true existentialist nursing encounter, the nurse must become an expert problem-solver, using a range of knowledge and skills to identify and respond to health need, while helping patients to choose and achieve their individual health goals. The solutions that the nurse and the patient negotiate will not necessarily be the safest or the best in scientific terms, although they will be the solutions chosen by the patient. The nurse's professional role is to calculate the extent of any risk, and to minimize it whenever possible. For many nurses, this is a style of care that they are not socialized to offer through the traditional educational preparation for their role, or through the hierarchies of accountability in which they have worked (Dobos, 1992). Nursing models and the nursing process tend to reinforce expectations that nursing is a predictable and organized activity, whereas, to be truly effective, nursing might have to be flexible, creative and responsive, and lack preconceived structure.

The distinguishing characteristics of nurse practitioners (NP) in primary health care are said to be that they are able to assess the health status of people who present with undiagnosed and undifferentiated health problems, and, using their clinical judgement, diagnose the condition and initiate appropriate treatment, or refer to another provider (Stilwell, 1988). This represents, for any health care provider, the ultimate challenge in problem solving and risk taking, because the patient's condition is completely unknown, and, in a primary health care setting, the patient is only present for a short period of time (Brykczynski, 1989).

As well as these important functions, NPs are also required to practise from a nursing framework, so that they would be concerned not only with an illness, but also with the patient's experience of the illness; they would pay attention to the relationship between themselves and their patient, and would seek to promote health as well as manage illness.

In considering the nature of autonomous practice for NPs, it became clear that a NP must take responsibility for assessing health status over time, rather than in 'snapshots' of the present. The implication of this is that a NP does not accept and carry out tasks delegated from others, but always makes an independent assessment of a patient, which includes a history as well as a future plan. Figure 3.1 shows how the dimensions of health can be integrated with time.

The 12 'boxes' in Figure 3.1 represent the broad dimensions of health within which NPs, and probably all nurse clinicians, must work with patients, if they are working as nurses. Nursing is, in this way, defined by its breadth of practice concerns. However, a diagram cannot represent the totality of what is happening in a nursing encounter, because it cannot represent the relationship between the nurse and the patient. It is this relationship that is the key to open each of the 'boxes' (the areas of practice represented in the diagram), and which 'puts together that which has been dissected by the cold hand of science' (Kitson, 1987). Clinicians in nursing and medicine have alluded to the need for developing consultation skills that encourage the patient to share concerns, to be truthful and to express

Components of health	Time		
	Past	Present	Future
Physical	Medical history Levels of fitness Physical status	Current physical status Physical examination	Optimum physical health prescription
Mental	Development of self Mental health history	Fears/anxiety Stress Health beliefs	Coping skills Appropriate health beliefs
Social	Role in society Perceptions of self	Effects of social status on health	Aware of need to adapt, accept or change
Emotional and spiritual	Has shown appropriate emotion Support in appropriate emotion	Ability to discuss emotion Insight into spiritual health	Understands emotion and health

RISKS AND THREATS · ASSESSING RISKS · PROMOTING HEALTH: ASSESSING RISKS

Figure 3.1. The dimensions of health

fears, although it has been less easy to be precise about what skills are optimally successful (Neighbour, 1987; Brykczynski, 1989). One reason for the lack of precision might be the elusive quality of what is necessary in an encounter to establish a relationship of such value between the health care provider and the patient in which it is safe to reveal feelings and fears. Martin Buber, a philosopher and rabbi, who was born in Vienna in 1878, believed that it was possible to view another person in two ways: in the first, the person was seen only as part of the existence of the viewer, rather than as a separate being; in the second, the person was genuinely acknowledged as exclusive and valued. Paterson and Zderad (1988) suggest that it is the presence of genuineness in caring that sets apart 'good' nurses, because it gives value to the patient and values what the patient is experiencing.

All patients are different, and have varying needs; every encounter with the same patient is also potentially different. No model of care or description of nursing practice can, therefore, ever be applicable to all situations. It is the skill of the expert nurse to select boxes that are appropriate for each encounter, not only through physical clues, but also by establishing relationships with patients that will 'open the boxes'. For example, a patient presenting with an acute emergency necessitating resuscitation would require a nurse to function in only the physical domain, and in the present. All other concerns could wait until later. On the other hand, a patient who is consulting about a medical problem, but who appeared to be depressed, requires the nurse to 'open the boxes' to past and present mental health, and probably social and spiritual or emotional concerns too. The expertise of nursing is in identifying the appropriate boxes, and in being able to open them, or, in other words, to give them meaning to the patient through the nurse personally seeing the possibilities of meanings in them. Meanings will change; for example, the meaning of open heart surgery for patients and nurses is different now from what it was 20 years ago. The experience of illness is affected by changing social factors (Goodwin, 1992) and so the meaning of nursing care changes also.

It is strongly suggested that this description of practice is appropriate in any field of nursing practice, although the exact nature of the knowledge needed for practice, and its application, will be dependent on the area of practice. A nurse specializing in the care of children, for example, will need specific knowledge and skills for that client group, but nevertheless as the nurse's practice becomes more expert, he or she will use that knowledge appropriately and understand how to work in every box shown in Figure 3.1.

The complex whole

Johnson (1994), in reviewing the work of 41 authors, suggests that there are five concepts of nursing art; these are the nurse's ability:

- to grasp meaning in patient encounters;
- to establish a meaningful connection with the patient;
- to perform nursing activities skilfully;
- to determine a course of action rationally;
- to conduct his or her nursing practice morally.

Although working in each of the boxes in Figure 3.1 demands depth and breadth of nursing knowledge as well as knowledge of assessment, diagnosis, and pharmacology, giving meaning to the boxes will be possible only if a 'meaningful connection' can be established with the patient. By the same token, nurses can plan rationally for the future only when there is an understanding between the nurse and the patient about each of their expectations. Nursing can be practised morally only when the nurse fully understands what the patient wants and acts as that person's advocate and support in achieving his or her personal goals.

Like the concert pianist, to be an advanced practitioner requires technical brilliance and sensitive interpretation. Models alone cannot express this, and neither can interpretations of caring; they must coexist. Holden (1991) asserts that:

> The caring role, intrinsic to the meaning of the word 'nurse', constrains nursing under the rubric of the arts, while nursing that embraces high technology constrains the discipline under the rubric of science.

Holden suggests that a hermeneutic approach to nursing theory and practice would unite the art and science of nursing, because hermeneutics is concerned with the subjective interpretation of events through phenomenology. This approach reinforces the notion that it is the total experience of a nursing encounter, for the patient and the nurse, which is important and filled with meaning for both. By losing the constraints of art and science in analysis, nursing is liberated and allowed to exist in its complex totality without being reduced in any way.

Conclusion

It is certainly possible to affirm the existence of nursing as a process and to observe the tasks that nurses do. It is possible to teach nurses the skills and knowledge required to make them competent; but it is not possible to know what will be the content of each nursing encounter, because it will be different every time, depending on the needs of the patient and the responses of the nurse. The success of the encounter for the patient and the nurse depends, too, on the ability of the nurse to find meaning in the encounter, opening up possibilities for himself or herself and for the patient. The most advanced practitioner will be the one who can, at every encounter, open the most appropriate boxes at the right time, in a way that is morally acceptable and offers safe and effective treatment. It is highly likely that a nurse will have to judge, at every patient encounter, which of the boxes should be explored.

Learning to be an expert practitioner in nursing must happen in myriad ways. It is undoubtedly important to be able critically to analyse and synthesize information in a number of fields, but the ability to discover and interpret the information in the first place is related not to cognitive ability but to self-awareness and awareness of others. It has been suggested that advanced practice differs from expert practice, but is this exploration of terms used to express what is happening in nursing practice merely another manifestation of the way in which nursing has been seduced by science into descriptions of models, which, because of the responsiveness of nursing to patients' needs and to societal changes, can never be truly accurate?

Supporting nurses in discovering themselves and the value of others, through helping them to reflect honestly on their practice, may be the most effective way of developing autonomous practitioners for new roles in a changing world.

References

Becher, T. (1989). *Academic Tribes and Territories: Intellectual Enquiry and the Cultures of Disciplines*. Milton Keynes: The Society for Research into Higher Education/Open University Press.

Benner, P. (1984). *From Novice to Expert: Excellence and Power in Clinical Nursing Practice*. Menlo Park, CA: Addison-Wesley.

Brown, R. A. (1995). The politics of specialist/advanced practice: conflict or confusion? *Br. J. Nurs.*, **4**, 944–948.

Brykczynski, K. A. (1989). An interpretive study describing the clinical judgement of nurse practitioners. *Scholarly Enquiry Nurs. Pract.*, **3**, 75–104.

Carper, B. A. (1978). Fundamental patterns of knowing in nursing. *Adv. Nurs. Sci.*, **1**(1), 13–23.

Dobos, C. (1992). Defining risk from the perspective of nurses in clinical roles. *J. Adv. Nurs.*, **17**, 1303–1309.

Gendron, D. (1994). The tapestry of care. *Adv. Nurs. Sci.*, **17**(1), 25–30.

Goodwin, S. (1991). Breaking the links between social deprivation and poor child health. *Health Visitor*, **64**, 376–380.

Holden, R. J. (1991). In defence of Cartesian dualism and the hermeneutic horizon. *J. Adv. Nurs.*, **16**, 1375–1391.

Holyoake, D. (1995). Advancing in confusion. *Nurs. Stand.*, **9**(51), 56.

Johnson, J. (1994). A dialectical examination of nursing art. *Adv. Nurs. Sci.*, **17**(1), 1–14.

Kitson, A. (1987). Raising standards of clinical practice: the fundamental issue of effective nursing practice. *J. Adv. Nurs.*, **12**, 321–329.

Lawler, J. (1991). *Behind the Screens; Nursing Somology and the Problem of the Body.* Edinburgh: Churchill Livingstone.

Neighbour, R. (1987). *The Inner Consultation.* Lancaster: MTP Press.

Paterson, J. G. and Zderad, L. T. (1988). *Humanistic Nursing.* New York: National League for Nursing.

Richardson, G. and Maynard, A. (1995). *Fewer Doctors? More Nurses? A Review of the Knowledge Base of Doctor–Nurse Substitution.* (Discussion paper 35.) York: Centre for Health Economics, University of York.

Robinson, J. (1994). Problems with paradigms in a caring profession. In *Models, Theories and Concepts.* (J. P. Smith, ed.) Oxford: Blackwell Scientific.

Salvage, J. (1993). Changing nursing practice. In *Nursing in Action: Strengthening Nursing and Midwifery to Support Health for All.* (WHO Regional Publications, European Series, no. 48.) (J. Salvage, ed.). Copenhagen: World Health Organisation.

Stilwell, B. (1988). Defining a role for nurse practitioners. In *Directions in Nursing Research.* (J. Wilson-Barnett and S. Robinson, eds.) pp. 76–84. London: Scutari Press.

Sutton, F. and Smith, C. (1995). Advanced Nursing Practice: new ideas and new perspectives. *Journal of Advanced Nursing*, **21**, 1037–1043.

4

Advanced practice in mental health nursing: developing the core

Phil Barker

Introduction

This chapter will address the concept of advanced practice in psychiatric nursing: how might individual nurses advance the collective activities assumed to represent this branch of practice? Before addressing this question it might be appropriate, however, to consider the territory of mental illness and mental health, as well as the province of psychiatric medicine, which has for so long served to define the characteristics of the domain of madness, if not also of the mad themselves.

Unlike most manifestations of physical distress or impairment, the world of mental distress is fraught with many conflicts. Not least among these is the dispute over the extent to which 'people with mental health problems' are *ill* (Szasz, 1961; Chamberlin, 1988; Rogers et al., 1993; Romme and Escher, 1993), or what functions the nurse should fulfil in meeting the needs of people who complain of mental health problems or have such problems attributed to them (Rudman, 1996).

The experience of illness

If the experience of psychiatric disorder possesses any distinctive quality, this may be the immediate, cumulative and ultimate effect of the putative disorder on the person's human identity. Most forms of illness effect some form of 'dis-ease' within the person, disrupting the sense of ordinary self. Illnesses that are physical in form are, however, often easier to objectify. The disease may be viewed as affecting only a part of the person ('I *have* lung cancer'); or the person may view the disorder as an affliction ('I *suffer* from epilepsy, multiple sclerosis or constipation'). In either case, the physical illness (despite its effect on the whole person) may be viewed, by the patient and others, as occupying a territory other than that of the 'person' themselves, or, at most, only a delimited part of that personal territory. This objectification of the disorder, illness or dysfunction is possible in mental illness (e.g. 'I suffer from depression'). Traditionally, however, people and their conditions have often been described as one and the same (e.g. (s)he *is* a schizophrenic, neurotic or personality disorder). The states of *having* and *being* a disorder tending to become regarded as synonymous.

Sociologists and social psychologists have made a strong case for the social construction of self or identity (Goffman, 1969; Gergen, 1985), illustrating how the person defined as 'a condition' might grow into the role, risking losing, at the same time, something of their human potential. Conversely, Wynne et al. (1992) noted that labelling a person as sick is a transactional process; a negotiation occurs in which the person experiencing distress is an active participant who may or may not accept an illness label. The analysis proposed by Wynne et al. is congruent with the growing activism of the user movement, some members of which reject the labels conferred by professionals, while others appear to negotiate the aetiological parameters of their diagnosis. Among those who reject the 'medicalization' of their experience are groups who emphasize the sociopolitical nature of mental distress (like 'Survivors Speak Out' in the UK), or those who perceive 'madness' as a form of enlightenment or 'human becoming' (like 'Crazy Folks' in the USA). In a related context, the American, Edward Cooper (1997), has written:

> Dennet and others [in cognitive science] are working hard to reduce the experience of being human to that of a computer. Psychiatry, trying to be a real science, is working right beside the folks who want to reduce us to mere machines. Well, damn them. I will keep my madness because I am more than a machine. I am fully human in the best illusionary sense.

People *in* physical and mental illness share one common feature: each includes a small proportion who somehow maintain a sense of personhood that is at variance with the self constructed, for them, by the diagnostic process (Wright, 1991). This may involve what professionals describe as *denial* of the disorder or a remarkable capacity to 'live with' the disorder, a vital expression of the notion of 'philosophical acceptance'. Edward Cooper may be a living example of someone who has explored his personhood through discovering the meaning of his madness. How people *relate* to their illness represents a key starting point for exploring how nurses might relate to the people defined as their patients.

The psychiatric enigma

Mental illness is a contradiction in terms. It is assumed generally to involve a disorder or disturbance of the mind. If one accepts that the mind does not occupy a space distinct from the body, then mental illness must be, and not be, an illness of the body at one and same time. The state of 'mental' ill-at-ease-ness is experienced *in* the body. This does not mean, necessarily, that this state is *of* the body, or at least not in the same sense that diabetes or carcinoma is *in* and *of* the body. The experience of anxiety, for example, is experienced in the body; we need a functioning autonomic nervous system to *be* anxious. If, however, we are to understand how the anxiety occurs and how it might be resolved, then we must look to the person who is (and is not) the body at one and the same time. 'Mental illnesses' appear, in this sense, to be *of the person*, or, rather, of the *human* 'self', as distinct from the *physical* 'self'. This is the 'territory' where beliefs, thoughts and emotions are constructed unceasingly in a seamless dialogue with the 'body' and its experience of the world and itself. The distress experienced by the person is somehow 'referred' to the body. Who (or what) is at the other end of this dialogue emanating from the mind, or whether it is no more than a self-referring 'loop' that passes through the body, remains unclear. If mental illness has a location, it is here, at the metaphorical interface between the body and what has traditionally been construed as the 'mind' (Gooch, 1980).

This perspective challenges the Cartesian tradition, upon which modern medicine was first based, which assumed a dualistic division of mind and body. The rejection of such dualism is, arguably, most evident in the growing interest in (w)holism, which, among other things, assumes that people are greater than the sum of their parts *and* benefit when treated as such. Some nurses have, however, expressed a reservation about the non-specificity of 'holistic' models of care and treatment, and have called for the restoration of the 'medical model' within nursing. One such view contends that the medical model assumes superior utility, being 'tried and tested, well understood ... orientated towards disease (the patient and the health worker's main concern), and decision-making is in the ambit of the doctor' (Lucas, 1993).

This plea derives from what used to be called 'general' nursing, but it has also found some echoes in psychiatric nursing (e.g. Gournay, 1995). Lucas' call to return, so to speak, to our medical roots recognizes the often absurd rhetoric that enshrouds many of the quasi-holistic nursing models that have been proposed to replace the medical model in a nursing context: '[the] host of "metaparadigms" and "concepts" deemed by some to be essential to nursing as it strives to "delineate its epistemological foundations"' (Lucas, 1993).

Lucas' concerns are justified, at least at the level of parsimony; why introduce more complex models of health/illness where simpler ones will suffice to explain the health problem? When we turn our attention, specifically, to the area of mental illness, however, we must ask whether the biomedical (or even biopsychosocial) model explains either what ails the person, or the means by which such life problems may be resolved. This is familiar territory, the so-called antipsychiatry critique. Over the past 10 years, however, this critique has been relocated within a lay context; the 'voices' of those who have suffered mental illness, or suffered the deficiencies of the psychiatric system, have reaffirmed the status of mental illness as a human crisis, challenging at the same time the notion that such human crises are psychic analogues of diabetes or influenza (cf. Chamberlin, 1988).

The shifting ground of mental health nursing

The reader might be excused for assuming that these considerations have little bearing on the concept of the advanced nurse practitioner. Yet, we cannot consider how the role of the nurse might be 'advanced' without considering how the subject of nursing, the person-in-care, might be changing, how the paradigms of 'patienthood' and professional advancement meet.

Arguably, psychiatric nursing is driven more by expediency than any other branch of nursing. In the mid-1990s, a number of policies and pieces of legislation emphasized the need for nurses to refocus their attention on people with 'serious (and/or enduring) mental illness' (e.g Department of Health, 1994), with the result that many nurses now assume that people who do not suffer from a psychosis are not 'seriously ill' (Repper et al., 1993; Barker and Jackson, 1997). This politically-driven emphasis might be viewed as, in part, a belated response to the failure of community care and, more likely, an attempt to convince hostile media that the 'threat' posed by people with psychotic disorders in the natural community is being addressed. Sadly, nurses' support for the concept of 'serious mental illness' has led, indirectly, to some patient groups such as those with an experience of self-harm, assuming that this means that they are no more than 'trivially mentally ill' (L. Pembroke, personal communication). The idea that a psychiatric nurse should discriminate the 'seriously mentally ill' from any other group may be the thin end of a dangerous wedge. It may be akin to ophthalmic nurses telling patients to go home on the grounds that cataracts are not, of themselves, life threatening.

At the same time, psychiatric nursing has been steered in the direction of a policing activity, by being required to 'ensure' that people deemed 'dangerous' or 'at risk' comply with treatment. Nurses appear to have been largely accepting of such directives, despite the ethical issues raised by assertions in the literature that, in some cases, neuroleptic medication may bring problems as great as those that it aims to treat (Breggin, 1991). Although some opposition has been expressed towards such policy initiatives, other nurses have readily seized the opportunity to emphasize the value of defining mental distress from a medical perspective and of narrowing the focus of nursing practice. Such a shift in professional philosophy is curious, to say the least, given that the branch has redefined itself, officially, as *mental health nursing*. The emphasis on pathology and illness implied by the terms 'mental' or 'psychiatric' nurse has been rejected in favour of an acknowledgement of the nurse's role in promoting adjustment, if not health itself.

Such developments may illustrate a concern expressed recently by Nolan in the conclusion to his history of British psychiatric nursing. Nurses, he argued, needed to be at the spearhead of changes, 'not lagging behind as has, sadly, been their traditional role' (Nolan, 1993). In Nolan's view, nurses could no longer afford to follow in the footsteps of other professional groups, who were 'more assertive than they [nurses] in defending their interests, since such lack of purpose could only lead to the obliteration of mental health nursing'.

The expectation that psychiatric nurses should refocus most, if not all, of their caring energies on serving one ill-defined group (serious mental illness), while at the same time trying to redefine the construct of caring as a health-promoting endeavour, may signal the lack of true purpose to which Nolan referred.

The advanced practitioner: in advance of whom or what?

Any discussion of the concept of the advanced practitioner in mental health nursing is dependent on clarifying what goes on between the nurse and the person-in-care. Some would argue that there is a need to recognize that the care that is proffered by nurses is no more, or less, than 'the reflection of self-understanding and a promotion of the best interests of another' (Brykczynska, 1997). Such an emphasis on the empathic basis of the interpersonal relationship between the nurse and the person-in-care may not be unique to nursing, but is undoubtedly a core characteristic of psychiatric nursing. The professional development of nursing might be dependent, at least in part, on the clarification or redefinition of the caring construct (Bradshaw, 1997). In psychiatric nursing, this need might not be located within some dichotomous notion of 'advanced' or 'basic' nursing practice. It may, however, be a need that might be addressed differently by those who are called advanced practitioners. The critical aspect of the role of those individual practitioners might be to advance practice, acting as a role model to all those defined, implicitly, as *basic* practitioners.

We live in an era increasingly 'wired' by developments in computing science, and it is popular to express awe and wonderment at every new pronouncement made by the neurosciences. Despite the new insights that biotechnology offers into the causes of mental distress, or its resolution, they are largely an irrelevance for psychiatric nurses. Brain imaging techniques, human genome mapping and developments in psychopharmacology tell us nothing of the human experience of mental distress (Barker, 1995). Although these developments might hold some significance for the eventual treatment or eradication of bodily dysfunctions, they are of little significance to the practice of nursing, which remains an interpersonal activity enacted within the human and moral context of 'everyday life'. People with mental health problems have a problem *with* their illness, disorder, dysfunction (or whatever). If nurses address any*thing*, it is the person's relationship with their illness (etc.). Adopting that perspective, the American Nurses Association defined the 'province' of nursing as 'the diagnosis and treatment of human *responses* to actual or potential health problems' (American Nurses Association, 1980; author's italics).

Following the lead of the person-in-care

The only possible source of true information about the 'mental' phenomena involved in a psychiatric disorder is the person who is the patient. It is assumed that the guiding paradigm of psychiatric nursing is that there exists a 'person' who, often, is overshadowed by a towering, diagnostic label (Barker, 1985, 1997a). This paradigm determines the nurse's core attitude (respect for the human experience of the person), and the nurse's core behavioural repertoire (exploring the experience of mental distress *with* the person). It would be folly to dismiss the importance of neuroscientific evidence about the influence of genetics or pathophysiology on human experience. However, it is assumed that persons are more than a function of some genetic stamping or marking, or the consequence of a complex biological machine. Such an assumption is central to the idea that 'we' might think about, reflect or otherwise decide upon our human behaviour. It is the 'I' who becomes 'we' within the context of the interpersonal relationship, which is the primary focus of nursing enquiry.

Alternatively, if we should rely over much on the knowledge gleaned from the neurosciences, at least philosophically, we would saw off the very branch on which we are sitting. It seems apparent that 'who' we are derives from an unceasing interaction between various levels of our 'internal' selves, and the myriad layers of experience that we call the world outside our skin. If I believe that this is true of me, then it must be true also of those who are my 'patients' (Barker, 1997a). This assumption appears to lead to the conclusion that we can only find out who are the people in our care by engaging in dialogue, although the nature of that dialogue may be translated into a wide range of forms. The challenge facing psychiatric nurses is not to become more conversant with psychotechnologies, but to develop more sophisticated ways of helping people to teach us about their experiences in mental distress and, through such teachings, reveal something of the human meaning of distress (see also Rogers et al., 1993). The emergence of meaning might change the whole context of distress, although it may not necessarily return the 'patient' to anything approaching 'normality'. This conundrum is not easily understood in our 'outcome-orientated' health service, in which 'outcome' often is interpreted as the 'curing', 'fixing' or the otherwise 'elimination' of the diagnosed illness. An example from Frankl may help to clarify the importance of 'searching for meaning' in a nursing context:

A young woman who had led an utterly pampered existence was one day unexpectedly thrown into a concentration camp. There she fell ill and was visibly wasting away. A few days before she died she said these very words: 'actually I am grateful to my fate for having treated me so harshly. In my former middle-class existence I had things a great deal too easy. I never was very serious about my literary ambitions.' She saw death coming and looked it squarely in the eye (Frankl, 1973).

The woman could just glimpse one twig and a few blossoms of a chestnut tree, which stood outside her window. Frankl noted:

She spoke of this tree often. 'This tree is my only friend in solitude ... I converse with it.' Was this an hallucination? Was she delirious? Did she think the tree was 'answering her'? What strange dialogue was this; what had the flowering tree 'said' to the dying woman? It says: 'I am here – I am life, eternal life' (Frankl, 1973).

Frankl reflected that this story illustrated how the patient, as the sufferer, is superior to the doctor when the suffering is incurable in nature. One might adopt the view that the patient is always superior, if only because of his or her (possible) access to the personal meaning of the suffering. We, intent only on healing the hurt, are mere witnesses to the illness state.

Increasingly, the view is taken that nursing is a collaborative venture, based on some kind of partnership. This was the basis for the recommendations in the Report of the Mental Health Nursing Review Team (Department of Health, 1994), which emphasized the need to develop more 'collaborative' forms of designing and implementing psychiatric nursing care. In other contexts, nurses have affirmed the importance of addressing the 'lived experience' of illness (or health) as the underpinning philosophy of nursing (Parse, 1995).

The sophistication of ordinariness

The concept of 'advanced practice' implies sophistication; in turn, the notion of the sophisticated nurse implies that the nurse needs to be 'extraordinary'. Although the advanced practitioner might have developed knowledge and skills to a degree that is far beyond that of the peer group, the core characteristic of the 'advanced' status might involve a paradoxical 'extraordinary ordinariness'. Morrison (1997) noted that: 'The positive effects of being an *ordinary person* who happens to be a nurse should not be underestimated. Patients need to know that those looking after them are human, too.' He illustrated this point by referring to the oft-cited study by Cowen (1982), who described how members of the public sought help for 'psychological problems' from hairdressers, lawyers, supervisors and bartenders, rather than traditional therapists. Cowen's sample group of 'informal helpers' not only used 'ordinary' and 'spontaneous' means of 'being helpful', but also were highly effective. Morrison concluded that nurses should try to develop such 'ordinary' and 'spontaneous' ways of responding to the human problems of patients within their nursing practice. Rogers et al.'s (1993) study of the users of psychiatric services led to a similar conclusion, that ordinary human responses were prized over formal offers of psychotherapy or counselling.

Towards a paradigm of collaborative caring in mental health nursing

Since 1994, a group of nurses in the North-east of England have been engaged in an extended course of reflection on the 'proper focus of psychiatric nursing'. This culminated in a 10-month long study using a 'co-operative inquiry' methodology (Heron, 1996). A set of philosophical propositions concerning the core activity of psychiatric and mental health nursing is currently being explored more widely across the range of clinical nursing contexts, hospital and community (Barker et al., 1995; Barker 1997b). The Tyneside Group has concluded that the psychiatric nursing paradigm is predicated on the following four core assumptions:

Premise 1

Psychiatric nursing is an interactive, developmental, human activity, more concerned with the future development of the person, than with the origins or causes of their present mental distress. It is concerned, therefore, to establish the conditions necessary for the promotion of the person's unique growth and development. Such growth and development will, of necessity, involve the person's adjustment to, or overcoming of the life-problems associated with, psychiatric disorder.

> The great thing in this world is not so much where we are but in what direction we are moving.   (Oliver Wendell Holmes)

Over a 10-year period working with people with major depression this nurse had worked with many who were considered suicidal. Over time he grew less interested in how the person had come to consider suicide as an option. Instead, he learned the truly 'vital' questions: 'How do you keep going?', or, 'What stops you from taking your life?', 'Tell me more about that!.' People are always 'going' somewhere in their lives. Such natural inquiry as underpins nursing practice should recognize that incessant movement down the life-path (Barker, 1996). The fundamental nature of nursing may involve accompanying people in their quest for the meaning of their experience of mental distress.

Premise 2

The experience of mental distress associated with psychiatric disorder is represented through public behavioural disturbance or reports of private events, and is known only to the individual concerned. Psychiatric nursing involves the provision of the conditions under which people may access and review those experiences. Such collaborative re-authoring of the person's life might involve the healing of past distress, the alleviation of present distress, and the opening of ways to further human development.

> However exquisitely human nature may have been described by writers, the true practical system can only be learned in the world.   (Henry Fielding)

A Community Psychiatric Nurse (CPN) was asked to see a woman whose GP described her as showing strange behaviour. Eleanor was visiting the supermarket and buying huge quantities of potatoes, scouring pads and bread. Despite her bulging cupboards at home, she continued with her purchasing. The GP thought that she was becoming demented, or developing a late onset 'psychotic illness'.

Eleanor could not account for her behaviour, and the conversation around the 'problem' seemed less interesting than that around other areas, such as what would she do now that her husband had retired? He was an organized and organizing man by his own definition, and had begun to take over the domestic domain, which had been sacred to his wife for 40 years. His housekeeping left her feeling useless. In addition to defining herself as a gifted housekeeper, the nurse learned that Eleanor was also a keen dancer. The opportunity to 'take to the floor' seemed to be limited to an annual New Year party. As she talked with the nurse, the possibility emerged that she could develop this interest, especially as she was now 'freed' from domestic routines. Eleanor was not told this directly, or prescribed this interest as a task for 'homework'. Rather, they agreed that expanding her interest in dancing was a helpful avenue to explore.

Premise 3

The nurse and the person-in-care are engaged in a relationship based on mutual influence. It is assumed that the reflective nature of the caring experience produces changes for the nurse, the person-in-care, and significant others. Nursing involves caring with, rather than caring for, people, irrespective of the context of care.

The least movement is of importance to all nature. The entire ocean is affected by a pebble.
(Blaise Pascal)

A student nurse needed to develop confidence in her own ability. Janet, one of the people on a ward where she was training, decided that she was ready to be a staff nurse. The nurse had not discussed her lack of confidence, but on reflection, she realized that Janet knew that she needed someone to endorse her.

The ward adjoined the training school. One day Janet went to find the tutor to demand a staff nurse's belt for the nurse, telling the tutor that she was ready to be qualified. She reported back at lunch time that she was unsuccessful, but unrepentant, and she made several further attempts.

Their paths crossed next when the nurse was working night duty. As she was growing older, Janet had begun to have more physical problems, which she could grumble about at length, confirming her reputation as a 'creaking gate'. Then it was discovered that she had a form of bone cancer. The nurse was on duty for the last week of Janet's life. Because of her reputation as a complainer, she felt that Janet was not having enough analgesia. Janet would talk about her pain, but there was something about how they could be together, talk together, that helped the nurse to 'just know' that her complaint was genuine. Reading small differences in her non-verbal communication, for example, a slightly different way of holding her body, a slightly different kind of frown, helped her to ask questions about the pain which she did not interpret as challenges. The nurse teased her about being an 'old wreck', and then asked her a serious question about what she needed. The relationship could be summarized as intimate.

The nurse often wondered whether she would have advocated quite as strongly for Janet if she had not taken on such a strong advocacy role for her in the past. In some ways it was Janet who prepared the nurse to be her advocate.

Premise 4

The experience of psychiatric disorder is translated into a variety of disturbances of everyday living. The practice of psychiatric nursing is located uniquely within the context of everyday life. As a result, nursing care is invariably an in vivo activity, focused on the person's relationship with self and others within the context of their interpersonal world. Nursing practice is focused on helping people to address their human responses to psychiatric disorder, rather than the disorders themselves, which are, by definition, professional constructs.

The web of our life is a mingled yarn.
(Shakespeare)

The nurse worked with Miriam for about nine months after she had been discharged from hospital. She had been diagnosed as suffering from manic depressive psychosis in her early 20s and by then she was aged over 70. Many protracted hospitalizations spanned the years. The nurse met Miriam's husband, Ted, who usually drove her the 20-odd miles to the clinic. He had bone cancer, which would soon prove fatal, although this was rarely discussed; his wife was the patient. After Ted's death, Miriam became seriously depressed and there was a concern that she might attempt suicide. Over the weeks, however, she became more philosophical, though no less depressed. Over several months the nurse listened to the account of her struggle to pick up the threads of her life. She was invited, from time to time, to say what that struggle meant for her, at which point she would fall silent and drop her head. One day, when asking the question again, the nurse added the request: 'Tell me what you're saying to yourself when you drop your head like that.' She looked up immediately and said, 'Why I'm not saying anything... all I can hear is my mother saying "self-praise is no praise at all"!'

It would be quaint if one could say that this was a 'cathartic experience', or that Miriam suddenly gained a profound insight. All that happened was that, over the next few weeks, Miriam talked more about her mother, the voice of whom, over 40 years, had turned into an auditory hallucination, which had from time to time fed her various delusions, and which now appeared to be growing fainter. As she related those tales she performed the ordinary magic which Hilda Peplau suggests lies at the heart of the interpersonal process: she made herself up as she talked (H. Peplau, personal communication). As a result, she gave her mother back 'her' voice as she settled down to the everyday business of finding her own. She began by recognizing that her last gift to her husband had been to help him toward his death. Now she needed to help herself to live *for* herself.

Advancing the proper focus of nursing

People with a diagnosis of mental illness have problems in their lives. These problems may involve their relations with the 'illness' or the diagnosis, but more often they involve *how* they live their lives, sharing their life with family, friends and the world in general. This assumption applies to people with mental illness in any context, hospital or community. The final vignette above illustrates how psychiatric nursing is enacted within the life of the person. What takes place between nurses and their clientele may be seen, from either side, as 'special'. The most special characteristic is perhaps how the short time nurses and the people in their care spend together is part of a wider whole, the person's whole life-path. In the related context of psychotherapy, Reynolds observed that:

> There is a myth in our culture that something magical occurs during an hour of psychotherapy... [people] believe that the other 167 hours of the week have less effect than that one hour. Even some therapists agree. To succumb to this myth is to relegate 167/168ths of life to meaninglessness. Life must be lived moment by moment. Each brings possibilities for purposeful activity. Each moment carries a message, a lesson for us. There are no golden hours, only ready people (Reynolds, 1985).

Many of the developments in health care provision have, at least at the level of rhetoric, involved the blurring of boundaries between the disciplines within the multidisciplinary team. The real challenge for nursing is, however, to clarify and develop further the proper focus of psychiatric nursing and the processes through which that focus might be addressed.

Given nursing's ambition to recognize the 'whole person' and to respect the personal, familial, social and cultural boundaries that define that person, more emphasis needs to be paid to understanding the person who experiences mental illness.

To date, there exists little consensus on the most appropriate models of nursing, or theories that might inform such models, for application across the range of distress addressed by mental health services. Indeed, the view has been adopted that models or theories of nursing are either redundant or anachronistic in contemporary health care (Gournay, 1996). Alternatively, it has been proposed that nurses should study and apply the theories and models that have informed medicine and psychology in an effort to develop 'evidence-based practice'. Although this proposition is not without value, it may not bring nursing closer to a clarification either of the *basic* or fundamental role and functions of the mental health nurse, or the possibilities for *advanced practice* (Barker and Reynolds, 1996). Perhaps, more importantly, it does not address the question: 'What do we need nurses for?'

Old wine in new bottles

Many developments in psychiatric nursing practice have involved nurses' acquisition of new roles, especially as therapists of one school or another. Such developments may demonstrate, among other things, nurses' capacity to join in the essentially masculine activity of 'tackling', 'challenging' or otherwise 'defeating' the phenomena that are called mental illnesses. The paradigm of psychiatric nursing that has been sketched here is essentially *feminine* in character, drawing on assumptions about the person's capacity for self-healing, adjustment or accommodation. As such, it might be viewed as belonging more to the *care* rather than to the *cure* continuum of intervention. Condon (1992) has suggested that caring provides a different, and indeed authentic, metaphor for nursing, one that is grounded in women's experience as mothers and care-givers. Such a metaphor draws its energy from the feminine persona, which lies within all people, and therefore has the potential to be represented also in men (Bly, 1990; Lee, 1991). In a more practical context, gender differences in the approach to 'care' or 'cure' may reflect differences of cognitive style, of men and women possessing quite differing world-views (Ve, 1989). Women tend to take responsibility, focusing on assisting the person to achieve maximal well-being, from a more overtly holistic perspective. Alternatively, the masculine style involves more of an efficiency–rational approach, which tends to narrow the emphasis on the individual, and on individual pathology (Ve, 1989). Dahlberg (1994) perceived this as a specific problem in Sweden, where 'medical care is one of the most patriarchal hierarchies in Swedish society'. That observation might be true of most Western societies, but may be a situation in transition.

Advanced roles and achieving goals

Mental health nursing is clearly a discipline in transition, searching for a specific role and set of functions in a health care system which is itself in a state of flux. Butterworth and Rushforth (1995) noted that the review of the roles and function of mental health nursing in the UK had taken place against a backdrop of 'breath-taking demands of policy ... added to concerns about the role of mental health nurses – perhaps an inevitable consequence of a period which had seen such dramatic change.

A common thread running through the 42 recommendations made in the 'working in partnership' report, was a need for nurses to:

> be honest about the limitations of mental health services and the uncertainty of solutions, they [nurses] should respond to people's expressed needs, taking them seriously and, whenever possible, providing choice ... [especially] real choice in matters of care. Choice should include the gender of the responsible nurse, types of treatment and the practicalities of daily living (Butterworth and Rushforth 1995).

The very *basic* nature of this philosophy suggests that the challenge that faces mental health nursing is to develop its core, emphasizing addressing the personal dimensions of the mental distress of people and their families, rather than the mere 'fixing' of illness or the compensation of disability. The primary goal of nursing appears to be the empowerment of people (and their families) who have been disempowered by the experience of illness, or the experience of inadequate care, or both.

Given the emphasis on this core 'empowerment' need, the role of the advanced nurse practitioner in mental health must be to *advance* the opportunities for achieving the goal of empowerment for the largest proportion of nurses deemed to be operating at the novice or *basic* level. The advanced nurse practitioner will, therefore, be someone with the capability of leading colleagues towards the realization of the goal of collaborative caring sketched in the 'working in partnership' report.

The function of such an advanced practitioner will differ little from a clinical leadership role in any other branch of nursing, midwifery or health visiting. The individual needs to be able to demonstrate the clinical skills, attitudes and knowledge necessary for empowering people-in-care and/or their families, to facilitate novice nurses' acquisition of such skills, attitudes and knowledge, and be able to lead, or participate in, research dedicated to clarifying the processes involved in, and the outcomes produced by, 'effective caring'.

This core leadership mission does not preclude the advanced nurse practitioner from developing 'new roles' involving, for example, prescribing medication, introducing innovative forms of psychotherapy, or engaging in preventive 'health promotion' activity in the wider community, but, such specific roles must, of necessity, be seen as an adjunct to the core activity of advancing the widespread empowerment of people and their families, rather than the main agenda item.

The wisdom that nurses might gain from the people in their care (what it means to be mentally ill, and what are the potentially infinite number of ways in which people might address and redress mental illness), represents the largely unexplored territory of mental health nursing. This is the territory that needs to be explored, mapped and charted, metaphorically speaking, by the *advanced* practitioner. The conceptual maps that they will produce will furnish the provisional knowledge that will help so-called novice (basic) nurses to find themselves within the caring relationship. If there is any higher consciousness for mental health nursing, this must be it.

Acknowledgement

I thank my colleague, Dr Chris Stevenson, for offering the lived examples of nursing illustrated in Premises 2 and 3.

References

American Nurses Association. (1980). *Nursing: A Social Policy Statement*. Kansas City, MO: ANA.

Barker, P. (1985). *Patient Assessment in Psychiatric Nursing*. London: Croom Helm.

Barker, P. (1995). Promoting growth through community mental health nursing. *Ment. Health Nurs.*, **15**(3), 12–15.

Barker, P. (1996). The logic of experience: Developing appropriate care through effective collaboration. *Aust. N. Z. J. Ment. Health Nurs.*, **5**, 3–12.

Barker, P. (1997a). *Assessment in Psychiatric and Mental Health Nursing: In Search of the Whole Person*. London: Stanley Thornes.

Barker, P. (1997b). A meta theory of nursing practice. *Mental Health Practice*, **1**(4), 18–21.

Barker, P. and Jackson, S. (1997). Mental health nursing: making it a primary concern. *Nurs. Stand.*, **11**(17), 39–41.

Barker, P. and Reynolds, W. (1996). Rediscovering the proper focus of nursing: a critique of Gournay's position on nursing theory and models. *J. Psychiatr. Ment. Health Nurs.*, **3**, 75–80.

Barker, P. J., Stevenson, C., Conway, E. et al. (1995). *Toward a Theory of Psychiatric Nursing Practice: The Tyneside View*. Newcastle: University of Newcastle upon Tyne.

Bly, R. (1990). *Iron John: A Book About Men*. New York: Addison-Wesley.

Bradshaw, A. (1997). The historical tradition of care. In *Caring: The Compassion and Wisdom of Nursing*. (G. Brykczynska, ed.) pp. 10–31. London: Edward Arnold.

Breggin, P. (1991). *Toxic Psychiatry*. New York: St Martin's Press.

Brykczynska, G. (1997). A brief overview of the epistemology of caring. In *Caring: The Compassion and Wisdom of Nursing*. (G. Brykczynska, ed.) pp. 1–9. London: Edward Arnold.

Butterworth, T. and Rushforth, D. (1995). Working in partnership with people who use services; reaffirming the foundations of practice for mental health nursing. *Int. J. Nurs. Stud.*, **32**, 373–385.

Chamberlin, J. (1988). On Our Own. London: MIND.

Condon, E. H. (1992). Nursing and the caring metaphor: gender and political influences on ethics of care. *Nursing Outlook*, **40**, 14–19.

Cooper, E. E. (1997). Dennet does it again. *Dream Again J.*, **3**(1), 7.

Cowen, E. L. (1982) Help where you find it – Four informal helping groups. *American Psychologist*, **37**, 385–395.

Dahlberg, K. (1994). The collision between caring theory and caring practice as a collision between feminine and masculine cognitive style. *J. Holistic Nurs.*, **12**, 391–401.

Department of Health. (1994). *Working in Partnership: A Collaborative Approach to Care*. (Report of the Mental Health Nursing Review Group.) London: HMSO.

Frankl, V. (1973). *The Doctor and the Soul: From Psychotherapy to Logotherapy*. Harmondsworth: Penguin.

Gergen, K. (1985). The social constructionist movement in modern psychology. *Am. Psychol.*, **40**, 266–275.

Goffman, E. (1969). *The presentation of self in everyday life*. Harmondsworth: Penguin.

Gooch, S. (1980). *The double helix of the mind.* London: Wildwood House.

Gournay, K. (1995). Mental health nurses working purposefully with people with serious and enduring mental illness – an international perspective. *Int. J. Nurs. Stud.*, **32**, 341–352.

Heron, J. (1996). *Co-operative Inquiry: Research into the Human Condition.* London: Sage.

Lee, J. (1991). *At My Father's Wedding: Reclaiming Our True Masculinity.* London: Piatkus.

Lucas, J. (1993). Nursing feature: In defence of the medical model. *Health Care Analysis*, **1**, 179–182.

Morrison, P. (1997). Patients' experience of being cared for. In *Caring: The Compassion and Wisdom of Nursing.* (G. Brykczynska, ed.) pp. 102–30. London: Edward Arnold.

Nolan, P. (1993). *A History of Mental Health Nursing.* London: Chapman and Hall.

Parse, R. R. (1981). Caring from a human science perspective. In *Caring an Essential Human Need* (M. Leininger, ed.). Proceedings from Three National Caring Conferences. Thorofore, NJ: Slack.

Parse, R. R. (ed.) (1995). *Illuminations: The Human Becoming Theory in Practice and Research.* New York: National League for Nursing.

Repper, J., Brooker, C. and Repper, D. (1993). Serious mental health problems: policy changes. *Nurs. Times*, **91**(25), 29–31.

Reynolds, D. (1985). *Playing Bull on Running Water.* London: Sheldon Press.

Rogers, A., Pilgrim, D. and Lacey, R. (1993). *Experiencing Psychiatry: Users' Views of Services.* London: Macmillan.

Romme, M. and Escher, S. (1993). *Accepting Voices.* London: MIND.

Rudman, M. J. (1996). User involvement in mental health nursing practice: rhetoric a reality? *J. Psych. and M. H. Nursing*, **3**, 385–390.

Szasz, T. S. (1961). *The Myth of Mental Illness: Foundations of a Theory of Personal Conduct.* New York: Hoeber Harper.

Ve, H. (1989). Gender difference in rationality. On the difference between technical limited and responsible rationality. Paper presented at NFPF Conference in Uppsala, Sweden. Cited in Dahlberg, K. (1994). The collision between caring theory and caring practice as a collision between feminine and masculine cognitive style. *J. Holistic Nurs.*, **12**, 391–401.

Wright, B. (1991). Labelling: The need for greater person–environment individuation. In *Handbook of Social and Clinical Psychology: The Health Perspective.* (C. R. Snyder and D. R. Forsyth, eds.) pp. 469–487. Oxford: Pergamon Press.

Wynne, L. C., Shields, C. G. and Sirkin, M. I. (1992). Illness, family theory and family therapy: 1. Conceptual issues. *Fam. Process*, **31**, 3–18.

Commentary: the theoretical perspective

As Castledine revealed in his 'Introduction' to this book, the UKCC '"fudged" the issue [of advanced nursing practice] somewhat and left nursing and midwifery to contemplate on the possibilities'. Albarran and Fulbrook, in the opening sentence of Chapter 1, reinforce this view, stating that: 'The nature of advanced practice is unclear. Furthermore, the role of the advanced practitioner...has yet to be made explicit in the literature.' The task that they set themselves is to clarify the nature of both advanced practice and the role of the advanced practitioner through an exploration of their historical development, and 'to place advanced practice within the context of contemporary nursing'. However, as we discover, the historical development of the role is far from straightforward, and probably adds to the current confusion rather than serving to clarify the situation.

Albarran and Fulbrook note that the role has its origins in the USA in the 1940s, but that it was only formally recognized in 1970 following the publication of a collection of papers in the *American Journal of Nursing*. Furthermore, although the Royal College of Nursing proposed the role of clinical nurse specialist/consultant in 1975, it failed to gain acceptance, and consequently there has been 'only limited development of advanced practice in terms of an advanced practitioner role in the UK over the last 20 years or so'. That is not to say that there have been no new advanced roles developed, but only that they have not been concerned with advanced *practice*. For example, the consultant nurse, as suggested by Wright, has been management-led, and the lecturer–practitioner is educationally-based.

It might seem on first sight that the clinical nurse specialist role fits the bill of advanced practice, but, as Albarran and Fulbrook point out, 'the role of the CNS appeared to develop on a somewhat individual basis, driven by local service demands, rather than according to a professional framework', resulting in many grey areas, confusion, and a lack of clarity. What is required, then, is clear guidelines for the role within a defined career structure, which distinguishes between the advanced practitioner, the clinical nurse specialist and the nurse practitioner.

However, this clarification of terminology is precisely what is missing, with the above-mentioned role titles being added to by the titles of 'clinical expert', 'clinical nurse manager', 'nurse consultant' and 'senior clinical nurse'. Thus, 'It is possible that although there are many different roles, they may all, in fact, be advanced practitioners. It is also possible that there are many practitioners who have a title that suggests they are advanced, when in fact they are not.' Albarran and Fulbrook continue: 'This source of confusion may be compounded as these titles are often used interchangeably. Thus, nurses can never be sure they are discussing the same concepts.

This can only add uncertainty about the broad nature of advanced nursing practice.'

The promise of a historical perspective has therefore not been realized, and although it is important to ground the search for the advanced practitioner role in a history of its development, Albarran and Fulbrook conclude that 'From the history outlined above, it is clear that there is still little real understanding about the nature of advanced practice and the role of the advanced practitioner ... Nursing has yet to answer two fundamental questions: "What is advanced practice?", and "What is an advanced practitioner?"'

In Chapter 2, Frost attempts to find answers to these questions by shifting the focus from history to politics, claiming that 'it is necessary to take a step back and consider what [and who] defines practice and how it is taken forward.' Her conclusion is that: 'Nursing is a self-regulated profession; decisions about new roles are derived from a creative tension between regulating bodies, employers, and practitioners and their professional organizations.' This view reinforces Albarran and Fulbrook's observation that the factors influencing the development of the role of advanced practitioner include professional developments, educational and health service reforms, a desire to retain clinical experts at the bedside, and a drive to advance excellence in the delivery of nursing services and strengthen the profile of clinical practice. The implication, which Frost develops later in her chapter, is that it is largely the responsibility of the profession itself to define and develop the role of advanced practitioner.

For Frost, 'nursing has reached a crossroads and must make a decision about how to move forward'. She poses the question of whether nursing should protect its core skills and retain its conventional role or develop into new areas and assume less traditional roles, and refers to these two possible routes as 'role expansion' and 'role extension'. Role expansion is concerned with 'skill and knowledge development within the concept of nursing as a separate therapeutic activity', and results from professional autonomy and self-determinism, whereas role extension 'generally refers to development that goes beyond conventional nursing boundaries' and leads to roles well outside of the conventional sphere of nursing practice.

Frost concludes that most nursing role developments included both role expansion and role extension, but, citing a study by Redshaw and Harris, suggests that *advanced* roles are qualitatively different from non-advanced roles. She then pursues this notion of a qualitative difference by claiming that: 'Advanced practice is concerned with leadership through knowledge and skill, and the advanced practitioner, in my view, is not someone who solely undertakes the most technical tasks, but who manages the delivery of nursing in ways that exploit all of the nurse's skills to collaborate with patients/clients and other members of the health team to achieve the best outcomes.' She then, significantly, adds that the role of undertaking technical tasks 'was what was intended by the UKCC in establishing the specialist practitioner specification'.

Thus, albeit by a circuitous route, Frost arrives at the central issue raised by Albarran and Fulbrook: the confusion over terminology, and in particular, over the differences between the advanced practitioner and the clinical specialist. She appears to be suggesting that advanced practice is more akin to role expansion, whereas clinical specialism is related more to role extension, although she is reluctant to push this distinction too far, since 'defining advanced practice is a bit like trying to secure jelly with drawing pins'. She therefore falls back on two mechanisms for clarifying and developing advanced practice: the first is UKCC's *The Scope of Professional Practice* document, which 'does enable nurses to take practice forward in many ways', and 'can give meaning and coherence to role development in ways that support rather than constrain initiative'. The second is education, which 'can contribute by ensuring that nurses develop the analytic thinking skills that enable practitioners to make decisions about the nature of their practice'. Frost appears to be implying, then, that we still do not have an answer to Albarran and Fulbrook's two questions, but that it is the task of practitioners themselves to move the debate forward through the framework of *The Scope of Professional Practice* document and through educational courses that attempt to facilitate discussion about the role rather than to impose it.

In the following chapter, Stilwell concurs with the lack of consensus and inability to define the role of the advanced practitioner, and suggests that the difficulty stems from problems inherent in the very nature of practice itself. Nursing, she claims, is not amenable to scientific analysis, since it is a series of unique encounters between unique individuals, and is therefore as much an art as a science. Thus, any attempt to classify practice according to what the practitioner knows or does is bound to fail: 'Nursing models and the nursing process tend to reinforce expectations that nursing is a predictable and organized activity, whereas, to be truly effective, nursing might have to be flexible, creative and responsive, and lack preconceived structure.'

For Stilwell, then, advanced practice is not defined by a specialist knowledge-base, or by the possession of specific specialist skills, but through the use of clinical judgement in a series of one-off encounters between the unique individuals who are the nurse and the patient: 'The most advanced practitioner will be the one who can, at every encounter, open the most appropriate boxes [that is, areas of practice] at the right time, in a way that is morally acceptable and offers safe and effective treatment. It is highly likely that a nurse will have to judge, at every patient encounter, which of the boxes should be explored.' Of course, unlike practice based on rules and protocols, this form of practice incurs a certain risk: 'The nurse's professional role is to calculate the extent of any risk, and to minimize it whenever possible', which is a view supported by Frost's claim that the prevailing ethos of safety can constrain and limit role development, and that 'the challenge of developing new roles is more likely to be addressed if nurses articulate the risk involved in developing new roles.'

However, Stilwell is careful not to be drawn in to the debate about titles such as advanced and specialist practitioners, or about models such as the extended and expanded roles, but asks 'is this exploration of terms used to express what is happening in nursing practice merely another manifestation of the way in which nursing has been seduced by science into descriptions of models, which, because of the responsiveness of nursing to patients' needs and to societal changes, can never be truly accurate?' Clearly, for Stilwell, advanced practice transcends labels and models.

In the final chapter of Part 1, Barker appears to be in substantial agreement with Stilwell about the nature of advanced practice as centring on the nurse–patient encounter. However, he reaches his conclusion from a slightly different perspective by cutting across the advanced/specialist and the expanded/extended role discussion with what amounts to a 'back to basics' campaign.

For Barker, advanced practice is neither about expanding nor extending what the nurse does, but rather about finding and developing the 'core' of nursing, the 'proper focus' from which nursing has strayed, particularly in its attempt to emulate the medical model. The core or proper focus of nursing entails a focus on the whole person of the patient, on 'what goes on between the nurse and the person-in-care'. Thus, advanced practitioners are concerned with 'advancing the proper focus of nursing', acting as an advance guard and mapping out the territory, and 'the conceptual maps that they will produce ... will help so-called novice (basic) nurses to find themselves within the caring relationship.'

What exactly is this 'proper focus of nursing', this 'going on' between nurse and patient, which the advanced practitioner is supposed to advance? According to Barker: 'The primary goal of nursing appears to be the empowerment of people (and their families) who have been disempowered by the experience of illness, or the experience of inadequate care, or both.' This is a powerful statement, which will ring true for many mental health nurses, but it is also a sentiment echoed by a number of writers from other branches of nursing. Thus, the role of the nurse is concerned as much with empowering, facilitating and advocating for the patient as it is with direct physical care; it is concerned as much with 'caring about' as it is with 'caring for' the patient.

Barker is not claiming that the development of new roles and technical skills should not be undertaken, but rather that 'such specific roles must, of necessity, be seen as an adjunct to the core activity of advancing the widespread empowerment of people and their families, rather than the main agenda item.' In this, he supports Frost's assertion that 'developing skills in one core area is not a threat to the core of nursing unless this replaces that core.' Specialist roles, including those that involve medical tasks, are acceptable as long as they do not reject the core or proper focus of nursing that is the empowering nurse–patient relationship.

Barker has moved us from the notion of *advanced* practice to that of *advancing* practice, such that: 'The critical aspect of the role of [advanced practitioners] might be to advance practice, acting as a role model to all those defined, implicitly, as *basic* practitioners.' However, the role is not just about acting as a role model. Barker also envisages a more direct role for the advanced practitioner in advancing basic practitioners. Thus, 'the role of the advanced nurse practitioner in mental health must be to *advance* the opportunities for achieving the goal of empowerment for ... nurses deemed to be operating at the novice or *basic* level.' If the proper focus of basic nurses is to empower patients, then the focus of advanced practitioners is to *enable* basic nurses to empower patients through the production of 'conceptual maps'. Quite what those conceptual maps are, and how they might be produced, is not elaborated, but will be the subject of much of Part 4 of this book.

Part 2

Exploring advanced practice:
the research perspective

5

Exploring new roles in nursing: a researcher's perspective

Susan M. Read

Introduction

It is a common complaint amongst researchers that we seldom have time to reflect on our work in sufficient depth. It is pleasing, then, to be given the opportunity to revisit some of my own research based explorations of new roles in nursing, and to re-examine my findings through a lens marked 'advanced practice'. This is not, therefore, a systematic review of the research literature on advanced practice; the lack of a common understanding of the term would make that a difficult exercise. I will, however, discuss varied perceptions of the component parts of advanced practice, and propose a check-list of criteria by which to assess whether a role exhibits characteristics of advanced practice. I will also explore briefly some of the pressures that have stimulated the introduction of new roles (understanding these pressures helps to explain why certain types of new role have become popular), and attempt to discern differences between what is new and advanced, and what is new but not advanced. New projects in this expanding area of research will also be mentioned.

What is a role in nursing?

The most common dictionary definition of 'role' is that it is a part played by an actor. That may be a useful analogy, as we think of an actor donning a costume, learning a script, relating to other characters, and moving about on a stage. Sometimes the part will be well known, and already have been played by a host of previous actors. Sometimes it will be brand new, with no role model to follow.

The role and function of the nurse have always been the subject of argument, ever since Nightingale subtitled her famous *Notes on Nursing* (1859) 'what it is and what it is not'. In the 1950s, when work-study methods were first applied to nursing, Goddard (1953) divided up nursing duties into basic and technical. This division, which led to a widespread delegation of bedside care to untrained staff, was later deplored by writers imbued with the ideal of holistic care (Williams, 1978; Pembrey, 1985). The policy document that first set out guidelines for certification of extended roles (Department of Health and Social Security (DHSS) 1977) maintained that nursing involved the promotion of health, the prevention of illness, the care of the sick, and rehabilitation. The core of the role was caring for people.

Nearly 20 years later, a consensus statement from professional leaders of nursing (Department of Health (DoH), 1994) said that caring was still the core, and that the role was built around skills and values, encompassing:

1. A co-ordinating function;
2. A teaching function;
3. Developing and maintaining programmes of care;
4. Technical expertise;
5. Concern for the ill and those who are currently well;
6. Special responsibility for the frail and vulnerable.

Different roles in nursing will contain these elements in varying quantities and constellations, and sometimes a nurse may be functioning in more than one role within a particular job, thus risking role confusion or role conflict. For instance, an experienced and well-trained nurse in an accident and emergency (A&E) department might move between the role of triage nurse (assessing urgency of arrivals), nurse practitioner (assessing, treating and discharging patients with minor injuries), major trauma nurse, and clinical shift manager.

What is new?

Any researcher setting out to explore new roles in nursing very soon becomes aware that what is new in one area of practice may be accepted as a normal activity in another, maybe not far away geographically, even in a different specialty in the same hospital. So decisions have to be taken early in a study about whether to adopt either a relative stance or an absolute one. The relative stance is typified by this definition of innovation used in a study of British hospital management:

> Innovation is the intentional introduction and application within a role, group or organization, of ideas, processes, products or procedures, *new to the relevant unit of adoption*, designed to significantly benefit the individual, group, organization or wider society (West and Farr, 1990) (my italics).

A similar stance is being taken in an ongoing research project 'Exploring new roles in practice', funded by the Department of Health, in which a team from Sheffield University is collaborating with colleagues at Bristol University and the King's Fund. The trusts taking part contribute information on any role that is *new to them*, or on specialist roles, which, although established for some time, are now breaking new ground.

Other research in which I have been involved has taken an absolute stance. For instance, a survey and census of nurse practitioner activity in A&E departments in England and Wales (Read et al., 1992a) took as its starting point the definition that an emergency nurse practitioner:

> is a nurse who is authorised to assess and treat patients attending an accident and emergency department, either as an alternative to the patient being seen by a

doctor, or in the absence of a doctor in a department where a continuous medical presence is not maintained.

However, even where a basic definition is given, there may be room within it for expression of variation. In the above A&E census and survey there were options for reply to clarify just how much authority was allowed. Some nurses function as nurse practitioners without actually holding the title, particularly in peripheral units where patients are assessed and treated by nurses acting on the authority of general practitioners. In some departments, nurses combine the process of triage (determining urgency) with the nurse practitioner role of assessing and treating certain categories of injury. Some nurses acting as nurse practitioners, whether or not they use that title, have authority to discharge patients from further attendance; others must advise patients to see a doctor within a stated period, either at the hospital or in a general practitioner's surgery.

Sometimes, the population for a research study on innovation is defined by the funding body who financed that innovation. The study might find that the level of innovation varies widely from site to site (e.g. Read and Graves, 1994), but all subjects defined by the funding body are still included.

What is advanced?

This reporting of variation in what is seen as 'new' between settings serves to illuminate the notion that advanced practice as an entity also varies in its expression. What is accepted as advanced in one place, like the idea of 'newness', may be standard practice in another. In this chapter, I therefore look in some detail at research in which I have been involved, and in less detail at several other reports, in an attempt to map a range of advanced practice in acute care. To do this, a number of criteria will be used as yardsticks to delineate what might in reality be termed advanced practice as opposed to more limited extensions to practice.

The first source of possible criteria is the United Kingdom Central Council for Nursing, Midwifery and Health Visiting (UKCC) statement on advanced practice in its document *PREP and You* (1995). Advanced practice is said to be concerned with:

- Adjusting the boundaries for the development of future practice;
- Pioneering and developing new roles that are responsive to changing needs;
- Advancing clinical practice, research and education to enrich nursing practice as a whole;
- Contributing to health policy and management and the determination of health needs;
- Continuing the development of the professions in the interests of patients, clients and health services.

Only the first two of these five areas of concern lend themselves to conversion into criteria by which to delineate advanced practice; the remaining three are so generalized that they cannot be converted easily into specific indicators.

Another source of criteria is a list of core attributes said, by two American leaders in these fields, to be needed by both nurse practitioners and clinical nurse specialists. They have compared curricula for the two streams of advanced practice nurses (Sparacino and Durand, 1986). The core attributes given are:

- A sophisticated use of clinical knowledge;
- A demonstration of a high level of accountability;
- Systematic assessment and intervention;
- Independent clinical decision making;
- Risk taking, autonomy and independence;
- Expansion of the boundaries of professional practice.

The defining attributes of the 'expert' nurse as postulated by Jasper (1994) can be added:

- Possession of a specialized body of knowledge or skill;
- Extensive experience in that field of practice;
- Highly developed levels of pattern recognition;
- Acknowledgement by others.

All the sources for criteria by which to delineate advanced practice used so far have taken it as read that what is under discussion is still nursing. However, the nursing press in recent years has reverberated to the sound of argument about whether certain new roles are legitimately nursing, or whether they are really a substitute for doctors (Castledine, 1996). For instance, Bowman and Thompson said in 1990:

> Many CNSs [clinical nurse specialists] are essentially medical assistants rather than CNSs; that is, they treat pathology, in which the doctor is the holder of knowledge on the subject and the purveyor of finer skills.

Bowman and Thompson go on to say that clinical nurse specialists' knowledge and skills should be steeped in nursing theory and practice, and that the clinical nurse specialist title should be reserved for those whose work is without doubt fixed in nursing. A colleague and I described our view of the difference between advanced nursing practice and being a medical assistant (Read and Graves, 1994):

> When nursing knowledge and experience continuously informs a practitioner's decision making, even though some parts of the role may overlap the medical role, then that may be said to be advanced nursing practice. Conversely, when a nurse is expected to perform routine technical tasks with no opportunity to exercise nursing knowledge or take autonomous decisions, then that is when a nurse becomes a doctor's assistant.

None of the quotations given so far has specified the level of education expected of a nurse in advanced practice. The American literature takes it for granted that both clinical nurse specialists and nurse practitioners will be educated at least to first degree level, and maybe to master's level. In the UK, opinion is moving that way, being particularly encouraged by a UKCC (1995) statement:

> The UKCC recognises that many practitioners are acquiring advanced skills and undertaking studies which are likely to be at Masters and PhD level. The UKCC

will review these regularly and may consider the recording of such qualifications in due course.

The Council stated that, until that happens, nurses may demonstrate through their professional profile that their practice and knowledge equates with the concept of advanced practice. In spite of the lack of a decision from the UKCC, it would be wise to add an educational criterion to any profile for an advanced practitioner.

A check-list of characteristics of advanced practice

If we aggregate the attributes listed, we may compile a check-list of questions to be asked in relation to a selection of new nursing roles described in research reports in the UK from 1992 onwards. The questions are as follows. Does this role entail the following?:

1. Expansion or adjustment of the boundaries of practice;
2. Pioneering in response to changing needs;
3. Sophisticated use of clinical knowledge and skill;
4. Possession of extensive experience in a particular field;
5. Systematic assessment of patients leading to the offering of some health care intervention;
6. Independent clinical decision making, using highly developed levels of pattern recognition;
7. Demonstration of a high level of accountability, autonomy and risk taking;
8. Recognition by colleagues of postholder expertise;
9. Grounding in the theory and practice of nursing, and opportunity to use nursing knowledge when making decisions;
10. An educational qualification beyond first level registration at certificate level, either through academic study or higher professional education.

Pressures stimulating the development of new roles

In 1995, I wrote *Catching the Tide: New Voyages in Nursing* (Read, 1995), extrapolating lessons for managers when creating new roles for nurses, drawn from research into Junior Doctors' Taskforce-funded posts in the Trent Region (Read and Graves, 1994). I likened the pressure for new roles to be developed to a rising tide, which might be seen either:

as a danger, threatening to wash away the sea defences of professional and disciplinary barriers. Alternatively, the tide may be seen as an opportunity to launch out on new voyages, where co-operation and collaboration between health care professions are essential... (Read, 1995).

This rising tide of pressure has a number of different sources. First, patients' needs for better co-ordinated care might be answered by the creation of new nursing roles. New nurse-led preoperative assessment clinics have arisen, not just to reduce junior doctors' hours, although they have contributed to that (Read and Graves, 1994), but to meet patients' needs for better information and a reduction in anxiety before surgery. Such patient need might be revealed in research studies or clinical audit, or expressed through the complaints mechanism in the NHS.

A second source of pressure is the reduced availability of junior doctors, through the 'new deal' initiative to cut their hours (National Health Service Management Executive (NHSME), 1991), and changes in specialist medical training (DoH, 1993) requiring more time to be spent in educational rather than service activity. Coupled with a shortage of doctors in particular specialties, for example, in anaesthetics and A&E (Special Workforce Advisory Group, 1996), these changes translate into specific gaps in service provision, which might possibly be met by nurses.

The increased freedom for trusts to determine their own staffing and skill-mix strategies (DoH, 1989a), combined with the issue in 1992 of the UKCC's *Scope of Professional Practice* statement allowing nurses greater discretion to decide whether to expand their practice, forms a third source of pressure for change.

A fourth source of pressure arises from new initiatives in the organization of care, such as 're-engineering' (Hammer and Champey, 1993; Humphreys, 1996), 'patient focused care' (Morgan, 1993; National Health Service Executive (NHSE), 1994) and case management (Petryshen and Petryshen, 1992; Hale, 1995). All these initiatives involve detailed examination of the processes of care for patients who have a range of problems, to try to streamline the service and make it more acceptable to the patient as well as more efficient and effective.

Linked with the concept of reconfiguring care processes is a greater willingness for the medical profession to see itself as part of the clinical team, and to be willing at least to consider greater sharing of skills and roles (Audit Commission, 1995; Moss and McNichol, 1995; Reilly et al., 1996; Royal College of Physicians and Royal College of Nursing, 1996).

A further range of pressures comes from the need to fulfil policy targets expressed in *The Health of the Nation* (DoH, 1991a), *Caring for People* (DoH, 1989b), *Primary Care: the Future* (NHSE, 1996a) and *The NHS – a Service with Ambitions* (NHSE, 1996b). These targets can only be achieved by good teamwork involving all health care professions. The pressures are increased by the drive to achieve greater clinical effectiveness within limited resources (NHSME, 1993; Drummond, 1994), to continue to reduce within-hospital waiting times, and to reach the standards set in *The Patient's Charter* (DoH, 1991b).

The final pressure recognized here is consideration of the future, when there will be greater patient demand from an ageing population, and comparatively less human and financial resource to meet the demand (DoH, 1994).

Using the check-list to search for advanced practice

Study 1: Triage in A&E

My own research into new roles in nursing began with a Department of Health funded study assessing the impact of triage by nurses in an A&E

department (George et al., 1992; Read et al., 1992b; Read et al., 1994). Although it was intended to compare the effect on waiting times for patients in different categories of urgency (assessed retrospectively from records) when triage was and was not in operation, in reality it was a comparison of the effect of formal and informal triage processes. When formal triage was not operating, a quicker, less bureaucratic assessment still took place, which turned out to be more effective at moving the really urgent patients more quickly through the department.

The role of a triage nurse is an example of a role that is not enacted exclusively by a very few people within an A&E department, but is shared out quite widely. It was a relatively new role when the research was carried out in 1990, introduced largely in response to patient need, and later adapted to help conform to 'Patients' Charter' standards. Four of the 10 check-list items set out above were definitely required for triage to be carried out properly (items 3, 4, 5 and 9), and possibly others would be recognizable in some triage nurses but not in all (items 1, 2, 6, 7, 8 and 10). One factor that would determine whether a particular department expected their triage nurses to practise at an advanced level was whether authority was given to direct certain patients to other sources of care, rather than admitting them to the A&E department.

Study 2: The nurse practitioner in A&E

The triage study was followed by a further Department of Health funded project, an exploration of the role of the nurse practitioner (NP) in A&E departments (Read et al., 1992a; Read and George, 1994). This study, too, did not unfold as originally intended. The planned randomized controlled trial comparing patients with minor injuries treated by either NPs or senior house officers (SHOs) could not take place for several reasons. First, the volume of patients managed by NPs was much lower than the number treated by SHOs, partly because the NPs were frequently diverted to other roles within the department. Secondly, the pathways of care were often the same for patients, whether initially assessed by a NP or a SHO. For example, instant X-ray reporting at the hospital in question from 9.00 a.m. to 5.00 p.m. on weekdays meant that patients with fractures went straight to the fracture clinic from the X-ray department, whoever had referred them. Patients with lacerations were often referred to nurses in the department for suturing, glueing or bandaging, by either SHOs or NPs. Thirdly, the relationship between treatment process and outcome was not by any means unequivocal. We, as researchers, reflected on this as follows:

> At the conclusion of the pilot studies we remained uncertain whether any delay in healing, or the occurrence of new problems during recovery, was due to shortcomings in diagnosis or treatment in the A&E department whether by NP or SHO, or whether these problems stemmed either from the nature of the original injury or from lack of compliance with instructions (Read and George, 1994).

It was also possible that due to the self-limiting nature of many minor injuries, the patients might have recovered equally well had they not attended the A&E department.

Because of all these difficulties, the randomized controlled trial was abandoned, and an extensive survey and census of A&E departments in

England and Wales was carried out. The objectives were to determine the distribution and scope of NP schemes in A&E departments, to describe the caseloads of doctors and NPs on two representative days, and to estimate the number of patients managed by NPs in the year from April 1990 to March 1991 (Read et al., 1992a).

All A&E departments in England and Wales were surveyed by post in 1991, including specialist departments (mainly paediatric and ophthalmic) and community hospitals with minor injury departments. A census of casenotes for the same two representative days (a weekday and a Sunday) was undertaken in 37 A&E departments (major, specialist and minor) scattered throughout the then 14 English NHS regions and Wales. Their survey returns indicated the likelihood of significant NP activity in terms of nurses taking responsibility for treatment decisions for patients with minor injuries. The definition of the NP used has already been quoted earlier in this chapter. The main findings were these:

- 27 (6%) of 465 responding departments had official NP schemes. Official NP schemes (where the title of NP is used and protocols are generally in place) were more common in specialist and major departments than in minor ones.
- 159 (34%) of the 465 departments reported unofficial NP schemes, where the NP title was not used, but experienced nurses fulfilled the function of NP through long-established custom and practice. Unofficial schemes were much more common in minor and specialist departments than in major ones.
- 279 (60%) of departments reported no NP scheme at all.
- 16 of 25 (64%) specialist (mainly ophthalmic and paediatric) A&E departments had either official or unofficial schemes. The majority of nurses working in these departments have postregistration qualifications in their specialty.
- Officially designated NPs usually exercised more authority and autonomy, particularly with respect to the right to discharge patients from further care, but for a somewhat more restricted group of patients than were treated by unofficial NPs. (Protocols often excluded official NPs from treating children, and patients with injuries above the elbow, or knee or on the face.)

Two major schools of thought about NPs were evident. The first believed that the NP role was an extension of triage, and the two roles were combined. The NP would do the triage assessment, treat a few patients within the protocol, and expedite the path of many more by referring them direct to the X-ray department and thence to a doctor. The second school saw the NP role as separate from triage; the NP was seen as a truly alternative provider of A&E care, to whom the triage nurse would refer suitable patients.

The census revealed few differences in the types of injury treated by official NPs in major departments and unofficial NPs in minor departments. Only 530 (9%) of the 5814 patients attending the 37 departments on the two census days were managed entirely by NPs. In both major and minor departments, open wounds, contusions and abrasions formed two-thirds of the NPs' workloads.

Survey respondents' perceptions of the levels of authority exercised by NPs in their departments were not always reflected in the census information. The observation that managers' concepts of what their staff do are not always borne out in reality recurs throughout my research experience in exploring new roles.

We need to remember that both the triage study and the A&E NP study were carried out before the issue of the UKCC's 'scope of practice' statement (1992) and the withdrawal of the regulations about certification of extended roles (DoH, 1992). Nevertheless, even in 1991, when the survey and census were carried out, many of the A&E NPs exhibited a majority of the characteristics listed in the check-list of features of advanced practice (items 1, 2, 3, 4, 5, 6, 8 and 9) and some NPs also showed the remainder.

Study 3: Junior doctors' hours: the nursing contribution. Year 1

My next opportunity to study new roles in nursing grew out of the 'new deal' initiative for junior doctors (NHSME, 1991). In 1993, Trent Regional Taskforce for Junior Doctors' Hours awarded funds to 18 different trusts or directly managed units within the region to pump–prime 32 nursing roles in 16 distinct clinical specialties. The nursing roles were created with the primary intention of reducing junior doctors' hours and intensity of work, and were to be evaluated in a study lasting one year and funded by the Taskforce (Read and Graves, 1994).

A multiple case-study design was chosen because of the complexity, variety and size of the research field, but making cross-case comparisons wherever possible. The postholders were interviewed on three occasions over the span of the study, contact was maintained with their related managers wherever possible, consultants and junior doctors were given questionnaires, and local documentation and audit data were used. Profiles were built up for each post, detailing specialty, grade and title of post (some were called 'nurse practitioner', some 'clinical nurse specialist', and there was a variety of other titles, both simple and complicated). Other features of the profiles were qualifications, experience, training for the post, objectives and their achievement, details of case-mix and audit, evidence of patient satisfaction, and perceptions of related consultants, junior doctors and managers.

Because of the difficulty of making exact measurements to ascertain the effect of the new nursing posts (some postholders liaised with large numbers of SHOs; the mean was four, and some rotations meant that SHOs changed every eight weeks), the notion of assessing trends towards effectiveness was used. The contributing factors to a positive trend were:

- Achievement of objectives for the role;
- Consensus among junior doctors and consultants that the junior doctor workload had been reduced (perceptions about intensity and hours);
- Improvement in junior doctor job satisfaction;
- Perception of patient service improvement.

Posts were assessed for trends towards effectiveness in groups. The most obviously effective roles were in the preoperative assessment group. Most nurses in this group worked to very clearly defined protocols and only exhibited some of the check-list characteristics associated with advanced practice (items 3, 4, 5, with possible additions of 1, 2, 8 and 9). They did, however, make an impact on junior doctor workload as well as improving service to patients and increasing efficiency.

Another clearly defined group was the A&E NPs. Here, the trend towards effectiveness was less clear, probably because in two of the three schemes studied, many of the experienced A&E nurses were being trained at the same time to take on the NP role. The result was gradual, with incremental change rather than a dramatic 'big-bang' approach. Frequently, the NP service was available only sporadically, when the department was well-staffed, so junior doctor workload and patient waiting times were not reduced consistently. Like the A&E NPs surveyed earlier, however, many were at least moving towards recognition according to the advanced practice check-list (items 1 to 6, 8 and 9), but it was a slow process because of training difficulties and the time needed to become confident in the role.

Another group of posts was much more task orientated. The group label we derived was 'the transfer of work group'. Nurses were very specifically taking over particular tasks from junior doctors, often with the strategy of cascading the skills training through a section of staff. For instance, in an integrated medicine unit, one nurse was given the job of training all the others to perform 12-lead electrocardiogram. Very few attributes of advanced practice were observed in this group (items 4 and 8), because the nurses were largely focused on particular tasks.

The research team grouped together most of the other roles studied under the heading of 'advanced practice/nurse-led care'. This grouping belies the presence of very great variety within the group, and the occurrence of many delaying factors, which prevented unequivocal recognition of effectiveness. Sometimes it was difficult for a trust to appoint a suitable postholder, or to arrange the necessary specialist training or supervised practice. Within this group, the three specialist gynaecology nurses appeared to be making the most impact. Each of them worked in a different trust. One spent most of her time co-ordinating the medical termination of pregnancy service. The other two spent a smaller proportion of their time in similar services and a greater proportion counselling infertile patients and those undergoing hysterectomy. The gynaecology specialist nurses developed very specific skills and expertise in their own field, and were definitely recognized as moving towards advanced practice.

Despite the problems that beset the establishment of posts in this group, in addition to the gynaecology nurses, others too were beginning to exhibit characteristics of advanced practice, particularly:

- A nurse specialist for analgesia, mainly for postoperative patients;
- Ear, nose and throat (ENT) specialist nurses/NPs;
- A cardiology day care nurse;
- Endocrinology specialist nurses/NPs;
- Psychiatric emergency liaison nurses.

The nurse specialist for analgesia had become a highly valued member of the pain relief team, teaching junior doctors and ward nurses about the safe use of patient-controlled analgesia pumps and the care and management of patients using epidural analgesia. Two trusts introduced expanded roles for nurses in ENT outpatients departments. In one trust, a sister and two staff nurses took over postoperative aural toilet procedures for myringotomy and mastoidectomy patients. In the other, three ENT NPs undertook preoperative clerking and preparation for ENT patients, as well as a wide range of postoperative procedures and general ENT care.

In a specialized cardiology unit, nurses co-ordinated all the care and investigations in the day-case ward, where patients attended for procedures such as cardiac catheterization and cardioversion. The necessary training for ward nurses was carried out by a nursing practice facilitator who pioneered the changing roles, and helped greatly to improve the continuity of care for patients.

In a similar way, two trusts introduced nurse-led care for endocrinology day patients so that, although the patients still needed some specialized procedures to be carried out by technical staff, the majority of their care was from their own primary nurse.

Most items on the advanced practice check-list are positive for these practitioners of nurse-led care, but items 6 and 7 are queried because independence and autonomy are not often appropriate in this acute care setting. However, interdependence and fully equal team membership are appropriate, and were present in most of the nurses in this 'nurse-led care' group.

The psychiatric liaison scheme, which began with one nurse working from 9.00 a.m. to 5.00 p.m. on weekdays was so effective that it quickly became a 24-hour, seven-day-a-week service. Experienced and qualified psychiatric nurses were on stand-by to assess the mental health needs of patients presenting in A&E, or showing signs of mental or emotional disturbance in the acute wards of a district general hospital. Not only were calls to junior doctors drastically reduced, but the patients received a speedier and more appropriate form of care.

Although this particular research project (Read and Graves, 1994) focused on posts designed to reduce junior doctors' hours and intensity of work, it did also help to further the identification of advanced practice.

Study 4: Junior doctors' hours: the nursing contribution. Year 2

A further group of Trent Regional Junior Doctors' Taskforce funded posts was studied during 1995 (Murray et al., 1995). The primary focus of this research was methodological. Trent Research and Development Directorate funded the project hoping that progress could be made in terms of improving the rigour of evaluating changing roles in the NHS. Unlike the first Trent Taskforce study, when all posts receiving funding were the subjects for case study, the researchers in this second study set up the criteria for inclusion early in the research process. Some criteria were based on the likelihood of obtaining adequate information for a rigorous study. Others, however, were clustered around the characteristics of the post, which made it likely that study of it would not only be feasible but also worth while. These criteria were that the postholder undertook some activities beyond the scope of normal nursing practice, that he or she provided direct patient care and managed a discrete caseload.

Prior to applying the criteria, however, one essential condition had to be met, and this eliminated a large number of posts from the study. The clinical manager for each post had to return a questionnaire giving basic information about the post. We sent questionnaires to the managers of 43 posts, and by the closing date six weeks later, had only received 17 replies. Of these, five were judged to be unsuitable for detailed study, either because the scope of practice was within usual limits, or because the likelihood of obtaining good data was remote. The remaining 12 were divided into a priority study group of eight posts and a secondary group of four.

On paper, from the information obtained through the questionnaires, the priority group of eight looked as though they would demonstrate most of the characteristics of advanced practice. A majority of the secondary group were planning to 'cascade' their skills to whole teams of nurses, but initially also appeared to be practising in an advanced way. Visits to the postholders, however, revealed a different perspective for some.

Three posts in the first group appeared, on paper, to be quite similar. All were nurse specialists in the field of anticoagulation, and were to become skilled at calculating and varying warfarin dosage in response to blood tests and following strict protocols. This was judged to be beyond the normal scope of nursing practice. All the NPs were meant to have their own caseloads and manage totally the long-term outpatient care of suitable patients. In practice, only one of the three nurses in this group actually had a discrete caseload of her own patients, the others were working in a fragmented, task-orientated way, which could not be called advanced practice.

The fourth post investigated in the priority group was of a NP in emergency ophthalmology, who was responsible for patients attending a 'walk-in' eye clinic, assessing and treating them within the framework of a protocol. The job description also covered plans for the same NP to be involved in preoperative assessment of ophthalmic surgery patients and screening for glaucoma. Neither of these intentions was being fulfilled. Most of the advanced practice characteristics were exhibited by this postholder in the course of assessing and treating emergency eye patients.

The fifth post, an A&E practitioner post, was being implemented only partially, due to staff shortages. The sixth one was in the field of paediatric urology and spanned the hospital/community interface; the postholder certainly carried out investigations that were not usually within nurses' scope of practice, and was a pioneer in spanning the hospital/community boundary. Although able to adjust dosage and timing of pre-prescribed medication, much of this postholder's expertise was rooted in her nursing background. She demonstrated many of the characteristics of advanced practice, and had been instrumental in setting up a special interest group for her particular specialty.

The remaining two posts in the priority study group were for night duty practitioners. The work was actually shared between three part-time staff, and it soon became evident that the posts were intended to cascade skills throughout the night staff. The work was task-orientated and fragmented but also involved teaching. These night duty practitioners could not really be classified as advanced practitioners.

I have already referred to a secondary group of four posts studied in this further evaluation of Trent Taskforce funded posts (Murray et al., 1995). They were assigned to the secondary group, either because the intention was to cascade the skills of other staff quite quickly, or because there were other reasons that made the prospect of rigorous research appear unlikely. Two of these posts involved preoperative assessment; one specialized in vascular surgery, the other's job description stated the intention to cover general surgery, gynaecology and orthopaedics. Site visits and further enquiries revealed that both posts were quite well focused; the second one was concentrating on general surgery, and awaiting further appointments to cover the other specialties. Both postholders were carrying out physical assessments and had a good deal of authority, both to request investigations and to make referrals, so fulfilling at least some of the characteristics of advanced practice.

A third post in the secondary group appeared on first sight to focus mainly on the cascading of skills to do with intravenous access. On closer investigation, it was clear that the postholder (whose title was 'intravenous access and nutrition sister') was intended to manage a small, but discrete, caseload spanning hospital and community patients who were receiving long-term parenteral nutrition through a central line. The sister would, in addition, teach nursing staff, junior doctors and medical students good practice in relation to intravenous therapy. This post, too, exhibited some characteristics of advanced practice.

The last post in this secondary group was for a NP in neurogenic urology. The job description covered a very broad range of activities in outpatients, the ward and theatre, including ultrasound scanning, ordering X-ray examinations and acting as first assistant to the surgeon. In practice, the NP was not able to undertake the latter two duties, due to unforeseen legal anxieties in the trust. However, the postholder did have a discrete caseload of patients and carried out quite complex patient assessments, and so appeared to be practising at an advanced level.

Towards the end of the second Trent funded project, the researchers gathered both sets of postholders for a study day and workshops. One observation made by one postholder received strong support from the rest of the audience, that advanced nursing practice was much more strongly related to a high level of clinical decision making for a discrete caseload of patients than to the carrying out of highly technical procedures.

Study 5: Nurse-led ear care service

One final study with which I have been associated should be mentioned, an evaluation of a nurse-led ear care service in primary care (Fall et al., 1997a; 1997b). Here again, the most significant aspect was the responsibility of the practice nurses who had been trained in ear care to discern whether the patient's ear condition could place them in danger (in the otologist's terms, whether the ear is 'safe' or 'unsafe'). The practice nurses had a number of technical skills at their disposal, but this decision was of primary concern to them (Rodgers, 1996).

Table 5.1 gives a summary of each of the roles mentioned.

Table 5.1. Nursing roles measured against a check-list of advanced practice

Nursing roles	Reference	Characteristics										Advanced practitioner?
		1	2	3	4	5	6	7	8	9	10	
Triage in A&E	George et al., 1992	?	?	✓	✓	✓	?	?	?	✓	?	Some triage nurses at this level
NPs in A&E	Read et al., 1992	✓	✓	✓	✓	✓	✓	?	✓	✓	?	Probably most A&E NPs
Trent Taskforce 1st Wave												
Preoperative assessment	Read and Graves, 1994	?	?	✓	✓	✓	−	−	?	?	?	Maybe a few at this level
NPs in A&E	Read and Graves, 1994	✓	?	✓	✓	✓	✓	?	✓	✓	?	Probably most A&E NPs
'Transfer of work' group	Read and Graves, 1994	−	−	?	✓	−	−	−	?	?	?	No
Gynae. CNSs/NPs	Read and Graves, 1994	✓	?✓	✓	✓	?✓	?✓	?	✓	✓	?	Probably yes
Preoperative pain CNS	Read and Graves, 1994	?	✓	✓	✓	✓	?	?	✓	✓	?	Probably yes
ENT CNSs/NPs	Read and Graves, 1994	?	✓	✓	✓	?	?	?	✓	✓	?	Probably yes
Cardiology CNS	Read and Graves, 1994	?	✓	✓	✓	✓	?	?	✓	✓	?	Probably yes
Endocrinology NPs	Read and Graves, 1994	?	✓	✓	✓	✓	?✓	✓	✓	✓	?	Probably yes
Psychiatric liaison	Read and Graves, 1994	−	✓	✓	✓	✓	?	?	✓	✓	?	Probably yes
Trent Taskforce 2nd Wave												
Anticoagulation nurse specialists	Murray et al., 1995	✓	✓	✓	✓	✓	?	?	?	?	?	Moving towards this level; one further forward than others
Emergency ophthalmology NP	Murray et al., 1995	✓	✓	✓	✓	✓	?	?	✓	✓	?	Probably yes
Paediatric urology NP	Murray et al., 1995	✓	✓	✓	✓	✓	?	?	✓	✓	?	Probably yes
Night NPs	Murray et al., 1995	✓	?	?	?	?	?	?	?	✓	?	No
Preoperative assessment × 2	Murray et al., 1995	✓	?	✓	✓	✓	?	?	✓	✓	?	Probably yes
Intravenous access and nutrition sister	Murray et al., 1995	✓	?	✓	✓	?	?	?	✓	✓	?	Probably yes
Neurogenic neurology NP	Murray et al., 1995	✓	✓	✓	✓	✓	?	?	✓	✓	?	Probably yes
Ear care trained practice nurses	Fall et al., 1997a; 1997b	✓	✓	✓	✓	✓	?	?	✓	✓	?	Some functioning at this level

Conclusion

I began this chapter by explaining that I would re-examine new roles in nursing, which had been the subject of my research over the last few years, looking at them through a lens marked 'advanced practice'. As we have seen, that lens itself is quite imprecise, because there is no consensus on what constitutes advanced practice. A group of nurses who have undertaken new roles felt strongly that the crucial factor is the level of decision making and responsibility for a caseload rather than the nature of the tasks undertaken. Another conclusion already observed is that independence and autonomy in decision making may not necessarily be appropriate for nurses in acute care, it would rather be interdependence and accountability within a team context.

One thing is certain; roles in nursing are not static. Current research funded under the Department of Health's 'Human Resources Initiative', including 'Exploring new roles in practice' and 'Realizing specialist and advanced nursing practice', with which I am involved, should shed some light on the development of advanced practice over the next few years.

References

Audit Commission. (1995). *The Doctor's Tale: the Work of Hospital Doctors in England and Wales.* London: HMSO.

Bowman, G. and Thompson, D. (1990). When is a specialist not a specialist? *Nurs. Times,* **86**(8), 48.

Castledine, G. (1996). Nurses must not become the mechanical hands of doctors. *Br. J. Nurs.,* **5**, 386.

Department of Health (1989a) *Working for Patients,* (Cm 555.) London: HMSO.

Department of Health. (1989b). *Caring for People: Community Care in the Next Decade and Beyond.* London: HMSO.

Department of Health. (1991a). *The Health of the Nation.* London: HMSO.

Department of Health. (1991b). *The Patient's Charter: Raising the Standard.* London: DoH.

Department of Health. (1992). *The Extended Role of the Nurse/Scope of Professional Practice.* (PL/CNO(92)4.) London: DoH.

Department of Health. (Calman Report, 1993). *Hospital Doctors: Training for the Future.* (The report of the Working Group on Specialist Medical Training.) London: DoH.

Department of Health. (1994). *The Challenges for Nursing and Midwifery in the 21st Century.* London: DoH.

Department of Health and Social Security. (1977). *The Extending Role of the Clinical Nurse.* (HL (77) 22.) London: DHSS.

Drummond, M. (1994). *Economic Analysis Alongside Controlled Clinical Trials: an Introduction for Clinical Researchers.* London: DoH.

Fall, M., Walters, S., Read, S. et al. (1997a). An evaluation of a nurse-led ear care service in primary care: benefits and costs. *Br. J. Gen. Pract.,* **47**, 699–703.

Fall, M., Read, S. M., Walters, S. and Deverill, M. (1997b). An evaluation of a nurse-led ear-care service in primary care: benefits and cost consequences. Sheffield University School of Health and Related Research: SCHARR Report to Research and Development directorate, NHS Executive (Trent).

George, S., Read, S., Westlake, L. et al. (1992). Evaluation of nurse triage in British A&E departments. *BMJ,* **304**, 876–878.

Goddard, H. (1953). *The Work of Nurses in Hospital Wards.* London: Nuffield Provincial Hospitals Trust.

Hale, C. (1995). Case management and managed care. *Nurs. Stand.,* **9**(19), 33–35.

Hammer, M. and Champey, J. (1993). *Re-engineering the Corporation – a Manifesto for Business Revolution.* London: Nicholas Brealey.

Humphreys, J. (1996). Old idea, new jargon. *Nurs. Stand.*, **10**, 16.

Jasper, M. A. (1994). Expert: a discussion of the implications of the concept as used in nursing. *J. Adv. Nurs.*, **20**, 769–776.

Morgan, G. (1993). The implications of patient focused care. *Nurs. Stand.*, **7**(52), 37–39.

Moss, F. and McNichol, M. (1995). Alternative models of organization are needed. *BMJ*, **310**, 925–928.

Murray, C., Read, S. M. and McCabe, C. (1995). Reduction of junior doctors' hours in Trent Region: the nursing contribution. Phase 2 A methodological study. Sheffield University School of Health and Related Research: SCHARR Report to Research and Development Directorate, NHS Executive (Trent).

National Health Service Executive (Value for Money Team). (1994). *The Patient's Progress – Towards a Better Service*. London: HMSO.

National Health Service Executive. (1996a). *Primary Care: the Future*. London: NHSME.

National Health Service Executive. (1996b). *A Service with Ambitions*. London: NHSME.

National Health Service Management Executive. (1991). *Junior Doctors: the New Deal*. London: NHSME.

National Health Service Management Executive. (1993). *Improving Clinical Effectiveness*. (EL (93) 115.) Leeds: NHSME.

Nightingale, F. (1859). *Notes on Nursing: What it is and What it is not*, 1974 edition. Glasgow: Blackie.

Pembrey, S. (1985). A framework for care. *Nurs. Times*, **81**(50), 47–49.

Petryshen, P. and Petryshen, P. (1992). The case management model: an innovative approach to the delivery of patient care. *J. Adv. Nurs.*, **17**, 1188–1194.

Read, S. M. (1995). *Catching the Tide: New Voyages in Nursing?* (SCHARR Occasional Paper no. 1.) Sheffield: Sheffield University School of Health and Related Research.

Read, S. M. and George, S. (1994). Nurse practitioners in A&E departments: reflections on a pilot study. *J. Adv. Nurs.*, **19**, 705–716.

Read, S. M. and Graves, K. (1994). *Reduction of Junior Doctors' Hours in Trent Region: the Nursing Contribution*. Sheffield: Trent RHA/NHSME.

Read, S. M., Jones, N. M. B. and Williams, B. T. (1992a). Nurse practitioners in A&E departments: what do they do? *BMJ*, **305**, 1466–1470.

Read, S. M., George, S., Westlake, L. et al. (1992b). Piloting an evaluation of triage. *Int. J. Nurs. Stud.*, **29**, 275–288.

Read, S. M., Broadbent, J. and George, S. (1994). Do formal controls always achieve control? The case of triage in A&E departments. *Health Serv. Manage. Res.*, **7**, 31–42.

Reilly, C., Barrett, A., Challands, A. et al. (1996). *Professional Roles in Anaesthetics: a Scoping Study*. Leeds: NHSME.

Rodgers, R. (1996). Life for ears. *Primary Health Care*, **6**(3), 18–21.

Royal College of Physicians and Royal College of Nursing. (1996). Skillsharing – a joint statement. *J. R. Coll. Physicians Lond.*, **30**, 1.

Sparacino, P. and Durand, B. A. (1986). Specialisation in advanced nursing practice [editorial]. *Momentum*, **4**(2), 2–3.

Specialist Workforce Advisory Group (SWAG). (1996). *Annual Report 1995/6*. London: Department of Health.

United Kingdom Central Council for Nursing, Midwifery and Health Visiting. (1992). *The Scope of Professional Practice*. London: UKCC.

United Kingdom Central Council for Nursing, Midwifery and Health Visiting. (1995). *PREP and You*. London: UKCC.

West, M. A. and Farr, J. L. (eds.) (1990). *Innovation and Creativity at Work: Psychological and Organisational Perspectives*. Chichester: Wiley. Cited in West, M. A. and Anderson, N. (1992). *Innovation, Cultural Values and the Management of Change in British Hospital Management*. (Discussion Paper 101.) p. 2. London: Centre for Economic Performance (LSE/ESRC).

Williams, K. (1978). Ideologies of nursing: their meanings and implications. In *Readings in the Sociology of Nursing*. (R. Dingwall and J. McIntosh, eds.) pp. 36–44 Edinburgh: Churchill Livingstone.

6

Advanced practice: the 'advanced practitioner' perspective

Paul Fulbrook

Introduction

This chapter presents the research findings of a study that investigated the nature of advanced practice and the advanced practitioner from the perspective of 'advanced practitioners' themselves. Herein lies the first problem. How does one identify 'advanced practitioners' when, as a profession, nursing has not yet quite come to grips with the concept? A starting point has to be identified, if only so that we might enter into debate from which (hopefully) a clarification of concepts emerges. For the purpose of this research, the starting point was the identification of a number of so-called 'advanced practitioners'. The key to their selection was that they were recognized as experts in their field of clinical practice by their peers. Whether they are in fact 'advanced practitioners' is an area that remains open for debate.

The subject of advanced practice was chosen for study because its very nature is unclear. Furthermore, at a time when the UK's nursing professional body, the United Kingdom Central Council for Nursing, Midwifery and Health Visiting (UKCC), was grappling with the idea of formalizing the role of the advanced practitioner, the literature had yet to make the concept explicit. The creation of the new role of advanced practitioner was undoubtedly envisaged as vital for the health care professions by the UKCC (1994) to enable 'pioneering clinical practice'. However, that this ideal was to be achieved in the absence of either a professional framework or a recognized career structure was ambitious to say the least.

It was a belief in the value of the art of nursing that guided the research method for this study. The hope was that data would be obtained which could be used to develop the concepts of advanced practice and the advanced practitioner for nursing practice, and that, by using an inductive approach, nursing knowledge would be generated in this respect: 'Inductive research starts with specific observations or events, moves to more generalised ideas regarding concepts and possible relationships and thence to generating theory' (Couchman and Dawson, 1980). It was anticipated that, by achieving an understanding of advanced practice from the perspective of advanced practitioners themselves, the advanced practitioner's role would become clearer. Thus, by pursuing an emic rather than etic perspective, a richer representation of advanced practice would result. Not until the concepts of 'advanced practice' and 'advanced practitioner' have been understood, and more widely explicated from the perspective of the practitioners themselves, can the role of advanced practitioner and its implications be considered in a more informed way by the profession.

The purpose of this research was to ask two questions: (1) what is advanced practice? and (2) what is an advanced practitioner? This chapter concentrates on the findings that relate to the first question, although the two are inter-related.

Study design

Naturalistic enquiry (Lincoln and Guba, 1985) utilizing focused interviews was used as a research approach to understand what 'advanced practice' and 'advanced practitioner' are from an emic perspective. An expert group of informants was selected from the clinical specialty of intensive care nursing. The group, all recognized clinical leaders in their field of practice, were purposefully chosen because they would be more likely to be informed of the nature of advanced practice. They are described as 'key' informants, that is, people who have 'more insight into the norms and values... than others' (Field and Morse, 1996). It was felt that in order to understand what advanced practice and the advanced practitioner are, it was necessary to ask people already recognized as advanced practitioners.

> Qualitative research is based on the rationale that human behaviour can only be understood by getting to know the perspective and interpretation of events of the person or the people being studied – by seeing things through their eyes (Couchman and Dawson, 1990).

It was because 'hard' science is characterized by 'reductionism, quantifiability, objectivity and operationalization' (Watson, 1981), that its rationalistic research methodology was rejected as unsuitable for this study, since it does not value personal opinion, personal experience and personal knowledge. Inherent in the rationalistic paradigm, knowledge is regarded as objective and acontextual as opposed to interpretative and context dependent, as found in the naturalistic paradigm. There is the danger when using rationalistic research approaches 'of missing a wealth of rich data of a softer nature; data which allow interpretative understanding of the phenomenon under study' (Melia, 1982).

Experiences throughout life shape one's personal identity and perspective on the world (Hospers, 1990). In the context of advanced practice, individuals will have different experiences that will have shaped their ideas and beliefs. Thus, it was necessary to employ a research method that both enabled the individual perspective to be recognized and assigned value to personal experience and knowledge. Inductive approaches are appropriate for studying areas where little is understood, and inductive theory is concerned with bringing knowledge into view (Field and Morse, 1996).

Inductive analysis...begins not with theories or hypotheses but with the data themselves, from which the theoretical categories and relational propositions may be arrived at by inductive reasoning processes (Lincoln and Guba, 1985).

Reductionist approaches may not be appropriate to understand the wholeness of nursing, which arguably should embrace all four of Carper's (1978) patterns of knowing: empirics, aesthetics, ethics, and personal knowledge. Thus, the guiding belief for this research was that, only through naturalistic enquiry, of which multiple realities and context dependence are part, and the use of congruent research methods that focus on knowledge as interpretive, could the wholeness and essence of nursing in relation to advanced practice be understood. The intention of this study was not to reduce advanced practice and the advanced practitioner to their component parts, but to attempt to describe them in their wholeness. Furthermore, since the naturalist has little interest in the generalizability of findings (Lincoln and Guba, 1985), the need to relate findings to a theoretical model was rejected. As Field and Morse (1996) state: 'the qualitative strength of validity [is lost] by "forcing" reality to fit the framework.'

Working within the naturalistic paradigm, it is necessary to obtain rich and freely given data, rather than responses directed along predetermined channels. Naturalistic enquiry methods for data collection from informants are given as interview (guided or open-ended), open-ended questionnaires, or participant observation (Field and Morse, 1996).

A focused interview method was used for this research. It was selected in preference to the questionnaire method primarily because it was felt that, to remain true to the guiding paradigm, it was necessary to obtain a richness of freely given data. The flexibility of the interview method is more likely to achieve this than a written questionnaire, which tends to generate superficial rather than in-depth material. A 'focused' interview was preferred over a standardized interview to enable informants the freedom to explore fully the issues that they felt were relevant. The diversity of informants' personal experience and knowledge precluded the use of a rigid format

In order to focus the interviews, a number of questions were devised. These questions were not asked verbatim, nor were they presented in any particular order:

1. Tell me what advanced practice means to you.
2. How does a nurse become an advanced practitioner?
3. Do all nurses have the potential to become an advanced practitioner?
4. How did you get to the stage of advanced practitioner?
5. What do advanced practitioners do that is different from other nurses?
6. How would you recognize an advanced practitioner?
7. Where should advanced practitioners spend most of their time?

The interview questions were intentionally vague and non-directive. Using a focused approach allows the interviewer the flexibility to phrase questions in any way that elicits the same meaning, thus 'acknowledging that not all words have the same meaning to all informants' (Treece and Treece, 1986). Reliability and validity depend upon the ability of the interviewer to convey equivalence of meaning (Denzin, 1989).

In the context of this research study, the aim was to facilitate an interview that enabled informants to articulate the meaning of advanced practice and advanced practitioner in such a way that I too was able to understand their meaning: what Mishler (1986) describes as the 'joint construction of meaning'.

The major strength of naturalistic research is its high validity because it employs methods of data collection and data analysis that remain true to the participants' perspective. One of the main questions to be asked of research is: does it measure what it purports to be measuring?; or, in the context of this study: does the focused interview achieve an appropriate response, that is, does it enable the informants to describe advanced practice/advanced practitioner? Predetermined questions enabled focusing of the interviews on the research topic, but the informal structure gave informants freedom to explore issues to whatever degree they felt necessary. In this way, questions were used as a 'springboard' for the informants to develop their ideas. As a result, a wide range of 'rich' data was collected.

Informant selection

The informants were a group of experienced intensive care nurses, selected for the purpose of this study. The criteria for inclusion were on the basis that informants were judged by their peers to be expert in intensive care nursing, were based in clinical practice, and had an educational component (not necessarily formalized) to their role. The inclusion criteria were based on Williams and Webb's (1994) model; that is, that the expert informant: has a proven professional track record; has considerable clinical experience in the field (in excess of 5 years was specified for this study) and is currently clinically based; demonstrates continuing professional interest; and makes an active educational contribution.

Thus, on the basis of an objective, though arguably personal, opinion, the assumption was made that these 'clinical experts' could themselves be regarded as advanced practitioners. It is acknowledged that the selection of informants according to criteria was likely to develop a certain perspective related to the experts' standing; for example, if the same research study was conducted using non-experts, different data might have been obtained. The eight informants in this study were selected on the basis that they were representative of clinical experts in intensive care nursing. They came from a wide geographical distribution and only one nurse was selected from each intensive care unit.

Subsequent to Benner's (1984) application to nursing of the Dreyfus model of skill acquisition (H. L. Dreyfus and S. Dreyfus, unpublished observations), nursing attention has increasingly focused on the concept of clinical expert. Benner (1984) describes an expert as someone who 'no longer relies on an analytic principle ... with an enormous background of experience' who has 'an intuitive grasp of each situation' and 'operates from a deep understanding of the total situation'. It is worth noting that Benner's work resulted from interviewing intensive care nurses about their practice. According to Benner, experts will have at least 5 years' experience in a particular clinical field (English, 1993).

The idea of using 'experts' for this research is contentious, since, as with the advanced practitioner, the issue of how an expert is defined is unresolved and arbitrary (Goodman, 1987). McKenna (1994) warns that the title 'expert' has the potential to mislead, and that the title alone does not qualify expertise. Bond and Bond (1982) concluded that in nursing there were no clearly identifiable clinical experts.

There are no criteria available to measure 'expertness', and, although peer assessment of expertise has been criticized (English, 1993), this is on the basis that it does not fit with first paradigm scientific theory. Since naturalistic research rejects the need to conform to such theory, the need to preset rigid definitions of expertise is also rejected. As Darbyshire (1994) argues in response to the critique by English, it is precisely because of the qualitative nature of expertise that it cannot be measured.

Data analysis followed the process of content analysis described by Burnard (1991), and was undertaken after checking and correction of the interview transcripts by the informants. It is suggested that each word, sentence or phrase extracted from the transcripts should have 'stand alone' meaning (Lincoln and Guba, 1985). However, this is to some extent contested by Mishler (1986), who describes a 'narrative clause' as the fundamental unit of meaning, which cannot be 'relocated to any other point in the account without a change in its "semantic interpretation"'. On this basis, 'narrative clauses' were extracted from the transcripts and coded accordingly. A detailed description of the procedure is outside the scope of this chapter, but is available elsewhere (Fulbrook, 1994).

Findings

Informants

Eight informants were interviewed. All were registered nurses, having qualified between 9 and 23 years previously. Their total sum of postregistration nursing experience amounted to 120 years. All were very experienced intensive care nurses employed in recognized roles in intensive care units, and their length of experience in the specialty of intensive care nursing ranged from 7 to 17 years, and totalled 99 years. Five of the informants had the job title of Clinical Nurse Specialist, the other three were titled Course Teacher, Lecturer–Practitioner, and Clinical Nurse Manager. Seven of the informants had undertaken English National Board Course 100 (intensive care nursing), four had completed a first degree, one of whom also had a masters degree. Two were currently studying for their masters degree, and one for a doctorate. Two were clinically based in the London area, two in the South, three in the Midlands, and one in the North.

Themes

From a total of 110 categories, 10 themes were generated: knowledge and education; getting there; what advanced practice is; core elements; constraints; based in clinical practice; roles; role attributes; personal qualities; and recognition. These themes were further categorized under three domains: achieving advanced practice; advanced practice; and advanced practitioner. The second domain of advanced practice comprised the themes: what advanced practice is; core elements; and constraints. This section will present the findings under these headings.

In order to remain credible to the informants, the findings are illustrated by the informants' own words (LeCompte and Goetz, 1982). Furthermore, it is of critical importance that sufficient primary material is included to support my interpretation of the data and subsequent conclusions (Field and Morse, 1985). Therefore, my contribution to the findings at this stage will be narrative rather than interpretive.

Advanced practice

What advanced practice is

It was apparent from all the informants that advanced practice is very difficult to describe because it is so complex. Some informants could only describe advanced practice by considering what an advanced practitioner does: 'It's amazing how much you take for granted that you understand until you are asked to explore it ... and I think it is much harder to actually explain.'

As the interviews progressed, informants had more time to reflect on the nature of advanced practice and were able to make their thoughts more explicit. One of the key issues that emerged on this theme was that advanced practitioners are expert clinical practitioners and therefore they deliver expert clinical care. The excellence of the care that they give is not measured in relation to their ability to perform tasks, but in their ability to assimilate a wide range of knowledge and understanding which they apply to their practice: 'It's a standard of practice that is informed by above average knowledge and insight.'

The informants were suggesting that, because advanced practitioners are able to function in this way, they operate at a higher level than non-advanced practitioners. Advanced practitioners are able to assimilate a multitude of information, which they process in relation to their expert knowledge. Thus, when they care for patients, what they do is determined by many factors. This informed approach to nursing care seems to describe advanced practice: 'Having a deeper understanding of what you are doing and why.'

Informants also argued that, because advanced practitioners are able to take on board all aspects of the patient and utilize a range of knowledge and expertise in their practice, they deliver more holistic care. Although clinical competence was considered to be extremely important in maintaining an advanced practitioner's credibility, the value assigned to the performance of tasks was minimalized: 'Advanced practice is not about being competent at tasks. It's about looking at nursing as a whole.'

Another area that, according to the informants, defines advanced practice, is the ability of advanced practitioners to operate not just autonomously but outside of 'rules'. It was suggested that part of advanced practice is the ability to respond to each situation individually, guided by instinct and experience. The advanced practitioner would not need to refer to rules or guidelines to determine what they do, and is quite happy to break rules if they feel it is in the interests of the patient. Some informants referred to the use of intuition. One informant described heurism: 'Sometimes acting on your instincts but knowing that it's got a solid foundation to it.' This was developed by another of the informants:

> One uses heuristic devices which may be the same as other people use but you use them for a purpose, knowing what their limitations are. So, they may be guiding – I wouldn't say rules – rules of thumb if you like, indicators you have perfected over a period of time and that you know have served you well.

Advanced practice is clearly a very complex concept, which requires a range of applied expertise. It is reasonable to suggest that most of this expertise has been gained through education and experience. However, there is a somewhat nebulous, intangible aspect of advanced practice, which is much more difficult to define. This area could be described as instinct or intuition. It is about the ability to act uniquely according to the complexities of each unique situation in a way that feels right: 'It does have a scientific base I'm sure, it's just that we can't articulate what it is.'

One aspect of advanced practice on which all informants agreed was that its focus is nursing. What they seemed to be saying was that advanced practice is really what nursing is. Advanced practice is nursing in its fullest sense: 'Nursing in more of its purest form.'

Advanced practice was also seen as an ideal, a goal to be achieved. As such, advanced practice should be considered as a continuum, a dynamic process: 'All connected to striving towards this ideal thing.'

Advanced practice was considered with respect to its outcomes. Because its focus is nursing, its outcomes are seen in patients. The aim of advanced practice is to achieve excellence through improving the standard and quality of nursing care. This may be achieved either directly through the care that advanced practitioners deliver, or indirectly through the way that they help to develop both the practice environment and their colleagues: 'It's important that if one is identified as an advanced practitioner then that person is used to advance practice in the area in which they are.'

Advanced practice, therefore, is more than nursing patients, more than 'hands on' care. It is about the advancement of nursing generally.

Core elements

This section of the findings focuses on the core elements of advanced practice, and the transferability of advanced practice skills to a different area of clinical practice. Most informants felt that there are core aspects of advanced practice, which are transferable. These core elements might be described as 'core nursing'. 'The principles of nursing are the same wherever you go, and the principles of advanced practice must be the same.'

However, it was felt that advanced practice relates to a specialist field of practice, and, although the ideal or principles of advanced practice might be the same wherever one practises, the actual practice itself is different. Therefore, an advanced practitioner in mental health nursing who moved to work in an intensive care unit would not be an advanced practitioner in intensive care nursing. There would be some areas of advanced practice that would be immediately transferable, such as research, education, personal knowledge and communication skills, and the ability to integrate a wide range of knowledge and experience into practice would also be there. What would be missing is specialist knowledge. Since clinical expertise requires specialist knowledge (however gained), informants generally felt that advanced practice as a whole was not transferable. Although it was felt that there are core elements of advanced practice that are transferable to a different clinical area, advanced practitioners might not be able to use them straight away. It would take time for advanced practitioners to gain the necessary experience and specialist knowledge base before they could practise effectively at an advanced level, utilizing their full range of expertise:

> I don't think that you could be described as an advanced practitioner in a practice area that you are new to, although you may have skills that are more advanced than [other] practitioners that are working in that field.

How quickly an advanced practitioner is able to function at an advanced level in a new area depends on how quickly they are able to gain the appropriate specialist knowledge and familiarize themselves with the new environment. The more different the environment to the advanced practitioner's previous area of practice, the longer it will take:

> I may have advanced practice skills but I may not be very competent at using those until I was more familiar and experienced with the context. So, potentially those could be transferable, but it would have to be after a period of refamiliarizing myself with the context and getting to know that...and that might take a long time depending on what the context was.

Familiarization with the practice context is also important for advanced practitioners' practical competence and thus their confidence. It was said that the environment itself had an impact upon the advanced practitioner's level of performance. However, it was felt that an advanced practitioner who moves to a different clinical area would achieve advanced practice more quickly than a non-advanced practitioner.

In summary, the principles of advanced practice were considered to be the same for any field of clinical nursing practice. The core elements of advanced practice are to do with nursing generally, and include areas of knowledge such as research and education. Some specialist knowledge is also transferable, depending on the field of practice. The highly developed abilities of advanced practitioners in such areas as the assimilation and application of knowledge and experience would still be there, although the lack of knowledge and familiarity with a new and unfamiliar context may limit their ability to practise at an advanced level. Because advanced practitioners have a core of skills and abilities, they can adapt more quickly to a new environment and will function at an advanced level more quickly than someone who has never achieved advanced practice.

Constraints

On the whole, advanced practice was seen as clinically based nursing practice, with the primary function of the advanced practitioner being the delivery of advanced nursing practice, that is, a clinical expert. Several subroles were also identified: change agent, consultant, educator, and researcher. Discussion of these subroles is outside the scope of this chapter; however, the issue of whether a formal management role should be part of the advanced practitioner's remit was raised.

Informants generally felt that advanced practitioners should not be managers, but that they should have a role in influencing and contributing to management decisions. It was apparent that if advanced practitioners were given too much management responsibility it would dilute their ability to perform effectively as clinical experts. Some informants felt that the management structure did not always support advanced practice, particularly when there were financial implications. It was also suggested that if advanced practitioners were 'managers' there might be a conflict of interests, which would limit the ability to pursue ideal practice: 'In this current climate the management role may overtake their advanced practice role.'

The advanced practitioner's role in relation to management was seen ideally as one of reciprocity, that is, mutually beneficial in the interests of patients. This sort of relationship depended upon the management structure sharing the values and beliefs of the advanced practitioner. There was some scepticism about whether managers placed as much value on advanced practice as they should.

Other identified constraints on advanced practice were time and finance. One informant felt that peers could sometimes block the efforts of advanced practitioners: 'Sometimes that commitment is stifled due to peer pressure.'

The lack of a recognized career structure for advanced practitioners was also lamented, the suggestion being that there was no external incentive for nurses to become advanced practitioners. Clearly, the main perceived constraint is with regard to the management structure. If advanced practitioners take on a management role, it could severely limit their advanced practice. Similarly, if the advanced practitioner's role is not valued by the organization, then their ability to practise effectively might be restricted.

Summary

Advanced practice is a complex concept, which is very difficult to describe. It is an ideal and its focus is nursing. The outcome of advanced practice is quality patient care, which is achieved both directly (through direct patient care) and indirectly (through development of colleagues and the practice environment). Advanced practice is expert clinical practice, which is at a higher level than that delivered by non-advanced practitioners. It is achieved through the assimilation of the context of practice with knowledge and experience, which is then applied to clinical practice. Competent clinical performance to a high standard is a hallmark of advanced practice, which is necessary for advanced practitioners' credibility. However, advanced practitioners minimalize the importance of the ability to perform tasks.

Advanced practitioners practise holistically and are able to utilize their experience and self-knowledge in their practice in a way that might be described as *developed* (rather than inherent) intuition. Advanced practice is also about the ability to practise outside of rules that govern non-advanced practitioners.

Advanced practice relates to a defined field of clinical practice, but its principles are the same wherever one practises. There is a core of advanced practice, which might be described as nursing and which is transferable across all areas of clinical practice. Because advanced practice relates to a specialist area, specialist knowledge and experience is also necessary. Therefore, an advanced practitioner who moves to a different clinical area would not be an advanced practitioner straight away.

Discussion

The informants in this study generally found the concept of advanced practice very difficult to explain. This was probably due to the complexity of what they each perceived advanced practice to be. Similarly, in defence of the phenomenological nature of expertise, Darbyshire (1994) asserts: 'It is simply not possible to explicate a complex human experience such as expert nursing in formal, representational propositions which will predict or identify the "criteria" of expertise.'

Each informant inevitably had a different perspective of advanced practice, although there were many areas of consensus. Advanced practice was primarily cited as being expert clinical care, the expertise having been gained from experience, formal education and a highly developed sense of self-awareness. Because the focus of advanced practice is clinical practice and patient care, it is nursing orientated. One informant even described it as 'pure' nursing. As such, advanced practice was regarded as an ideal.

It was stated that advanced practitioners practise at a higher level than other nurses. What characterizes advanced practice is the way that advanced practitioners apply a wide range of knowledge and a deep understanding of nursing in their practice. In addition to such application is their ability to assimilate information pertaining to the context of each situation they encounter. They tend not to react to single stimuli and are more likely to weigh up the whole situation before deciding what to do. Their knowledge and experience gives them heightened analytical ability and foresight, which enables them to predict the consequences of their decision making. Because advanced practitioners have a wealth of experience to draw upon, they utilize experiential knowledge in their everyday practice. This might sometimes take the form of intuition or heurism. Advanced practice is therefore the result of a complex composite of knowledge and experience applied in a unique way according to each situation and through the medium of the self of the advanced practitioner.

The concept of advanced practice as expressed in this study, particularly because of its central theme of clinical expertise, has many similarities to Benner's (1984) expert. It is also relevant because Benner's work was based on a study of intensive care nurses. Benner characterizes an expert as being an 'expert performer' who 'no longer relies on analytic principle,' has 'an enormous background of experience . . . an intuitive grasp of each situation' and operates 'from a deep understanding of the total situation' (Benner, 1984). Similar views were expressed by the informants. However, one area where the informants would seem to disagree with Benner is regarding the use of analytical principles. Although intuition and heurism were considered part of advanced practice, informants did not reject analytical ability. In fact, on the contrary, it was frequently mentioned as an important factor that was necessary for advanced practice. In Benner's statement above, she at first appears to reject analytical ability. However, on further reading, she explains that 'highly skilled analytic ability is necessary for those situations with which the nurse has had no previous experience' (Benner, 1984). The informants in this study did not specify how analytical ability was used. They simply stated that it was necessary.

The theme of expert or expertise arose on many occasions in this research, but was most commonly linked with knowledge from clinical experience rather than with knowledge from formal education. This is somewhat in contrast with the American models of advanced practice, which tend to place a higher value on theoretical knowledge. Harper (1985), however, is an American who believes advanced practitioners to be primarily clinical experts and states that 'clinical expertise is developed through the integration of theoretical knowledge and highly refined practice skills in expert nursing situations'.

As described above, advanced practice was seen as multidimensional, as a complex composite of different types of knowledge applied in practice. As such, the model of advanced practice described by the informants is reflective of Carper's (1978) 'patterns of knowing'. Carper describes four patterns of knowledge in nursing: empirics, aesthetics, ethics, and personal knowledge, all of which are necessary for 'achieving mastery in a discipline' (Carper, 1978). It is possible to equate mastery with expertise in the context of advanced practice, since mastery is 'a human response...in which competency, control and dominion have been gained' (Younger, 1991). It is also useful to consider mastery in relation to art. An art can never be mastered, one can only get better, like a dancer or a painter. Similarly, if advanced nursing practice is to be regarded as an artistic process, then it too can never be mastered. One can only continually strive for improvement. As such, advanced practice is dynamic.

Carper (1978) suggests that all of her patterns of knowing are inter-related and states that nursing:

depends on the scientific knowledge of human behaviour...the esthetic perception of significant human experiences, a personal understanding of the unique individuality of the self and the capacity to make choices...involving particular moral judgements (Carper, 1978).

Her ideas are similar to those expressed by the informants regarding the complexity of knowledge, which is integrated in order to achieve advanced practice. Although not explicitly mentioning aesthetic or ethical knowledge, they are certainly implied in many of their descriptions of how an advanced practitioner operates. Scientific (empiric) knowledge and personal knowledge were frequently referred to by informants.

Several informants referred to advanced practitioners' autonomy and their ability to operate beyond the rules and procedures that govern non-advanced practitioners. Because advanced practitioners are self-aware and conscious of their limitations, they know how far they can go. They are also confident in their ability to apply experiential knowledge to their practice.

Although they are usually able to articulate the basis for their actions with reference to theory, they may not always be able to explain what they do. However, they are confident to base their actions on previous similar experiences and intuitive feel. Benner (1984) described the confidence experts have for rule-breaking, and in a later study identified the way expert knowledge is shaped by learning from clinical experience (Benner et al., 1992).

The informants believed advanced practice to be located in a specialist field of clinical practice, and therefore an advanced practitioner could not transfer to a different clinical area and immediately continue to practise at an advanced level. In describing the transferability of advanced practice to different clinical areas, informants were able to identify a core of advanced practice. This core comprised mostly the type of knowledge possessed by advanced practitioners. Components of the core were: research, education, general knowledge, nursing knowledge and personal knowledge. Along with theoretical knowledge and self-knowledge, were abilities such as critiquing, analysing and synthesizing. These aspects were deemed transferable to a different area of clinical practice.

Because there is a transferable core, it was expected that advanced practitioners would not take long to gain the relevant specialist knowledge and experience in a new specialty to enable them again to practise at an advanced level. It was also stated that the more different the clinical area from the advanced practitioner's previous area, the longer it would take. For example, the transition from intensive care to coronary care advanced practice would not take very long when compared with a move to, for example, community nursing. Castledine (1991) also considers advanced practice to have a core, and suggests four core competencies of the advanced practitioner: communication, problem solving, academic, and practical nursing. In terms of competencies, his core elements are comparable with the findings in this study, since problem solving and communication skills are considered to be at the forefront of the advanced practitioner's role attributes (Fulbrook, 1994). However, in terms of a transferable core, problem solving, communication and practical nursing may be dependent upon the possession of relevant specialist knowledge and experience for successful advanced practice. The idea that advanced practice has a core is also supported by Kitzman (1989) in relation to the clinical nurse specialist. She states that in order to be able to deliver comprehensive holistic care, nurses engaged in advanced practice 'will need to draw upon core knowledge that will permit them to address the interaction of a patient's sub-systems'.

The most common factor described by the informants that might impair the advanced practitioner's ability to practise at an advanced level was considered to be the management structure. It was considered from two perspectives. Primarily, it was felt that formal management was not a component of advanced practice, and, if it was to become so, there would inevitably be role restrictions and moral conflicts. However, the advanced practitioner should liaise with management. It was felt that the advanced practitioner has a key role in relation to management, but that this role was one of liaison and collaboration. Secondly, it was felt that, to achieve advanced practice, the management structure and the advanced practitioner should share common values, and there were some feelings expressed that organizational issues such as cost might take precedence.

Gournic (1989) discusses the clinical nurse specialist in a management position and highlights the potential danger of loss of the clinical practice component of the role. This concern is echoed by Castledine (1991), who states that it is imperative that line management positions for advanced practitioners 'do not impede their ability to function in the clinical setting'.

Conclusions

There are several conclusions that can be drawn from this research study. However, their generalizability is limited, due to the fact that they represent the perspectives of intensive care nurses only, and it is possible that the findings would have been significantly different had a cross-section of advanced practitioners been interviewed. Furthermore, all the informants were senior intensive care nurses, and, as such, their perspective may not be congruent with that of junior nurses or non-advanced practitioners. There may be other areas regarding advanced practice that have yet to be explored. It is thus important to consider the findings and conclusions in this light.

Informants were selected for this research on the basis of their expertise and the assumption that they were all advanced practitioners. The possibility that some personal bias might have influenced the selection of informants is acknowledged.

Advanced practice is a complex concept, which is very difficult to articulate. It is practice based in a specific clinical area and therefore requires experience in that specialty before it can be achieved. As such, advanced practice is not immediately transferable when an advanced practitioner moves to a different field of clinical practice.

Although the transferability of advanced practice is questioned, the components of advanced practice have been identified. The main role of the advanced practitioner is that of expert clinical practitioner. This role is not transferable, since it is dependent on the acquisition of specialist knowledge and specialist expertise. However, there will be many areas of knowledge and expertise within the main role which *are* transferable. Thus, should an advanced practitioner transfer to a different specialty, it is expected that it would not take him or her very long to gain the relevant specialist knowledge and clinical expertise. On the basis of the findings of this study, one could not say: 'once an advanced practitioner always an advanced practitioner', and there is potential for advanced practitioners to move away from their specialty, never to regain advanced practice in a new field. Such a possibility might arise because the new specialty is too different, or as a result of internal motivational factors.

If 'advanced practitioner' was ever to become a registrable qualification, it would require regulation to ensure that all registered advanced practitioners are actually practising at an advanced level. This would be extremely difficult to ensure.

Titling for advanced practice needs careful consideration. The term 'clinical nurse specialist' is cumbersome and has obvious connotations with the American model, which, although similar, is not congruent with the model of advanced practice proposed by the informants. The UKCC recommend that the term 'nurse practitioner' is no longer used since it has no identifiable role (Foundation of Nursing Studies, 1993). However, many such roles are currently being developed, and are often described in terms of advanced practice. Titles such as 'clinical expert' seem rather elitist and do not reflect adequately the practice element of advanced practice or the advanced level of knowledge that is necessary.

Advanced practice is very difficult to describe. Informants found it very challenging to articulate what their ideas of advanced practice were, and frequently had to revert to describing what the advanced practitioner does and how they do it to clarify what they meant. It is clear from this study that advanced practice arises from a background of clinical experience in a clinical specialty. Through a period of time, which is individual in nature and therefore cannot be specified, the advanced practitioner develops a comprehensive knowledge and a high degree of skill relating to a particular specialty. This experiential background develops an 'expert by experience', and gives the advanced practitioner clinical credibility with peers.

Clinical expertise alone is insufficient to earn the status of advanced practitioner; expert knowledge is also required. Clinical expertise and knowledge expertise are the foundations of advanced practice. However, according to the informants, the two together do not necessarily qualify practice. The advanced practitioner must also develop personally (Fulbrook, 1994). The development of communication skills, the use of reflection, and, in particular, a heightened self-awareness, is stressed. Thus advanced practice is a complex composite of knowledge and experience applied in a unique way according to each situation through the medium of the self.

Advanced practice was described by one informant as 'pure' nursing, and is congruent with the informants' shared belief in the value of nursing and their assertion that the focus of advanced practice is nursing. It would seem that the informants are describing advanced nursing as an art form in which many facets of nursing expertise are brought together. This advanced 'art form' was frequently described as being the 'higher level' at which advanced practitioners practise. This 'higher level' is characterized by several abilities that merit their advanced status and define them as clinical experts. Advanced practitioners have the ability to practise autonomously, and are not bound by the rules of practice that are there to govern others. Because they have a wealth of knowledge and experience, they are able to rationalize and justify their actions, and are not afraid to make decisions based on past experiences rather than acknowledged theory. When advanced practitioners make decisions, they do so having acknowledged all the factors that impinge on a particular situation and having weighed up the possible consequences of a variety of possible interventions. They tend not to react to single stimuli, and are more likely to reserve their judgement until they are in possession of all the facts that relate to the context. They are able to do this because they have a deeper understanding of the situation. Having established the full context of a situation, advanced practitioners are very good at prioritizing their interventions. This is enhanced by their ability to predict outcomes, which is further enhanced by their intuitive grasp of the situation.

Advanced practitioners are articulate and skilled in presenting the nursing perspective in any situation. This ability is borne out of their wealth of nursing knowledge and experience, and the fact that the focus of their practice is, and always has been, nursing itself.

In conclusion, if the concept of advanced practice is to become a professional reality, much more work is required to make its components explicit. The danger is that the development of advanced practice might be driven more by government policies than by professional motivation. One concern in this respect is the reduction of junior doctors' hours (Department of Health, 1993) and the expectation that nurses take on tasks that were previously considered to be the doctor's domain. This is quite clearly not what the informants in this study consider to be advanced practice; it is not even role extension; it is simply the performance of additional tasks. It is a cynical, though plausible, view that professional advancements such as the UKCC's *Scope of Professional Practice* (UKCC, 1992), which offer professional support to the expansion of the nursing role, were allowed to advance by the Department of Health only because of the impending reduction of doctors' hours. As Christine Hancock states, the extension of the nursing role 'has been particularly evident since the reduction of junior doctors' hours' (Foundation of Nursing Studies, 1993).

On a more positive note, the development of advanced practice is a challenge for the profession. With the right framework, the role could be properly developed. The development of a recognized structure for advanced practice should enable expert clinical nurses to remain in the clinical area, doing what they do best: advancing practice in the interests of patients.

References

Benner, P. (1984). *From Novice to Expert: Excellence and Power in Clinical Nursing Practice.* Menlo Park, CA: Addison-Wesley.

Benner, P., Tanner, C. and Chesla, C. (1992). From beginner to expert: gaining a differentiated clinical world in critical care nursing. *Adv. Nurs. Sci.*, **14**(3), 13–28.

Bond, S. and Bond, J. (1982). A Delphi survey of clinical nursing research priorities. *J. Adv. Nurs.*, **7**, 565 576.

Burnard, P. (1991). A method of analysing interview transcripts in qualitative research. *Nurse Educ. Today*, **11**, 461–466.

Carper, B. A. (1978). Fundamental patterns of knowing in nursing. *Adv. Nurs. Sci.*, **1**(1), 13–23.

Castledine, G. (1991). The advanced nurse practitioner, part 2. *Nurs. Stand.*, **5**(44), 33–35.

Couchman, W. and Dawson, J. (1990). *Nursing and Health Care Research: A Practical Guide.* London: Scutari Press.

Darbyshire, P. (1994). Skilled expert practice: is it 'all in the mind'? A response to English's critique of Benner's novice to expert model. *J. Adv. Nurs.*, **19**, 755–761.

Denzin, N. K. (1989). *The Research Act: A Theoretical Introduction to Sociological Methods*, 3rd ed. Englewood Cliffs, NJ: Prentice Hall. Cited in Barriball, K. L. and While, A. (1994). Collecting data using a semi-structured interview: a discussion paper. *J. Adv. Nurs.*, **19**, 328–335.

Department of Health. (Calman Report, 1993). *Hospital Doctors: Training for the Future.* (The report of the Working Group on Specialist Medical Training). London: DoH.

English, I. (1993). Intuition as a function of the expert nurse: a critique of Benner's novice to expert model. *J. Adv. Nurs.*, **18**, 387–393.

Field, P. A. and Morse, J. M. (1985). *Nursing Research: The Application of Qualitative Approaches.* London: Chapman and Hall.

Field, P. A. and Morse, J. M. (1996). *Nursing Research: The Application of Qualitative Approaches,* 2nd ed. London: Chapman and Hall.

Foundation of Nursing Studies. (1993). *Annual Report: Better Practice. Annual Report (1993).* London: Foundation of Nursing Studies.

Fulbrook, P. (1994). *Advanced Practice and the Advanced Practitioner: An Emic Perspective* [dissertation]. Manchester: Royal College of Nursing/University of Manchester.

Goodman, C. M. (1987). The Delphi technique: a critique. *J. Adv. Nurs.*, **12**, 729–734.

Gournic, J. L. (1989). Clinical leadership, management and the CNS. In *The Clinical Nurse Specialist in Theory and Practice,* 2nd ed. (A. B. Hamric and J. A. Spross, eds.) pp. 227–248. London: Saunders.

Harper, D. C. (1985). The process of advanced nursing practice. *J. Prof. Nurs.*, **1**, 323, 385.

Hospers, J. (1990). *An Introduction to Philosophical Analysis.* 3rd ed. London: Routledge.

Kitzman, H. J. (1989). The CNS and the nurse practitioner. In *The Clinical Nurse Specialist in Theory and Practice,* 2nd ed. (A. B. Hamric and J. A. Spross, eds.) pp. 379–394. London: Saunders.

LeCompte, M. D. and Goetz, J. P. (1982). Problems of reliability and validity in ethnographic research. *Rev. Educ. Res.*, **52**(1), 31–60.

Lincoln, Y. S. and Guba, E. G. (1985). *Naturalistic Inquiry.* Newbury Park, CA: Sage.

McKenna, H. P. (1994). The Delphi technique: a worthwhile research approach for nursing? *J. Adv. Nurs.*, **19**, 1221–1225.

Melia, K. M. (1982). 'Tell it as it is' – qualitative methodology and nursing research: understanding the student nurse's world. *J. Adv. Nurs.*, **7**, 327–336.

Mishler, E. G. (1986). *Research Interviewing: Context and Narrative.* Cambridge, MA: Harvard University Press.

Treece, E. W. and Treece, J. W. (1986). *Elements of Research in Nursing,* 4th ed. St Louis, MO: Mosby.

United Kingdom Central Council for Nursing, Midwifery and Health Visiting. (1992). *The Scope of Professional Practice.* London: UKCC.

United Kingdom Central Council for Nursing, Midwifery and Health Visiting. (1994). *The Future of Professional Practice – the Council's Standards for Education and Practice Following Registration.* London: UKCC.

Watson, J. (1981). Nursing's scientific quest. *Nurs. Outlook,* **29**, 413–416.

Williams, P. L. and Webb, C. (1994). The Delphi technique: a methodological discussion. *J. Adv. Nurs.*, **19**, 180–186.

Younger, J. B. (1991). A theory of mastery. *Adv. Nurs. Sci.*, **14**(1), 76–89.

7

Advanced nursing practice: lessons from the province of Ontario, Canada

Marie Roberts-Davis

This chapter outlines developments in the advanced practice role, as it pertains to the primary health care and acute care nurse practitioners, which are taking place in the province of Ontario in Canada. It is based on a study sponsored by the Florence Nightingale Foundation in 1995 and the follow-up in 1996. The study comprised a literature review, interviews and observation of the role. The impetus for this investigation was the need, as a nurse and educator, to enter as an informed participant in discussion and debate concerning the future role of nurses within the 'new NHS'. The aim was to investigate specialist and advanced practice roles from the basis of the understanding of these roles within the UK. The study was initially undertaken as a preliminary to personal research concerning the role and preparation of nurses working at the interface with medical practice. It has subsequently been invaluable in informing a funded national research project evaluating the educational preparation of nurse practitioners (NPs).

Context in which the study was undertaken

The future of nursing in the UK lies very firmly in policy and professional contexts (Department of Health, 1993, 1994a, 1994b; NHSME, 1991; Read and Graves, 1994; United Kingdom Central Council for Nursing, Midwifery and Health Visiting (UKCC), 1992, 1994). Views may differ about which is the more influential.

Policy changes emphasizing the efficiency and effectiveness of the market economy in delivering public services have resulted in the creation of the 'purchaser–provider' structure within the NHS. This change moves the organization of health care delivery closer to that of Canada and the USA. The 'new NHS' is concerned with the 'quality' of service, defined as efficiency and effectiveness, and with meeting consumer needs in the National Health Service and Community Care Act, 1990. The resource to provide this service is limited, and various measures to improve the cost effectiveness of health care, such as 'skill-mix' exercises with a reanalysis of the skills required to deliver a given service, have been undertaken. The extension of skill and task reanalysis across the nursing/medicine interface is deemed necessary by many (Richardson and Maynard, 1995). This has meant the creation of 'new roles' for many health care professionals.

A further factor is the changes in medical education as it pertains to the 'junior doctor' (National Health Service Management Executive, 1991). A considerable cash injection has been put into the system through the Regional Junior Doctors' Hours Taskforce Working Groups to fill the deficit left by the removal of the services of the junior doctors to allow them 'an education-driven experience'. The allocation of these resources in the way that it was done is, perhaps, regrettable, as it allowed a very ad hoc creation of nursing posts. Read and Graves (1994), and Read (1995) have found that the creation of new posts involved very little clear identification of the function and planned educational preparation for those appointed.

This initiative has given rise to what, for lack of an agreed definition, can be described as 'innovative nursing roles'. These new roles, which often extend across the interface with medical practice, are being undertaken within the *Scope of Professional Practice* (UKCC, 1992). This must be viewed in the context of nursing legislation in the UK. This legislation comprises Statutory Instruments 875 (1983) and 1456 (1989), which outline the educational requirements for registration. The principle of education specifying practice is very important where the scope of professional practice is not prescribed in law as it is in both the USA and Canada. It is of great concern to some that individuals are practising within roles where the accepted boundary of what is defined as nursing is being moved forward, with no means of controlling the quality of practice through the establishment of standards for education at what *might* be 'advanced practice'. On the other hand, there is justification for the statutory body to move carefully. There are two issues. First, there is the belief that the principle of individual professional accountability and responsibility for practice enshrined in the UK 'Scope of Practice' should be sufficient to guide practitioners during this period of role development and expansion or extension. The second is that the setting of educational standards in support of 'expanded' roles at this point may delimit the future of what is now innovative, making it static and inappropriate for future needs, particularly when the full scope of the practitioner role is as yet undefined.

The original intention to look at 'specialist' and 'advanced' practice roles became redundant once the Canadian definition of these terms was understood by the author. It was clear from the beginning of the study that 'specialist' referred only to the area of practice, not to the level. The clinical nurse specialist (CNS) and NP are both considered to be 'advanced' practice nurses (Fenton and Brykcynski, 1993). Attention was, therefore, concentrated on the NP role that is re-emerging after many years in a static state (Mitchell et al., 1993) and on the new educational programmes Consortium of Ontario Universities with Programs in Nursing (COUPN) Nurse Practitioner Curriculum Committee, 1994; Pringle, 1994) being developed to prepare these practitioners.

Why Canada?

Although outwardly there appear to be many differences, both politically and socially, Canadian structures and legislative processes are based on the same principles as the UK, and, although there is some variation between provinces, all provinces operate legislatively along similar lines.

As a dominion comprising 10 provinces and two territories, Canada has a federal government with two houses, mirroring the British Parliament. Each province has a legislature that governs health, welfare and educational issues. Because of formalized legislative powers, tensions may be acute at times, especially because one province, Quebec, has a unique cultural identity.

Early Canadian social welfare developments (pensions, public assistance, national insurance, industrial injury) paralleled those in the UK. Government-funded universal health insurance was introduced gradually, on a provincial basis, following the end of World War II (Raffel, 1984).

Nursing education is similar to that in the UK. The usual preregistration programme is a 3-year diploma, with a small number (20–25%) of nurses qualifying through 4-year bachelor of nursing courses in universities. An essential difference is that all students completing either diploma or graduate programmes must sit the same examinations set by the statutory body in order to become registered.

The NP movement, which began in the early 1970s to provide health care to underserviced areas, did not develop as in the USA, mainly because of problems with remuneration, an oversupply of physicians in urban areas, and lack of career opportunities. About 250 NPs have continued to practise in Ontario and have demonstrated their value in a variety of settings (Ontario Ministry of Health, 1994). In response to perceived need, 'innovative' roles developed, mirroring many of the issues we are facing in the UK: the variety of titles used by such nurses (Alcock, 1994); the need to formalize educational preparation; and public protection. Much of this is in the context of changes brought on by a crisis in the cost of health care, as described later.

The issues: health care systems and resources

By 1960, all the Canadian provinces had introduced universal *hospital insurance* programmes, the principles of which were universal access, comprehensiveness of benefit, public administration, and portability between the provinces. By 1971, the provinces had introduced parallel universal *medical insurance*. Both are funded from provincial and federal taxation. Private insurance exists to extend the cover for drugs, 'out of province' cover, dental care, optical care, etc., usually through 'group' plans at the place of employment.

The dominant hospital 'system' in Canada comprises around 1000 independent 'public' hospitals (privately or municipally owned, or managed by medical schools). The income for hospitals is derived primarily from provincial hospital insurance programmes. Although managed by local hospital boards, all must operate under provincial regulations. Provincial governments set standards for hospital facilities and staffing through their procedures for approving new capital construction grants and their annual review of each hospital's operating budget under hospital insurance. This can be compared with the situation of NHS trusts in the UK.

There is an essential difference, however, in how medical care is provided within hospitals. General practitioners as well as specialists (consultants) can have 'hospital privileges'. This allows them to admit patients and provide their medical care during their hospital stay, carry out minor surgery, deliver babies and carry out a range of other activities. Only large teaching hospitals resemble the UK system, with a hierarchy of specialists, medical students, and interns and residents (junior doctors). Medical services in non-teaching hospitals are generally provided by local general practitioners and a few 'specialists'.

The health care system has one major problem: escalating health care costs. Encouraged by the federal government and the introduction of the hospital insurance schemes from the 1960s, too many acute beds were established during this period. Hospital beds are labour intensive and expensive. Some of the current cost has been attributed to extensive fraudulent use of the insurance scheme by individuals outside the province, and, indeed, the country. This has resulted in intense scrutiny of the use of services. Other contributors to the problem are: the high use of technology; the 'fee for service' reimbursement system; an oversupply of physicians; and maldistribution of physicians in terms of specialist/generalist provision (Barer and Stoddart, 1991). The need to contain cost led the authors of this report to recommend a reduction in medical school intakes and residency programmes, as well as consideration of options for increased scope of practice for other health care professionals (Barer and Stoddart, 1991).

Since the late 1980s, considerable reduction has taken place both in the numbers of beds and the length of hospital stay. Controls have been placed on the pool of physician specialists, with rationalization or regionalization of certain specialisms and services (Raffel, 1984). Controls have also been placed on hospital rates, on physicians' fees, and on utilization of services.

As in the UK, community services have been expanded. Many long-term and chronically ill individuals are supported in the community through a combination of welfare, health and voluntary services, and through their own resources. The government's contribution to care is often time limited and means tested. 'Care packages' are provided to support patients in their own homes, with services being purchased from nursing agencies, visiting homemaker agencies, and commercial health care equipment and technical service providers, as well as being provided in a market system by the hospital itself.

One outcome of this cost constraint, focus on prevention and community care, and maldistribution of services, has been the growth of 'new' nursing roles in acute care: the acute care nurse practitioner (ACNP), and, in primary care, the revitalization of the NP role.

The issues: registration of nurses

In Canada, nurse registration is a provincial matter, with approaches to, and forms of, regulation varying between provinces. Statutory powers are designated, as in the UK, under an act passed by each provincial legislature. Generally, there are similarities in the legislative authority (or power) granted to the regulatory body across the provinces. Differences, however, exist in structure and specific mechanisms by which that authority is carried out. The responsibilities of the statutory bodies are similar to that of the UKCC.

The registration of nurses in Ontario is governed by the Regulated Health Professions Act, 1991, and the Nursing Act, 1991. Each health profession has a 'college', which registers and regulates the profession. The College of Nurses of Ontario (CNO) is the equivalent of the UKCC. There are two categories of registration: registered nurse and registered practical nurse. Both are 'generic' qualifications. As stated earlier, legislation states prescriptively the scope of practice for all health professionals. The prescriptive nature of the scope of practice has led to a complication: the need to amend legislation to allow NPs to practise autonomously.

The quality and competence of nursing practice at registration and during the lifetime of practice is ensured through a 'dual' system referred to as 'credentializing'. Licensure (credentialing) to protect the public, which is maintained by statute, is carried out by the College through registration examinations, which they set. A nurse must be credentialed through this process in order to practise, and the CNO, like the UKCC, monitors and reviews professional conduct of registered practitioners. Credentialing for 'other than the public protection' is organized through professional organizations such as the Canadian Nurses Association, which maintains a credentialing process. The latter is primarily for employment purposes and is recognized by employers for 'specialist' status, but may also be used by the CNO as a guide, both for education and practice.

In relation to education, the monitoring of the quality of educational programmes is rather complex. The ultimate responsibility in Ontario rests with the Ministry of Universities and Colleges. The Ministry devolves this responsibility in the case of university courses to the Canadian Association of University Schools of Nursing, and, for college courses, to the College of Nurses of Ontario.

The issues: the nurse practitioner – role and scope of practice

In 1993, in the context of a concerted drive for efficiency and economy in health care, the Minister of Health identified the NP role as a potentially important component of the health care system in the primary care setting, and in areas poorly serviced by general practitioners. She commissioned a report from McMaster University on the use of the NPs in Ontario. This report, *Utilization of Nurse Practitioners in Ontario* (Mitchell et al., 1993), which, from a survey of the literature over the previous 25 years, documented that nurse practitioners are effective, efficient and economic health care providers, encouraged the incumbent Minister of Health to take on the development of the NP role as a 'personal' project. Unfortunately, the party of the minister in question was voted out of office in the middle stages of this development. During her tenure, however, this minister managed to precipitate discussion and shape thinking about the NP role in both acute and primary care.

In Ontario, a nurse practitioner (NP) is a registered nurse who holds a current certificate of competence with the College of Nurses of Ontario, has a nurse practitioner certificate or equivalent from an approved programme and has demonstrated advanced knowledge and decision-making skills in assessment, diagnosis and health care management in a defined area of practice. NPs are responsible for their practice and may undertake only those activities that they have the education and competence to perform safely, ethically and effectively (Ontario Ministry of Health, 1994).

The NP, states the Ministry of Health, brings the dimension of care to the patient or client that his or her nursing background has enabled him or her to develop. NPs take a holistic approach, looking at all of a patient's or client's needs, abilities and resources. They focus on giving people the information, care, advice and support they need to be healthier and prevent illness and injury. They help to ensure that the public receives all the therapeutic benefits of nursing, while providing a service that overlaps medicine and involves such activities as the diagnosis and treatment of common illnesses and physical examinations.

The Government drive for this development was viewed by nurses as a double-edged sword; it was an opportunity for development, but one that might be controlled and moulded by political rather than professional imperatives.

In recognizing this fact, the Nurse Practitioners Association of Ontario (NPAO) defined and documented their *Standards of Practice for Nurse Practitioners* in Ontario (Nurse Practitioners Association of Ontario, 1994). The five standards that are articulated in 'process criteria' (relating to the practitioner) and 'outcome criteria' (pertaining to the client or patient and family) concern the areas of knowledge, professional accountability and quality assurance, assessment, planning, implementation and evaluation (NPAO, 1994).

Returning to the issue of nursing legislation in Ontario, the defined scope of practice made necessary a change in legislation. Existing NPs had practised using extensive protocols and with the support of decision trees. To allow the 'new' role NPs to practise autonomously as service need appeared to demand, amendments to the Regulated Health Professions Act (Government of Ontario, 1991a), and the Nursing Act (Government of Ontario, 1991b), were required. To inform the necessary changes, a survey was undertaken amongst NPs and physicians to identify the common conditions seen, when nurses made diagnoses, and how these conditions were managed. The outcome is an extensive list of diseases and disorders that may be diagnosed, laboratory tests that may be ordered and drugs that may be prescribed by NPs, which are documented in the 'Controlled Acts' legislation, and which will be made addenda to the Nursing Act (Office of the Nursing Coordinator, 1995).

A new category of registration, access to which will be controlled by the statutory body, will also be created. Nurse practitioners will then be able to register with the CNO under the 'extended class status'. Nurses may achieve this in three ways: entirely through demonstration that he or she meets the criteria (including possessing a bachelor of nursing degree) for extended class status; through a combination of prior learning assessment (PLA – similar to Accreditation of Prior Experiential Leasing/Accreditation of Prior Leasing) and demonstration of meeting criteria; or through undertaking the NP programme (see Figure 7.1).

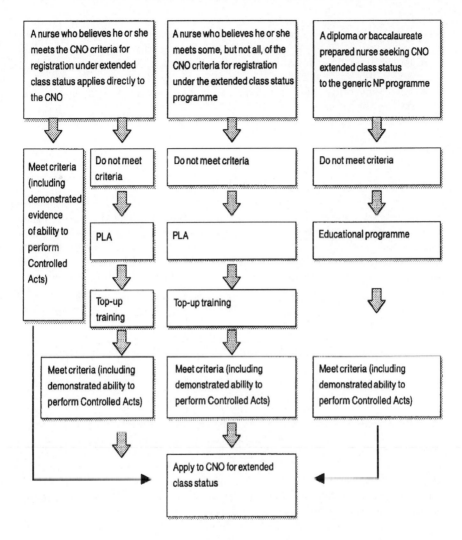

Figure 7.1. Foundation for Prior Learning Assessment. The COUPN Nurse Practitioner Programme

Unfortunately, because of the demise of the initiating governing party, this legislation is 'stuck' in the system and other stakeholders are beginning to exert pressure against its passage.

The issues: educational preparation of the nurse practitioner

There are two initiatives relating to the development of the NP within the province. One concerns those who will practise in the primary care setting, the other concerns those intending to work in acute care. Both programmes cover similar material:

- Advanced health assessment and diagnosis (history-taking, physical examination, laboratory tests and screening tools);
- Roles, relationships and responsibilities of the NP (professional, legal, policy and ethical context of the NP role);
- Pathophysiology for the NP (advanced anatomy, physiology and pathophysiology);
- Therapeutics (pharmacology, nursing therapeutics, counselling and technical skills);
- Integrative practicum (taken only after successful completion of all other components).

In both courses, students are preceptored by a medical practitioner in their specialist area, with whom they negotiate specific learning objectives. The physician is integral to the evaluation (assessment) of their competence in the range of knowledge and skills required to practise in the field (Pringle, 1994).

To prepare NPs for primary care, the 10 universities in Ontario with nursing programmes formed a consortium (COUPN) for the delivery of the certificate programme. This initiative was in response to government directives as described earlier. Selected universities have taken responsibility for developing courses. All universities will offer the 'integrated practicum' (clinical experience) for students registered locally.

The programme is designed primarily for public health nurses, who, like health visitors in the UK, have for many years been prepared through postregistration programmes in higher education. Any registered nurse may, however, apply. Those entering as diplomats will be required to undertake 2 years of full-time study (or part-time equivalent) to gain a bachelor's degree as well as the NP certificate. Graduates will access the NP programme directly for a 1-year course of study. The NP programme is, in effect, a *postgraduate* programme. Innovative means of offering the programme in a distance learning format using multimedia technology is being developed.

The second initiative, the 'Toronto initiative', which is the first part of a phased programme offered by the Faculty of Nursing at the University of Toronto, in partnership with eight large acute teaching hospitals in the city, is designed to prepare NPs for the acute sector. The project was designed to prepare already masters-prepared CNSs to become ACNPs by a 'fast track' method. The strategy planned was in recognition of the fact that, while their present masters programme enabled nurses practising in specialist areas to enhance and enrich their practice, it did not prepare nurses for the role of the NP.

The Toronto hospitals are regional centres for specialties and university teaching hospitals. They provide care to the most complex and critically ill patients, and are affected by the same pressures as all hospitals. In addition, they are facing severe budget restrictions. Their situation is further complicated by the policies recently adopted by the Ontario Ministry of Health, which is directed at controlling the size and cost of the medical workforce, including the Barer–Stoddart Report (1991) on physician resource policy, which indicated a need for a 10 per cent reduction in the number of physicians being produced. The implementation of this recommendation has resulted in a reduction in the number of medical students since 1993. This will have an impact on residency (junior doctors') positions by the end of the decade, and is additional to reductions already made in an attempt to reduce numbers in medical specialisms and subspecialisms. As their numbers are cut back and more attention is paid to enhancing their education rather than exploiting their service provision, a gap has been created in the care of acutely ill patients across the entire spectrum of medical specialties (Pringle, 1994).

The Toronto project has been designed deliberately in phases to allow the evaluation of its adequacy in preparing ACNPs. The nurses prepared through the 3-month ACNP post-masters programme (the fast track) were used in the evaluation of the preparation and role development, and the information gathered is being used to inform the next step: the development of a NP programme dedicated to the preparation of ACNPs. It is already felt that the economic climate would not sustain the ACNP programme of a 2-year full-time masters course as in the USA. Thus, a more innovative, shorter, but certainly graduate (postgraduate) level preparation is en- visaged.

The issues: the reality of the nurse practitioner role

The NPs and physician (consultant) interviewed were all working in the acute care sector. Unfortunately, time and access did not allow for contact with any who were presently working in primary care, although the NP programme organizers at McMaster University and the University of Western Ontario maintained close clinical contact.

Regarding the latter, the indications are that, where primary care NPs are established, they are working well and are well supported by physician colleagues (Mitchell et al., 1993; Way and Jones, 1994). This is particularly the case where they are part of the team in a community health centre. It is also noteworthy that the 'Burlington trial' (Spitzer et al., 1974) is the only recorded randomized controlled trial of the NP role. In this context, rather than a 'fee for service' system, a 'block contract' for services is placed by the government. Within this system, the NP can provide a high quality and cost effective service.

The development of either the primary care NP or the ACNP role outside this context, that is, in 'privately' provided family practice or in smaller general hospitals, has not been well received according to those interviewed. This is because of the potential for infringement on, or competition with, medical practice both in primary care and where general practitioners supply the medical care in local general hospitals. This is reflected in comments reported in the press (Van Brenk, 1994). It is also perceived that opposition from the medical community has been the reason for the slowness in the progress of legislation to enable more autonomous practice.

The ACNP (called an 'expanded role nurse' (ERN)) and the physician interviewed worked in a large university teaching hospital within a regional specialty unit. The ACNP holds a bachelor of nursing degree and a master's degree in nurse education and had completed the 'Toronto programme' just described. She had worked for several years in the specialist area as a CNS.

There follows a description of her role as outlined by her employer.

Her 'position description' defines her as 'an advanced practitioner whose role encompasses expert nursing practice and crosses boundaries into traditional medical practice'. The document goes on to say that 'the role was introduced in response to increasing patient acuity with greater demands for specialized care and cut-backs in residency training programs and house staff available'. The ERN role 'includes components of clinical practice, education, consultation and research'. The prerequisites for her role are:

Qualifications
- Completion of a clinical masters degree in nursing in a clinical specialty or a recognized postgraduate programme
- Current certification or eligibility for certification with the CNO
- A minimum of 5 years of relevant experience

Personal characteristics
- Critical thinking and problem-solving skills
- Flexibility and adaptability
- Capability of assuming responsibility for clinical decisions beyond the scope of nursing
- Advanced interpersonal and communication skills (oral and written)
- Leadership skills

More specifically, her role involves:

Clinical practice (70–80%)
The ERN is a self-directed practitioner who directs, provides and evaluates inpatients, outpatients and community based patients, founded on medical and nursing practice models. The ERN:

- Performs and documents comprehensive patient assessments based on completing a medical history and physical examination to arrive at a nursing and medical diagnosis
- Identifies, orders and prioritizes, and interprets specific diagnostic tests and procedures
- Prescribes specific pharmacological and other therapeutic interventions
- Independently performs selected invasive/non-invasive medical procedures
- Authorizes/co-ordinates admission, discharge, transfers; determines need for medical follow-up
- Communicates with patients/families, hospital and community health care members, results/diagnosis/treatment plan and related implications

Education (5–10%)
The ERN is a clinical expert and has advanced knowledge about educational theory. The incumbent directs and develops innovative educational programmes (formal and informal) for health care professionals, patients, families and students. She attends regional, national and international conferences at which she presents papers and disseminates, in this way and through publication, her research findings.

Consultation (5–10%)
The ERN provides expert knowledge and guidance about medical/nursing practice and health care issues. Both formal and informal consultation is provided to internal and external health care professionals, patients and families. Through consultation and committee membership, she influences decision making relative to clinical and nursing policies and procedures.

Research (5–10%)
The ERN provides leadership by advancing nursing knowledge and practice through research-related activities. She critically analyses current research, and models and facilitates the incorporation of appropriate research findings into practice. She conducts clinical unidisciplinary and multidisciplinary research as a collaborator and principal investigator, and oversees and guides nursing staff in the research process.

When interviewed, both she and the consultant for the unit were very positive about her role and how it had developed. When asked about potential barriers to her role, she emphasized that the role development must be co-operative and supported by the physicians in the specialist area. A trust must be gradually developed, which gives the nurse the confidence to perform the role fully and the physician the confidence to 'let go'. She identified, also, that, because of issues of liability, this relationship was being more formalized. Although they were legal 'delegated' activities, the system of her making care decisions within this fiduciary relationship and recording them as 'verbal orders' from the physician was gradually being developed into protocols. This has been necessitated because of the failure, as yet, of the passage of the 'Controlled Acts' legislation.

Her main function, she felt, was to ensure continuity of care for the patients within her unit in the face of a reduction in junior doctor cover and rotation of consultant coverage. The need to ensure that the individual practising in this role possessed the skills of advanced practice nursing was emphasized. She saw the difference between herself and a CNS as primarily in her allocation of time between practitioner, educator, researcher, consultant and leader/change agent activities and the nature of her practitioner role. Because her 'practitioner' activities included the 'expanded activities' (medical functions enhanced by nursing knowledge and skills), she has not had the time to devote to the educational activities. She manages, however, to maintain a considerable commitment to consultancy and research, and has demonstrated her leadership and change agent abilities (according to her physician colleague). The educational role, she felt, was the particular strength of the CNS. A CNS was about to be appointed to work with her.

The second ACNP interviewed works in a non-teaching district general hospital in a pre-admission clinic. There are no resident medical staff. Medical services are provided by general practitioners and 'specialists' with visiting privileges. She is a Canadian 'trained' nurse who did a postregistration bachelors degree in public health and administration and a masters NP programme (Health Nurse Clinician Course) in the USA. She worked for 5 years as an ACNP in a large hospital in the USA.

As an NP in this setting, where, as there had never been any 'junior doctors', they were not missed, she has had great difficulty in establishing her role. It should be borne in mind that the majority of nurses working within this hospital would not be degree-prepared, and few would hold masters degrees. She felt that her problems stemmed from 'control issues', where traditional medical roles were very entrenched, and family practitioners can claim payment for medical care that they give to patients within the hospital. She has, however, received considerable support from 'specialist' physicians and surgeons in the hospital, who see her as a positive addition, enabling them to provide a more efficient and effective service. Personal knowledge of this care setting suggests that she must be performing very effectively if she has 'won over' some of the individuals mentioned!

In respect of preparation for the role, all those interviewed concurred that the ability to think critically, and the skills to plan and organize, not only patient care but also service development, are essential. The consultant was particularly at pains to make the point that he originally felt that masters-level preparation was an unnecessary (and expensive) frill. He has changed his mind, however, from thinking that any nurse could be trained for an extended role, and he now fully appreciates that the ACNP role can only be developed through someone who possesses the abilities honed by masters-level study.

Any programme of preparation, according to both ACNPs, is only the first step: the motivation and ability to identify continuing educational needs, and set and achieve educational objectives, is essential. The ACNP who studied in the USA felt, in addition, that far more was needed to prepare nurses for the role than could be found in present Canadian masters programmes (very similar to those in the UK). She advised that the high level of skills needed to undertake a physical assessment and history is not to be underrated. Lack of knowledge of the extent of the role, she felt, was often a failing of educationalists who plan these programmes. On the positive side, however, she suggested a physical examination and history done by a competent nurse was far better than one done by a physician: 'Nurses don't think they already know everything and are much more thorough because of this; they also include social and psychological aspects in the assessment.'

The level of skills required was borne out by the other ACNP, who despite working about 55 hours per week, selects and attends relevant classes within the Faculty of Medicine and undertakes assessments of the knowledge and clinical skills gained alongside the medical students.

The lessons

The issues raised by the re-emergence of the NP role in the province of Ontario provide valuable lessons for us in the UK. Whether in the 1960s or today, the NP role is inexorably tied to economic and political issues. At any one time these may be working for or against the development of the role.

In Ontario, the current pressures of financial constraints on health care provision, the removal of junior doctors from the workforce, and the emergence of new health care systems and types of services, are creating a 'new' role for nurses. These pressures have been viewed as an opportunity by nursing leaders who have worked with service providers and the Government to try to ensure that, although driven by economic and political forces, the patient has been the focus of developments.

Opposition to the role from the medical profession is being eroded in Ontario, not by government pressure or policy change, but on an individual basis, as these practitioners prove their worth, both in the quality of care provided and in its cost effectiveness. The key barrier has been that of remuneration; the fact that nurses, if they become autonomous practitioners, will be able to compete in a 'fee for service' system. In planning for service in the UK, politicians and managers must ensure that the system for remuneration for health services does not create barriers to nurses practising in this role.

One of the key issues in the success of this role is the educational and clinical preparation of individuals for practice. It is essential that this is seen as being of the highest quality and aimed at fitting the individual for 'purpose and practice'. The creation of the confident decision maker and life-long learner is central to any programme, and, although ideally, according to nursing leaders, this preparation should be at masters level, practicality and economics may determine otherwise. Nurse practitioners will, however, be prepared to a point beyond graduate level, both extending the range of skills and developing the individual holistically in the practice of nursing.

In Ontario, public protection has become a central issue. This must be assured through legislative change, which is a difficult process made necessary by the prescriptive scope of practice enshrined in legislation. Within the UK, this is not necessary. Because of the nature of the UK *Scope of Professional Practice* (UKCC, 1992), there is no need to create an 'extended class status' part of the register. There *are* other models of credentializing and regulation that are working successfully, and professional bodies *may* undertake to establish standards for a role, as indeed the Royal College of Nursing has recently done (Royal College of Nursing, 1996), and to set up credentialing mechanisms. The developments in Ontario demonstrate, however, that every system has its drawbacks. Perhaps we in the UK should be concentrating more on developing an attitude within practitioners that will enable them to practise within the *Scope of Professional Practice*, rather than seeking the security of prescriptive 'dos and don'ts'.

Note

Nurse practitioner legislation (e.g. creation of the extended role status) was enacted in the summer of 1997 in Ontario. It is worth noting that the legislation applies only to NPs working in the community and that the title 'nurse practitioner' has not been protected.

References

Alcock, D. (1994). *The Clinical Nurse Specialist, Clinical Nurse Specialist/Nurse Practitioner and Other Titled Nurse in Ontario*, prepared for The Ministry of Health of Ontario. Ottawa: Faculty of Health Sciences, University of Ottawa.

Barer, M. and Stoddart, G. (1991). *Towards integrated medical resource policies for Canada* [background document]. Report prepared for the Federal/Provincial/Territorial Conference of Deputy Ministers of Health. Cited in D. Pringle (1994). *A Proposal to Develop Acute Care Nurse Practitioners*. Toronto: Faculty of Nursing, University of Toronto.

COUPN Nurse Practitioner Curriculum Committee. (1994). *Draft Nurse Practitioner Program Outline* [internal document].

Department of Health. (1993). *Hospital Doctors: Training for the Future*. London: DoH.

Department of Health. (1995). *Planning the Medical Workforce*. (Medical Workforce Standing Advisory Committee: Second Report.) London: DoH.

Department of Health. (1994a). *The Challenges for Nursing and Midwifery in the 21st Century: the Heathrow Debate, May 1993*. (Nursing Strategy Workshop: Health and Social Care 2010 – Shaping the Future.) London: DoH.

Department of Health. (1994b). *Nursing, Midwifery and Health Visiting Education: A Statement of Strategic Intent*. (Nursing, Midwifery and Health Visiting Forum.) London: DoH.

Fenton, M. and Brykczynski, K. (1993). Qualitative distinctions and similarites in the practice of Clinical Nurse Specialists and Nurse Practitioners. *Journal of Professional Nursing*, **9**(6), 322.

Government of Ontario. (1991a). *The Nursing Act*. (An Act respecting the regulation of the Profession of Nursing.) Toronto: Queen's Printers.

Government of Ontario. (1991b). *Regulated Health Professions Act*. Toronto: Queen's Printers.

Mitchell, A., Pinelli, J. and Patterson, C. (1993). *Utilization of nurse practitioners in Ontario: A discussion paper requested by the Ministry of Health*. Hamilton: Quality of Nursing Worklife Research Unit, University of Toronto–McMaster University.

Nurse Practitioners' Association of Ontario. (1994). *Standards of Practice for Nurse Practitioners in Ontario*. Toronto: NPAO.

Ontario Ministry of Health. (1994). *Nurse Practitioners in Ontario: A Plan for Their Education and Employment*. Toronto: Ministry of Health.

Ontario Ministry of Health. (1995). *Letter to the Council of Ontario Universities, 1, 19 April, 1995*. Toronto: Office of the Nursing Co-ordinator, Ministry of Health.

Pringle, D. (1994). *A Proposal to Develop Acute Care Nurse Practitioners*. Toronto: Faculty of Nursing, University of Toronto.

Raffel, M. ed. (1984). *Comparative Health Systems: Descriptive Analyses of Fourteen National Health Systems*. University Park: Pennsylvania State University Press.

Read, S. (1995). *Catching the Tide: New Voyages in Nursing*. Sheffield: Sheffield Centre for Health and Related Research.

Read, S. and Graves, K. (1994). *Reduction of Junior Doctor's Hours in Trent Region: the Nursing Contribution*. Sheffield: NHS Executive (Trent).

Richardson, G. and Maynard, A. (1995). *Fewer Doctors? – More Nurses? A Review of the Knowledge Base of Doctor–Nurse Substitution*. York: University of York, Centre for Health Economics.

Royal College of Nursing Council. (1996). *The Royal College of Nursing of the United Kingdom: Statement on the Role and Scope of Nurse Practitioner Practice*. London: RCN.

Spitzer, W. O., Sackett, D. L., Sibley, J. C. et al. (1974). The Burlington randomised trial of the nurse practitioner. *N. Engl. J. Med.*, **290**, 251–256.

Statutory Instrument 875. (1983). *Nurses Midwives and Health Visitors Rules Approval Order*. London: HMSO.

Statutory Instrument 1456. (1989). *Nurses Midwives and Health Visitors Rules Approval Order*. London: HMSO.

United Kingdom Central Council for Nursing, Midwifery and Health Visiting. (1992). *Scope of*

Professional Practice. London: UKCC.

United Kingdom Central Council for Nursing, Midwifery and Health Visiting. (1994). *The Future of Professional Practice – the Council's Standards for Education and Practice following Registration*. London: UKCC.

Van Brenk, D. (1994). Nursing plan aid to patients says pioneer. *London Free Press*, November 14, B1–B2.

Way, D. and Jones, L. (1994). The family physician–nurse practitioner dyad: indications and guidelines. *Can. Med. Assoc. J.*, **151**, 29–34.

8

A conceptual framework for advanced practice: an action research project operationalizing an advanced practitioner/consultant nurse role

Kim Manley

Introduction

This chapter presents a preliminary conceptual model for advanced practice developed in the process of analysing data from a 3-year action research study involving the operationalization of an advanced practice/consultant nurse role, in which I was the action researcher. One of the hallmarks of action research is that analysis occurs in practice during each phase in the action research cycle. Hence, this is a preliminary conceptual framework resulting from the early research. A deeper analysis of data collected to inform action will be used further to refine the model at a later date.

The terms 'advanced practitioner' and 'consultant nurse' are used interchangeably in this chapter. The reason for this is that, currently, there appear to be two schools of thought concerning the essence of advanced practice (Manley, 1996a). One school sees advanced practice as relating to the new clinical posts developing at the nursing–medicine interface. Many of these, although retaining nursing values, are associated with taking on what were previously considered to be medical tasks. Such posts serve an important function in enabling nursing to respond to changing health care needs, but I see them as primarily specialist posts, rather than advanced practitioner posts. The other school of thought (to which I subscribe) is associated with advancing nursing practice, rather than medical practice. This view encompasses expert nursing practice (as a generalist or a specialist), but it is more than that, as it also integrates the subroles of educator, researcher and consultant. Such posts are multidimensional and their purpose is to promote and develop clinical nursing from clinical to strategic and policy levels, whilst simultaneously creating and maintaining a culture in which nurses and nursing strive for more effective patient and health care services.

Background: the context in which the post was developed, and related contemporary issues

The post developed within the context of the early nursing development unit (NDU) movement and followed 2 years of developmental work in 1989–1991 (Manley, 1990; Warfield and Manley, 1990; Clayton and McCabe, 1991; Jenkins, 1991). I facilitated this development work using a values clarification approach with the all-qualified nursing staff of a five-bedded intensive care unit. A number of practice developments resulted, which were congruent with the values and beliefs shared. These core values and beliefs centred on:

• Nursing
• Collaboration
• Change
• The value of the individual
• Teamwork

An open and non-hierarchical management approach further facilitated an environment for development (Salvage, 1989; Jenkins, 1991).

In 1991, a second values clarification exercise was undertaken in preparation for the unit's application to the King's Fund for financial support. This resulted in staff identifying what they wanted to achieve in the forthcoming years, and also how they wished any funding to be used. The priority areas identified included staff development, education, research, practice development and quality assurance activities. Staff perceived the need for someone to help them with these areas and decided that any financial support obtained should be used for that purpose.

At the time, a number of posts designed to achieve similar objectives existed in the UK and the USA. Within the UK, there was the consultant nurse (Wright, 1991) and the lecturer–practitioner (Vaughan, 1987, 1989). In 1991, both of these lacked detailed role descriptions, although both roles have subsequently developed. Within the USA, the clinical nurse specialist and nurse practitioner roles predominated, both being promoted as advanced practice roles (Kitzman, 1989). The role description for the clinical nurse specialist was the most developed in terms of its explicit four subroles, skills and competencies, and the primary criteria required by the postholder. These are outlined in Figure 1 (Hamric, 1989). Nurse practitioners were considered to have primarily a unidimensional focus to their role (providing direct services), whereas the clinical nurse specialist was multidimensional (providing both direct and indirect services as represented by a combination of direct and indirect practice and the other subroles) (Kitzman, 1989). Kitzman considered that the differing role dimensions of the clinical nurse specialist and nurse practitioner reflected their respective purposes. For nurse practitioners, their stated purpose was 'to provide patient care' (Ford and Silver, 1967), and for clinical nurse specialists it was 'to improve patient care' (Crabtree, 1979; Holt, 1984). Today, in contemporary American practice, there has been some amalgamation of the two roles (Hickey et al., 1996). Both are beginning to share similar attributes, with the nurse practitioner moving towards the multidimensional focus of the clinical nurse specialist.

```
Subroles
   Expert practitioner
   Educator
   Researcher
   Consultant

Skills and competencies
   Change agent
   Collaborator
   Clinical leader
   Role model
   Patient advocate

Primary criteria
   Master's/doctorate prepared
   Client based practice
   Certification through meeting expert criteria in practice
```

Figure 8.1 The subroles, skills and competencies and primary criteria of the American clinical nurse specialist adapted from by Hamric (1989)

In the UK, the title 'clinical nurse specialist' was beginning to be used in the late 1980s and early 1990s, but roles in the UK were very different to the American roles, and the title was inconsistently applied (Manley, 1993). UK nurses with the title of clinical nurse specialist fulfilled primarily a specialist practice role in the areas of stoma nursing, diabetic nursing and infection control (Wade and Moyer, 1989). Some aspects of the educator and consultant roles were evident, but these were superficial and under-developed compared with their American counterparts. Nurse practitioners, who were also beginning to develop in the UK in similar ways to the USA, tended in contrast to encompass direct practice totally, with little involvement with the other subroles.

Contemporary views on the nature of advanced practice in Britain are reflected in the United Kingdom Central Council of Nursing, Midwifery and Health Visiting's (UKCC) statement on advanced practice, which seems to suggest a multidimensional rather than unidimensional focus to such posts:

> Advanced nursing practice is concerned with adjusting the boundaries for the development of future practice, pioneering and developing new roles responsive to changing needs, and with advancing clinical practice, research and education to enrich professional practice as a whole (UKCC, 1994).

Such a view seems to imply achievement as an expert practitioner within an area of nursing, be that generalist or specialist, and highlights the other dimensions of the role that are necessary to facilitate the development of other practitioners and nursing practice.

The post and its evaluation

Through values clarification, the staff of the NDU discussed in this article had identified the need for an advanced practice-type post. They also identified eight future objectives, one of which reflected their wish to fulfil what they considered an important responsibility: the evaluation of such a post. This objective was particularly important, as the proposal was being developed at a time when other senior clinical posts were being lost within NHS restructuring exercises throughout the UK, and the value of a clinical career structure for nursing needed to be demonstrated, particularly to senior managers nationally.

The funding proposal was successful and unit staff asked me to undertake the new role in order to continue the work already collaboratively achieved. The role description outlined by Hamric (1989) was used as a starting point to develop what was then a unique role in the UK. The job description was structured around the four subroles identified by Hamric (1989) for 4 days a week, and then combined with the responsibilities of a lecturer in higher education (course tutor to the MSc in nursing) for the remaining day.

I fulfilled all the primary criteria outlined by Hamric (1989), but their relevance to the UK context had not yet been established. There had, however, been European moves for master's prepared nurses in practice (Casey, 1990).

In relation to evaluation, the possession of theoretical and practical knowledge implied by the primary criteria, skills competencies and subroles (Figure 8.1) had already been linked to quality outcome indicators (Georgopoulos and Christman, 1990). Georgopoulos and Christman, in a 2-year longitudinal study, compared practitioners who possessed these criteria with two other groups: those attributed the same title but not possessing all of the identified skills and competencies, and those who were conventional nurse ward managers. A significant impact on over 100 outcome indicators was demonstrated in practitioners who possessed all the criteria, compared with the other two groups who did not. This seems to suggest that practitioners with both theoretical and practical knowledge to at least the academic level of master's degree within the four subroles, can have a major impact on outcomes when they are based in practice. What is not so explicit are the processes that such practitioners use. It is this area that subsequently became the focus of the action research project, as reflected by the research question: How does the advanced practitioner/consultant nurse facilitate the development of nurses and nursing to provide a quality nursing service?

Methodology

In light of the values held by staff and myself, as well as the objectives aspired to and the processes used to date (namely values clarification and reflection), it was important to choose a methodology that would be congruent, valuing staff as coresearchers and recognizing the messiness and complexity of both practice and the context in which practice takes place (Greenwood, 1984), which was so well described by Schön (1983) as 'the swampy lowlands'. Action research was therefore selected, specifically the approach underpinned by critical science (McCutcheon and Jung, 1990) and associated with staff participation, collaboration and emancipation. To differentiate this approach from action research from other perspectives,

Grundy (1982) named it 'emancipatory action research' in education. In nursing it has been called the 'enhancement approach' (Holter and Schwartz-Barcott, 1993), and in health and social care, the 'empowering type' (Hart and Bond, 1995).

With hindsight, the 3-year action project can be considered as falling within three broad but interconnected areas, each associated with innumerable action research cycles. The first area was at the macro/ strategic level, where my role was linked inextricably with the stated purpose of the unit and facilitation of that purpose, namely developing a quality patient service. The second area was more concrete and middle in scope, as represented by action research cycles linked to each of the unit's eight objectives. Again, my actions were inextricably linked with both the facilitation of, and collaboration with, staff in achieving these objectives. The third area concerned my personal actions and reflections during the time the role was undertaken. This paper draws mainly on work within the middle area, specifically the staff's objective concerned with evaluating the post.

Data analysis

A very crude analysis of my working diary was undertaken for the type of work activity performed during the first 2 years of the project (July 1992– June 1994). The work diary was, and continued to be, used to record all appointments, daily objectives and daily achievements in note form. More detailed field notes were also kept during the project.

Each member of staff was provided with a detailed itemized list of activities grouped under some loose thematic headings. Focused group discussions with each primary nursing team were used to explore how staff felt this advanced practitioner/consultant nurse post was working, whether more or less of different aspects were desired, and whether refinements were required. This also provided an opportunity for staff to participate in my performance review. Minor refinements were incorporated into the role, in relation to aspects such as clinical rounds, primary nurse reviews, and the timing of such activities.

The conceptual framework presented here has resulted from re-analysing the 2 years' data in more depth, something that was not possible to do at the time. One hundred and ninety-five different work items were identified, 77 from year one, and 118 from year two. The analysis was undertaken in two stages: first, a thematic analysis of the work activities resulting in 22 categories and seven themes (Figure 8.2); and, secondly, a cross-analysis of the 22 categories for the types of processes used and the knowledge base drawn upon.

From this, the following further nine themes were derived:

- Role modeller
- Catalyst
- Facilitator
- Staff development
- Practice development
- Change agent

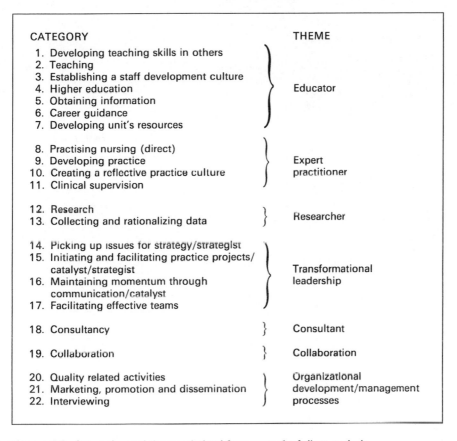

CATEGORY	THEME
1. Developing teaching skills in others 2. Teaching 3. Establishing a staff development culture 4. Higher education 5. Obtaining information 6. Career guidance 7. Developing unit's resources	Educator
8. Practising nursing (direct) 9. Developing practice 10. Creating a reflective practice culture 11. Clinical supervision	Expert practitioner
12. Research 13. Collecting and rationalizing data	Researcher
14. Picking up issues for strategy/strategist 15. Initiating and facilitating practice projects/ catalyst/strategist 16. Maintaining momentum through communication/catalyst 17. Facilitating effective teams	Transformational leadership
18. Consultancy	Consultant
19. Collaboration	Collaboration
20. Quality related activities 21. Marketing, promotion and dissemination 22. Interviewing	Organizational development/management processes

Figure 8.2. Categories and themes derived from stage 1 of diary analysis

- Change manager
- Infrastructure development
- Strategist

The combined 16 themes were then used to construct a conceptual framework, which identifies the roles and skills necessary for operationalizing an advanced practitioner/consultant nurse role, linked to essential contextual prerequisites and outcomes (Figure 8.3).

The conceptual framework

The conceptual framework has three parts: the advanced practitioner/consultant nurse, characterized by four integrated subroles and a set of skills and processes; the context in which the advanced practitioner/consultant nurse operates; and the outcomes in practice, which result when such roles, processes and contexts are combined.

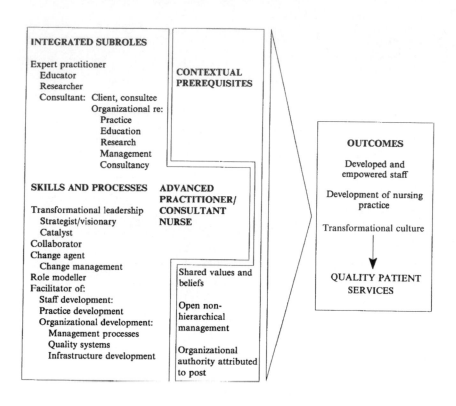

Figure 8.3. A conceptual framework for the advanced practitioner/consultant nurse

Context

The context in which all practitioners operate will have an influence on their practice, a premise underpinning naturalistic inquiry: 'realities are wholes which cannot be understood in isolation from their contexts' (Lincoln and Guba, 1985). In this study, three influences were identified as essential prerequisites for successful operationalization of the advanced practitioner/consultant nurse role:

- Shared values and beliefs;
- Open non-hierarchical unit management;
- Organizational authority attributed to the post.

The first two influences particularly characterized the NDU culture in which the post was established. These are also factors identified by the King's Fund (Salvage, 1989) as conducive to establishing a NDU. The third prerequisite emerged as important, particularly if (as in this study) the postholder does not possess the positional power of a traditional management post. The post therefore requires senior status recognition, and hence legitimate authority from the senior management board, with the postholder being recognized as an important contributor to trust strategy and a partner in the senior management nursing team.

Subroles

The four subroles previously identified by Hamric (1989) clearly emerged from the data, but have been further expanded. They are presented as separate entities within the conceptual framework. In practice, the subroles demonstrate considerable overlap, each informing the other in terms of their respective knowledge bases and processes. The emphasis given to any one subrole varied according to the issues and needs being addressed, the changing needs of the service and the unit's purpose.

The *expert practitioner role* encompassed both direct and indirect practice. Direct practice involved caring for patients and their families, whereas indirect practice involved, amongst other activities, working with staff in planning care for their patients and developing practice protocols that were evidence based, supervising staff in guided structured reflection, facilitating reflective primary reviews, and exploring practice issues. The role also involved creating a culture for staff to reflect on their own practice and on nursing generally. This was achieved by being based in practice, through practising nursing, and using strategies that facilitate practice development.

Although I was working within the specific field of intensive care nursing, the knowledge base, skills and values central to nursing generally were drawn on to inform both direct and indirect practice as much as those of intensive care nursing. Both knowledge bases complemented each other, and were manifested in both the 'know-how' and 'know-that' (Polanyi, 1958) of nursing practice. It was through expertise in nursing practice and the practice of nursing that credibility was accorded to the post. This credibility made it easier to introduce and manage change. Direct practice also provided opportunities to be exposed to (and be reminded of) the realities of practice, and the daily issues and struggles that exist for staff, patients and their families. This acted as a motivator for action.

The *educator role* clearly emerged as involving a broad view of education, encompassing the development of others, including their teaching skills, providing opportunities for others to learn, establishing a staff development culture, and developing and facilitating the maintenance of the unit as a learning environment. Besides the skills and knowledge necessary to provide a positive learning environment in practice, knowledge and skills relating to higher education and career development were also used. My experience in higher education was repeatedly drawn on by staff to help them to gain access to, and to progress within, the higher education system, to optimize their higher education experience to benefit practice, and to gain credit and recognition for their practice from higher education.

Other aspects of this subrole included providing opportunities for staff to develop new knowledge and skills, and developing and maintaining the unit's educational resources. Both staff development and practice development were therefore interlinked with the educator subrole.

The *researcher role* emerged clearly, as described by Hodgman (1983), who identified the three levels outlined in Figure 8.4. From the data, examples of level 1 working included establishing a research culture and journal review group, critiquing and helping others to critique research, exploring the implications for the practice of research, updating practice protocols in the light of research, and facilitating the rationalization of data collection and its implications. As the unit was a critical care unit, many data were routinely collected. With the development of audit tools and ongoing research projects, this potentially placed increasing demands on staff.

Level 1: Utilizing, interpreting, evaluating, communicating research and deriving implications

Level 2: Testing and applying; translating into protocols; acting as a research co-ordinator and research generator

Level 3: Replicating; generating original ideas; supervising research projects; undertaking collaborative research

---

Figure 8.4. The Three Levels of Researcher Activity (after Hodgman, 1983)

At level 2, examples of activity included developing research based and evidence based protocols for both quality assurance and educational purposes. Other activities included co-ordinating research, highlighting research questions, providing consultancy, and teaching on research methodology and methods.

Client centred case consultation (case-direct)
The problem is case focused, that is, client/patient focused and involves the consultant making direct recommendations to the consultee on how the client should be treated or managed. A spin-off may be that the consultee might improve his or her knowledge and skills, but this is secondary to the primary aim of focusing on the client. This is the traditional medical approach to consultation, referred to as the clinical approach (Gallessich, 1982).
    Examples of activities from the data are responding to nurses' requests for help concerning:

• How to care for a patient who is experiencing hopelessness or powerlessness, or manifesting the signs of sleep deprivation;
• How to help patients and their families make difficult decisions;
• Clarifying the ethical issues within a particular patient situation.

Consultee centred case consultation (case-indirect)
The problem is again case focused, but this time the consultant's primary focus is on the consultee's difficulty, which Caplan considers may be in the following four areas:

• Lack of knowledge;
• Lack of skill in making use of the knowledge;
• Lack of self-confidence;
• Lack of professional objectivity.

Examples of activities from the data are

• Helping nurses to develop their family assessment skills or their psychological and physical assessment skills;
• Working through ethical frameworks to help nurses to analyse and make sense of ethical dilemmas generally.

Program centred administrative consultation (administration-direct)
The problem focus is on the organization rather than on the client or group of clients; otherwise it is similar to client centred case consultation. A consultant may be invited by a group of administrators to help with a problem concerning, perhaps, some area of service provision, or to help with the planning and implementation of organizational policy. It would involve assessing the problem and then writing a report with the consultant's assessment and recommendations. The purpose is the improved understanding and operation of the consultees, it is therefore direct and usually short term.

Caplan makes parallels between this type of consultancy and management consultancy. He suggests that mental health consultancy is a competitor to the traditional management consultant because of the special expertise that mental health consultants have in relation to interpersonal skills and communication. He does recognize the need to have additional knowledge and experience in the areas of organizational theory, practice and planning, fiscal and personnel management, and general administration, to operate in this type of consultancy.
Examples of activities from the data are:

• Providing guidance on how to implement both a marketing strategy and a research strategy;
• Helping to develop, plan, and evaluate programmes for the orientation of new staff or for developing essential competencies in inexperienced staff;
• Providing expertise in skill-mix and establishment review.

Consultee centred administrative consultation (administration-indirect)
Again, the focus is on the organization, but the methods are indirect in that the primary focus is on increasing the skills of the consultee(s), which will, in return, benefit the organisation. In Caplan's words:

> Consultee-centred administrative consultation is probably the most complicated, interest-ing, and demanding type of mental health consultation. The consultant is called in by the administrative staff of an organization to help them deal with current problems in organizational planning, programme development, personnel management, and other aspects of the implementation of organizational policies. It is expected that he will help them to improve their capacity to handle such problems on their own in the future. The consultant centres his attention primarily on the work difficulties of the consultees and attempts to help them improve their problem-solving skills and overcome their short comings. He is interested in collecting information about the organization, its goals, programmes, policies and administrative structure and functioning, not in order to work out his own recommendations or a collaborative plan for improving these, but as an aid in assessing the problems that impede the operations of the consultees and as a vehicle for assisting them to improve their ways of overcoming their work difficulties (Caplan, 1970).

Examples of activities from the data are:
• Facilitating the development of a philosophy, mission statement, strategy;
• Working with team co-ordinators to develop their teambuilding and leadership skills or approaches to group clinical supervision;
• Helping staff to develop skills in developing role definitions, quality assurance programmes, change management strategies.

Figure 8.5. Caplan's model of mental health consultation (1970) with examples of activities from the work of advanced practitioner/consultant nurse. (Adapted from Manley, K, 1996b)

At level 3, collaborative research was undertaken to help others with no previous research experience to participate in and experience the research process.

To undertake such a role in practice requires a knowledge base that has a firm foundation in all ways of knowing in nursing, related and appropriate methodologies, and the assumptions underpinning all three research paradigms: postpositivist, interpretive, and critical science (Lucock, 1996).

The data supporting the *consultant role* demonstrated that the content of the consultancy was drawn from all subroles: nursing practice, practice development, education in practice, educational theory, higher education, research methodology and methods, data collection, the nature of knowledge and theory development in nursing, and consultancy skills.

Caplan's model (1970), based on mental health consultation, provides an appropriate framework for illustrating the types of consultancy undertaken in this study: client-centred, consultee centred, programme centred, and organization centred. Figure 8.5 illustrates the main characteristics of each and provides examples from the work activities highlighted in the diary analysis.

In practice, several types of consultancy may be used simultaneously. This point is further supported by Hendrix and LaGodna (1982), who consider that, for maximal effectiveness, consultants would be using all four types at various times.

In addition to levels of consultancy, the study data also demonstrated specific consultancy approaches. Schein (1988) labelled three models representing these approaches as the purchase of expertise model, the doctor–patient model, and the process model. Each is underpinned by different assumptions. The study data demonstrated that two of these approaches were used extensively: the expert model and the process model. The expert model encompasses giving advice and guidance, while the process model is more concerned with developing the skills and problem-solving activities of others. Process consultancy is underpinned by values about collaboration and how others develop.

Caplan's model therefore offers a way of understanding the potential for different levels of consultancy within nursing. The ability to operate within all four types would be a fundamental function of advanced practitioners/consultant nurses if the potential of nursing practice was to be realized at strategic level as well as at the clinical level (Manley, 1996b). The specialist practitioner, in contrast, would be involved predominantly in client centred consultancy and occasionally consultee centred consultancy. To operate within the other two types of consultancy requires an understanding of organizational behaviour, as well as culture and the other skills and knowledge alluded to by Caplan.

Thus, it is when the skills and knowledge base of consultancy, underpinned by a strong nursing foundation and augmented by strong leadership, are combined with the educator and researcher functions that the attributes of the advanced practitioner/consultant nurse begin to become evident. This demonstrates the reason for linking the title of advanced practitioner to that of consultant nurse. To fulfil the function of consultant, however, requires more than expertise in one's area of nursing and the ability to give advice:

> Many professionals, in fact, assume that experience in a particular field – for example, social work or communications – is adequate preparation for consultation. But helping others with their work is a far more intricate process than working directly on one's own task. Moreover the organisational milieu is fraught with conflicts that may ensnare consultants and leave them impotent (Gallessich, 1982).

Skills and processes

Some of the skills possessed and the processes used by the advanced practitioner/consultant nurse have been implied by the subroles described. Again, the skills and processes are inextricably linked with each other.

The processes I used focused on facilitating a culture in which staff could become leaders themselves. These processes reflected both my own values and those of the unit staff. It is only with hindsight and on reading the literature that the processes can be recognized as being of a transformational leadership nature (Sashkin and Rosenbach, 1993). From the study data, the following processes emerged, which have also been identified by a number of writers and researchers on transformational leadership:

- *Developing a shared vision* Providing a sense of mission, vision, excitement and pride (Bass, 1985). Inspiring a shared vision (Kouzes and Posner, 1987).
- *Inspiring and communicating* Inspiring, setting high expectations, expressing important purposes simply, communicating a vision (Bass, 1985). Clarity, focusing the attention of others on key ideas, active listening and providing feedback (Sashkin and Burke, 1990). Communication (Sashkin and Burke, 1990).
- *Valuing others* Valuing the individual, focusing on the individual's needs, encouraging personal responsibility (Bass, 1985). Caring about others, unconditional positive regard (Sashkin and Burke, 1990). Encouraging, recognizing others' contributions and celebrating them (Kouzes and Posner, 1987).
- *Challenging and stimulating* Providing intellectual stimulation and a flow of new ideas that challenge others to rethink old ways of doing things, stimulating others to develop their own structures and problem solving ability (Bass, 1985). Challenging the process: searching for opportunities and experimenting (Kouzes and Posner, 1987).
- *Developing trust* By acting consistently over time, between words and actions (Sashkin and Burke, 1990). Developing respect and trust (Bass, 1985).
- *Enabling* Creating opportunities, supporting others in taking on challenges, and by minimizing the risks (Sashkin and Burke, 1990). Enabling others to act through collaboration, supporting the development of others (Kouzes and Posner, 1987). Fostering collaboration, modelling the way (Kouzes and Posner, 1987).

Linked to the processes of transformational leadership were those of being a strategist and a catalyst. Being a strategist included activities that involved actively looking for and raising awareness of potential future issues, developments, and opportunities that nurses needed to explore and develop. Acting as a catalyst encapsulates those activities that are necessary to 'get things going'. Through facilitating and initiating developments, through supporting them and participating in them, it was possible for those with potential interest to become involved, to get started, to feel supported, and to maintain momentum. Being a catalyst involved a great deal of communication, including getting people together, organizing somewhere for them to meet, co-ordinating diaries and off-duties, and helping groups to clarify and formulate their purpose and frames of reference.

In operationalizing the advanced practitioner/consultant nurse role and working towards a common purpose and vision, collaboration was the predominant way of working with staff. Collaboration is pivotal to: process consultancy; transformational leadership; being an educator; being a partner with patients, families and the multidisciplinary team; and facilitating change. The concept analysis by Henneman et al. (1995) conveys the attributes that represent what is meant by collaboration.

The management of change and helping others with change permeated almost every activity undertaken. Again, the values underpinning change management were congruent with the values underpinning collaborative ways of working, transformational leadership, and process consultancy, and reflected a normative–re-educative change strategy (Chin and Benne, 1985).

All activities provided opportunities for role modelling. Individual interviews with staff indicated that some began to aspire to similar roles for themselves within clinical practice, representing a clinical career ladder that they valued, and one they had not before thought possible.

All the subroles and processes facilitated staff development, practice development and organizational development. The organization and its infrastructure provided the context for practice and staff development. Knowledge of management processes was, therefore, essential, not just in nurturing and fostering a transformational culture, but also in supporting staff in their own management development. Activities in this area related to developing the organization and the infrastructure. This was reflected in activities concerned with facilitating staff in:

- Development of policies and practices regarding:
  - skill-mix, staff establishment;
  - individual performance review;
  - staff development and orientation.
- Protocols and guidelines concerning:
  - role definitions;
  - interviewing;
  - staff study leave and funding.
- Reports and proposals for expanding and improving the service.

Many activities involved the introduction of quality systems. Such systems linked management processes to the development of practice, quality patient services, educational strategies and research evidence, to support effective practice. Simultaneously, this involved working with staff to develop their own skills in the area of quality. Many of the management processes were therefore about establishing a sound infrastructure, where staff were able to optimize their practice for patients, enhanced by working in a culture that supported them.

Outcomes

The final part of the conceptual framework identifies the desired outcomes. Evidence from the study data also suggests these were achieved. The ultimate purpose of advanced practice/consultant nurse posts is to improve the quality of care experienced by patients and their families. Such posts and the processes used must therefore be linked to the effect they have on this purpose if they are to be supported and valued by stakeholders. The key to achieving this purpose is the role of the advanced practitioner/consultant nurse in developing a transformational culture. Such a culture will also facilitate staff empowerment and nursing practice development.

Discussion and implications

The relationship of the conceptual framework presented here to Hamric's model (1989) will first be discussed. Implications will be considered in relation to refining the framework and to the future preparation and accreditation of advanced practitioners/consultant nurses.

This conceptual framework has resulted from experiences of operationalizing an advanced practitioner/consultant nurse role in a UK context. The original job description was initially guided by the model and four subroles identified by Hamric (1989) in the absence of any other available framework of sufficient detail. This study identifies some similarities with Hamric's model, namely the four subroles themselves. However, there are a number of differences, for example, the role of transformational leadership and its associated skills and processes.

Similarities relate to the existence of the four subroles in both models. The subroles in this study have, however, been derived from data obtained in the process of an action research project, in contrast with the policy and professional consensus informing Hamric's model (1989). The subroles are, by their nature, broad, and reflect the need for both practical and theoretical expertise in areas of nursing practice, education, research and consultancy. This study particularly emphasizes the integration of the four subroles with one another, and also further expands on the nature of the consultant and educator roles. It additionally highlights the benefits of having one foot in the higher education camp. Uniquely, all roles are linked to the skills and processes that facilitate the development of a transformational culture, staff development, practice development and organizational development. An understanding of, and expertise in, related management processes is therefore also emphasized.

Greater differences exist between the conceptual framework presented here and Hamric's model in relation to the skills and processes used. Several processes in this study are completely new, while some are made more explicit or expanded. The processes of transformational leadership is one such example, and is central to the conceptual model presented. Transformational processes derived from the data are congruent with those in the literature. The importance of these processes has been linked to creating and sustaining a transformational culture. Transformational processes are also linked to being a strategist and a catalyst, and to using a number of other management processes (those concerned, for example, with quality systems and infrastructure development).

I feel that a particular strength in this conceptual framework, which differentiates it from Hamric's model, is the explicit link between the advanced practitioner/consultant nurse role, its context and its outcomes.

This serves to acknowledge that, however much practical and theoretical expertise an advanced practitioner/consultant nurse possesses, this, on its own, is of little value. The context has to be conducive and the basic ingredients need to exist (namely, shared values and a non-hierarchical, open management style). Similarly, such posts always need to be linked to their ultimate purpose, that of facilitating quality services to patients and their families. The other strength of the conceptual framework is that it reflects more appropriately the culture in which it has developed (i.e. a UK rather than an American one).

Future analysis will need to focus on explicating the links between the three components of the conceptual framework, and developing further understanding of the processes used and their relationship to the outcomes. This is vital if both nursing and advanced practitioner/consultant nurse posts are to be valued by executive management, the Government and the public.

The conceptual framework presented raises a number of implications for practice, particularly in relation to the preparation and accreditation of advanced practitioners/consultant nurses.

To operate successfully within all four subroles, and to develop the expertise, skills and processes required, will involve more than merely undertaking a theoretical course. All four subroles are practice based, requiring both practical and theoretical knowledge. It is likely, therefore, that practitioners en route to such posts will have followed diverse and individual pathways, in which extensive and varied experience, as well as formal study, will be necessary components. The biggest challenge will be the identification of practice outcomes of the advanced practitioner/consultant nurse as a basis for accreditation. From this study, it is easy to argue that one needs preparation as educator, consultant and researcher, built on a foundation of expertise in the practice of nursing, underpinned by a strong theoretical base and an understanding of all ways of knowing in nursing. Theoretical and academic outcomes are much easier to state and recognize, but it is the 'know-how' of expert practice within the four subroles that is much more difficult to explicate. Furthermore, a list of behaviourally stated competencies would be incongruent, as advanced practitioners/consultant nurses would autonomously decide which strategies and subroles they need to focus on at any one point in time, depending on the needs of practice, practitioners, the organization, and the service; this is a complex process. However, from the processes and frameworks discussed in this chapter, some guiding principles for recognizing outcomes in practice could be developed.

With regard to the level of academic preparation, it is probably the researcher role that is the determinant, since, to operate at all three levels as a researcher (Hodgman, 1983) and be able to work with the premises underpinning all three paradigms, requires preparation to at least master's level; in the future this is likely to be to doctoral level. This is because, increasingly, the role of interpreting and using research has been separated from that of doing research. Additionally, the opportunities to do research are not now provided formally until studying at master's level. Therefore, to develop confidence in the three research paradigms, their underlying premises, and their appropriateness for different ways of knowing within nursing, will probably only develop during post-master's level study.

In relation to accreditation, academic frameworks are well established, but what does not exist (except in its infancy at the graduate level via the Higher Award (English National Board, 1991)) are mechanisms for accrediting expertise in practice. This, of course, begs the question: Who will accredit such practitioners, even if outcomes can be made explicit? In relation to the conceptual framework presented here, it would seem that the best judges are those affected by the outcomes, namely, practitioners, organizations, and, most importantly, the patients and their families themselves. It is likely that any accreditation of practice would therefore involve multiple sources of evidence.

Conclusion

The conceptual framework presented here has resulted from a study that attempted to operationalize the advanced practitioner/consultant nurse role. The post developed from staff's own values and beliefs and aspirations for the future. The original job description was guided by the four subroles identified by Hamric (1989). This model was chosen only in the absence of any other detailed guidance. Although some similarities with Hamric's model have resulted, namely the four subroles, there are several differences, particularly the skills and processes necessary for creating a transformational culture. The resulting conceptual framework has also highlighted implications to be considered regarding the preparation of advanced practitioners/consultant nurses. Those aspiring to advanced practice/consultant nurse posts will be guided in their career progression by this framework, in the sense that specific theoretical and practical expertise needs to be developed.

Future work on analysing data arising from the action research project is proposed, to make the links between the three components within the conceptual framework more explicit and to expand on the processes used. In the meantime, it is hoped that the conceptual framework presented here will go some way to making explicit the multidimensional nature of advanced practice and the potential and powerful impact that such posts can have on the future advancement of nursing for the benefit of patients, clients and their loved ones.

Acknowledgements

I would like to acknowledge the role and contribution of the coresearchers in this project, namely all the staff of the Chelsea and Westminster Intensive Care and Nursing Development Unit, and, additionally, the valuable support provided by Ricky Lucock and Carolyn Mills.

References

Bass, B. M. (1985). *Leadership and Performance Beyond Expectations*. New York: Free Press.
Caplan, G. (1970). *The Theory and Practice of Mental Health Consultation*. London: Tavistock.

Casey, N. (1990). The specialist debate. *Nurs. Stand.*, **4**(31), 18–19.

Chin, R. and Benne, K. D. (1985). General strategies for effecting change in human systems. In *The Planning of Change*, 4th ed. (W. G. Bennis and K. D. Benne, eds.) pp. 22–43. New York: Holt, Rinehart and Winston.

Clayton, J. and McCabe, S. (1991). Continuing education in the NDU. *Nurs. Stand.*, **6**(9), 28–31.

Crabtree, M. (1979). Effective utilization of clinical specialists within the organizational structure of hospital nursing service. *Nurs. Admin. Q.*, **4**(1), 1–11.

English National Board. (1991). *Framework for Continuing Professional Education for Nurses, Midwives and Health Visitors. Guide to Implementation.* London: ENB.

Ford, L. and Silver, H. (1967). Expanded role of the nurse in child care. *Nurs. Outlook*, **15**, 43–45.

Gallessich, J. (1982). *The Profession and Practice of Consultation.* San Francisco: Jossey-Bass.

Georgopoulos, B. and Christman, L. (1990). *Effects of Clinical Nursing Specialization.* New York: Edwin Melson.

Greenwood, J. (1984). Nursing research: a position paper. *J. Adv. Nurs.*, **9**, 77–82.

Grundy, S. (1982). Three modes of action research. *Curriculum Perspect.*, **2**(3), 23–34.

Hamric, A. (1989). A model for CNS evaluation. In *The Clinical Nurse Specialist in Theory and Practice*, 2nd ed. (A. Hamric and J. Spross, eds.) pp. 83–104. Philadelphia, PA: Saunders.

Hart, E. and Bond, M. (1995). *Action Research for Health and Social Care.* Buckingham: Open University Press.

Hendrix, M. J. and LaGodna, G. E. (1982). Consultation: a political process aimed at change. In *The nurse as a change agent.* (J. Lancaster and W. Lancaster, eds.) pp. 387–412. St Louis, MO: Mosby.

Henneman, E. A., Lee, J. L. and Cohen, J. I. (1995). Collaboration: a concept analysis. *J. Adv. Nurs.*, **21**, 103–109.

Hickey, J., Ouimette, R. M. and Venegoni, S. (1996). *Advanced Practice Nursing: Changing Roles and Clinical Applications.* Philadelphia, PA: Lippincott.

Hodgman, E. C. (1983). The CNS as researcher. In *The Clinical Nurse Specialist in Theory and Practice.* (A. Hamric and J. Spross, eds.) pp. 73–82. New York: Grune and Stratton.

Holt, F. (1984). A theoretical model for clinical specialist practice. *Nurs. Health Care*, **5**, 445–449.

Holter, M. and Schwartz-Barcott, D. (1993). Action research: what is it? How has it been used and how can it be used in nursing? *J. Adv. Nurs.*, **18**, 298–304.

Jenkins, D. (1991). Developing an NDU: the manager's role. *Nurs. Stand.*, **6**(8), 36–39.

Kitzman, H. J. (1989). The CNS and the nurse practitioner. In *The Clinical Nurse Specialist in Theory and Practice*, 2nd ed. (A. Hamric and J. Spross, eds.) pp. 379–394. Philadelphia, PA: Saunders.

Kouzes, J. M. and Posner, B. Z. (1987). *The Leadership Challenge.* San Francisco: Jossey-Bass.

Lincoln, Y. S. and Guba, E. G. (1985). *Naturalistic Inquiry.* London: Sage.

Lucock, R. (1996) *Research Methodology* [dissertation]. London: Royal College of Nursing Institute.

Manley, K. (1990). The birth of a nursing development unit. *Nurs. Stand.*, **4**(26), 36–38.

Manley, K. (1993). The clinical nurse specialist. *Surg. Nurse*, **6**(3), 21–25.

Manley, K. (1996a). Advanced practice is not about medicalising nursing roles [editorial]. *Nurs. Crit. Care*, **1**, 2.

Manley, K. (1996b). *Consultancy* [Distance Learning Module]. London: Royal College of Nursing Institute.

McCutcheon Jung, B. (1990). Alternative perspectives on action research. *Theory Into Pract.*, **XXIX**(3), Summer, 144–151.

Polanyi, M. (1958). *Personal Knowledge.* London: Routledge and Kegan Paul.

Salvage, J. (1989). Nursing development. *Nurs. Stand.*, **3**(22), 25–28.

Sashkin, M. E. and Burke, W. W. (1990). Understanding and assessing organisational leadership. In *Measures of Leadership.* (K. Clark and M. B. Clark, eds.) pp. 297–325. West Orange, NJ: Leadership Library of America/Centre for Creative Leadership.

Sashkin, M. E. and Rosenbach, W. E. (1993). A new leadership paradigm. In *Contemporary Issues in Leadership*, 3rd ed. (W. E. Rosenbach and R. Taylor, eds.) pp. 87–108. Westview Press: Colorado.

Schein, E. H. (1988). *Process Consultation (Volume I): Its Role in Organizational Development*, 2nd ed. Reading, MA: Addison-Wesley.

Schön, D. (1983). *The Reflective Practitioner*. San Francisco, CA: Jossey-Bass.

United Kingdom Central Council for Nursing, Midwifery and Health Visting. (1994). *The Future of Professional Practice – the Council's Standards for Education and Practice following Registration. Position Statement on Policy and Implementation*. London: UKCC.

Vaughan, B. (1987). Bridging the gap. *Sen Nurse*, **6**(5), 30–31.

Vaughan, B. (1989). Two roles – one job. *Nurs. Times*, **85**(11), 52.

Wade, B. and Moyer, A. (1989) An evaluation of clinical nurse specialists: implications for education and the organisation of care. *Sen. Nurse*, **9**(9), 11–15.

Warfield, C. and Manley, K. (1990). Developing a new philosophy in the NDU. *Nurs. Stand.*, **4**(41), 27–30.

Wright, S. (1991). The nurse as a consultant. *Nurs. Stand.*, **5**(20), 31–34.

Commentary: the research perspective

Part 2 shifted the focus of this book from a theoretical perspective to an empirical one. It included four research studies that explored the nature of advanced practice and the role of the advanced practitioner, using four different research methodologies and four different theoretical frameworks.

Methodologies

Part 2 opened with Read providing a retrospective analysis of a number of studies, which she had undertaken over a period of several years. As she points out, this gave her 'the opportunity to revisit some of [her] own research-based explorations of new roles in nursing, and to re-examine [her] findings through a lens marked "advanced practice"'. This reinterpretation is, she fully admits, not a systematic review of the literature, but turns out to be a partial meta-analysis in which 19 nursing roles from five studies are re-analysed in respect of a number of criteria for advanced practice. This meta-analysis provides not only a typological description of these roles, but also an analysis and discussion of the extent to which they meet Read's criteria for advanced practice. It is therefore a research study in its own right, deductively applying a set of general criteria to a number of individual roles.

Fulbrook's chapter, in contrast, takes an inductive approach by attempting to build an understanding of the role 'from the perspective of "advanced practitioners" themselves', a perspective that he describes as 'emic' and 'naturalistic'. For Fulbrook, 'it was felt that in order to understand what advanced practice and the advanced practitioner are, it was necessary to ask people already recognized as advanced practitioners.' This, of course, is the very opposite of the approach taken by Read, who devised the criteria of advanced practice at the outset and examined the extent to which existing roles fitted those criteria. As we shall see, both approaches have advantages and disadvantages, and each produced distinctive findings.

Roberts-Davis takes what might be described as an in-depth case study approach to the question of what is advanced practice, using a combination of literature review, interviews and observations to produce a descriptive study of the historical development of an existing role. She chose to study the Canadian experience, since 'Although outwardly there appear to be many differences, politically and socially, Canadian structures and legislative processes are based on the same principles as the UK.' She was particularly concerned with how political issues and policy decisions shape the development of the role of the advanced practitioner, and: 'The impetus for this investigation was the need, as a nurse and educator, to enter as an informed participant in discussion and debate concerning the future role of nurses within the "new NHS".' It is in a sense, then, prospective rather than retrospective, since it attempts to explore the possible implications for the UK of a particular political initiative.

Finally, Manley takes yet another methodological approach, that of action research. This entails exploring the role of the advanced practitioner as it developed rather than taking a retrospective or prospective view, and of using her findings reflectively to influence the continuing development of the role. Furthermore, unlike the other researchers in Part 2, she was exploring the development of her own role rather than the roles of others, which inevitably added a subjective element to her findings. The outcome of the study was a conceptual framework for advanced practice and, of course, an actual role grounded directly in the data that it helped to generate. On the one hand, then, Manley is interested in the local application of her findings. Indeed, the application cannot be separated from the findings, since each informs the other, but she also wishes to generalize, such that: 'Those aspiring to advanced practice/consultant nurse posts will be guided in their career progression by this framework, in the sense that specific theoretical and practical expertise needs to be developed.'

Theoretical frameworks

As might be expected from four methodologically distinct studies, each also starts from a different theoretical framework in its exploration of advanced practice.

As we have already seen, Read developed a list of criteria from the literature, against which she attempted to judge a variety of new roles. This approach raises two difficulties. First, there is the question of who decides on the chosen criteria. This, loosely speaking, is the issue of the construct validity of the study, the extent to which it measures the construct that it claims to measure, since clearly the selection of 10 criteria from a possible choice of dozens, if not hundreds, will determine the shape that the role takes. Secondly, there is the issue of necessary and sufficient criteria, that is, of content validity, or the extent to which the chosen criteria represent the full range and scope of the role. Thus, the criteria can be said to be *necessary* if an advanced practitioner role needs to include all of them, and they can be said to be *sufficient* if those criteria, and those alone, are enough to warrant the title of advanced practitioner. We can see from the table at the end of Read's chapter that none of the 19 roles she examines meets the standards of necessity and sufficiency. This raises difficult questions about relative merit, about whether each of her criteria has equal standing or whether some are more important than others, and, in particular, which, if any, are necessary for advanced practice.

Fulbrook attempts to avoid this problem by asking the practitioners to devise their own criteria for advanced practice. However, as Fulbrook himself points out, this introduces a different problem of who decides on who are advanced practitioners. Thus: 'The key to their selection was that they were recognized as experts in their field of clinical practice by their peers.' He continued: 'Whether they are in fact "advanced practitioners" is an area which remains open for debate.'

We can see, then, that for Fulbrook, the question of validity relates not to the selection of the criteria for advanced practice but to the selection of the advanced practitioners themselves; that is, to sampling issues. More specifically, the content validity of his study (whether he has explored the full scope and extent of the role) is limited by the fact that his respondents were drawn from a single specialism, and the construct validity (whether he was actually exploring what he claimed to be) is limited by the fact that his respondents were identified by their peers as advanced practitioners, rather than selected through research based criteria.

In fact, Fulbrook and Read both recognized the limitations of their respective studies, but could find no way around them. It would seem, then, that we appear to have stumbled upon a nursing version of Heisenberg's uncertainty principle in atomic physics, which states that we cannot measure both the position and the velocity of a subatomic particle at the same time. We can either measure where it is, or where it is going, but not both. Thus, empirical investigation can only take us so far, and we can never really 'know' a subatomic particle. Similarly, it would appear that in order to explore what the advanced practitioner does, we must first identify who the advanced practitioner is; and, in order to identify who he or she is, we need to determine what it is that he or she does. Thus, in order to explore one of the variables, we have to make assumptions about the other in order to pin it down. There will always be a degree of uncertainty in our empirical knowledge of advanced practice.

Read pinned down the nature of the role by defining it in terms of 10 criteria, which she herself chose, and was thereby able to measure the extent to which performers of the role met those criteria. Fulbrook, on the other hand, pinned down the nature of the performer in terms of practitioners recognized by their peers as advanced, and was thereby able to measure the elements of advanced practice. In each case, the researcher has to make certain assumptions that are not entirely research based.

Roberts-Davis went one step further and pinned down both variables, in that she was examining an existing predefined role and existing practitioners in order to learn some important lessons for the UK. Whereas Read and Fulbrook were both concerned with a practice perspective, Roberts-Davis views advanced practice through a political lens to examine how practice might be shaped by government policy. This is particularly relevant to a developing role such as advanced practice, and Roberts-Davis paints a vivid picture of one particular course that the role could take if it is allowed to be influenced by wider political needs (for example, the gap left by shorter hours for junior doctors) rather than by the needs and wishes of the profession.

In contrast, the framework adopted by Manley starts from the same foundation of the four subroles of practice, education, consultation and research, but develops the role along nursing rather than medical lines to reach a very different conclusion. Thus, whereas for Roberts-Davis, the creation of new roles has stemmed from: 'The extension of skill and task reanalysis across the nursing/medicine interface', Manley prefers to focus on 'advancing nursing practice, rather than medical practice'. We should not be surprised, therefore, that the emerging roles are so very different, since the Canadian 'expanded role nurse' and the 'nurse practitioner' were both devised as a result of government initiatives, whereas Manley's advanced practitioner role came about through an action research study 'associated with staff participation, collaboration and emancipation'.

Furthermore, Manley started neither by pinning down the theoretical framework in order to examine the qualities of the practitioner, as Read did, nor by pinning down the definition of the practitioner in order to explore the nature of the role, as Fulbrook did, but rather by partially defining both and letting each develop alongside the other. As a local action research study, issues of content and construct validity are to some extent irrelevant, and it is only when the findings are generalized beyond the scope of the setting in which they were generated that validity becomes an issue, although arguably it is an issue for the reader of the study to resolve rather than for the writer.

Findings

Having discussed the methodologies and theoretical frameworks of the four studies in some detail, we will now turn briefly to the findings. As we might expect from four contrasting studies, the findings of each tend to have a specific focus, although there are several areas of agreement, some of which cover issues already discussed from a theoretical perspective in Part 1. The most pressing of these relates to the future development of the role, and as in the earlier theoretical discussion, two possible routes have been identified. First, there is the possible medicalization of the role (what Frost earlier referred to as 'role extension'), and the merging of the role of the nurse with that of the junior doctor, as described by Roberts-Davis from the Canadian perspective; and, second, there is the 'nursification' of the role (Frost's 'role expansion'), with the emphasis on what the nurse does differently from the other professions, as typified by Fulbrook's emic perspective.

As Frost pointed out earlier: 'It could be argued that nursing has reached a crossroads and must make a decision about how to move forward.' Thus, advanced practice could develop in either of the two ways, depending on the relative strength of the push from the Government on the one hand and the profession on the other. As Roberts-Davis observed: 'The future of nursing in the UK lies very firmly in policy and professional contexts. Views may differ about which is the more influential.'

What makes Roberts-Davis' study so important and valuable is that it offers us a clear vision of the likely outcomes of taking one of those routes, in this case, the route driven by government policy rather than by practitioners at grass-roots level, as well as describing the antecedent factors that led up to the decision to move in that particular direction. In contrast, Manley produces a parallel vision of a role driven almost entirely by practitioners themselves, and although superficially the roles appear to be similar, particularly in terms of their component subroles, a closer inspection reveals some fundamental differences.

The most important difference is in the clear medical focus of the Canadian role, with its emphasis on history taking, physical examination, diagnostic tests and medical procedures, in contrast with Manley's more facilitative and enabling role which aims to 'promote and develop clinical nursing from clinical to strategic and policy levels, whilst simultaneously creating and maintaining a culture in which nurses and nursing strive for more effective patient and health care services.'

Roberts-Davis takes a fairly neutral stance on the direction that advanced practice in the UK should take, pointing out only that 'the... role is inexorably tied to economic and political issues'. Fulbrook, on the other hand, is quite clear which way he wishes to see the role develop, stating that: 'The danger is that the development of advanced practice might be driven more by government policies than by professional motivation.' This comment echoes Frost's earlier observation that 'the more cynical would indeed see the issue of role extension as part of an overt move to undermine professional autonomy and control.' Fulbrook is clearly concerned about the lack of professional leadership being offered by the UKCC, citing in particular the *Scope of Professional Practice* document, which, unlike Frost, he believes is driving the nursing profession in a medical direction, and the implicit concern is that the failure of the UKCC to give a professional lead will leave the door open to the Government to exert an influence based not so much on the wishes of practitioners as on economics and political expediency. He points to the reduction in junior doctors' hours as an example of a government-driven initiative, claiming that there is 'the expectation that nurses take on tasks that were previously considered to be the doctor's domain'. Thus, in contrast to the Canadian view of the advanced practitioner, which takes its very identity from its extension into the medical domain, Fulbrook claims that, 'This is quite clearly not what the informants in this study consider to be advanced practice; it is not even role extension; it is simply the performance of additional tasks.'

This last statement relates to another of the general findings from Part 2. Fulbrook's rejection of the medical role of the nurse as 'simply the performance of additional tasks' rather than advanced practice or even role extension, stems from the general agreement that advanced practice is concerned with process rather than with content, with the 'how' rather than with the 'what' of practice. Thus, for Fulbrook, advanced practice 'is not measured in relation to [the nurse's] ability to perform tasks', for Read, 'advanced nursing practice was much more strongly related to a high level of clinical decision making... than to the carrying out of highly technical procedures'; and for Stilwell, 'protocols of care cannot account for every situation'. Even Roberts-Davis acknowledges that, 'Perhaps we in the UK should be concentrating more on developing an attitude within practitioners that will enable them to practice within the *Scope of Professional Practice*, rather than seeking the security of prescriptive "dos and don'ts".'

If we delve slightly deeper into exactly what these advanced processes are, we again find that there is a broad agreement. We have already seen that, in Read's study, the practitioners felt that a high level of clinical decision making was the most crucial factor in determining advanced practice, a view partly supported by Manley, who emphasized the importance of the underlying 'know how' of expert practice. Fulbrook explored the issue in far greater depth, and found that the processes that make practice 'advanced' are closely linked to the personal development of the practitioner him or herself, echoing Stilwell's earlier assertion that 'to practice successfully, nurses must be highly self-aware, as well as open to the singularity of each person'. In particular, Fulbrook's study found that the advanced practitioner was considered to possess high-level communication skills, the ability to reflect on practice, and a heightened self-awareness. As with Manley's work, Fulbrook's study emphasized experiential 'know how', such that advanced practitioners 'are not afraid to make decisions based on past experiences rather than acknowledged theory'.

It is interesting that Roberts-Davis arrived at very similar process criteria, although the role she was describing was, of course, very different. Like Read, she found that critical thinking and problem solving were essential prerequisites for the advanced practitioner, and, like Fulbrook, she found that the personal characteristics of flexibility, autonomy, communication skills and leadership skills were stressed as being essential to the role. It would appear, then, that these core process skills cut across discussions and disputes about the content and focus of the role, and represent what Fulbrook's respondents called the 'art', which takes nursing to a 'higher level'.

Part 3

Developing advanced practice: the practice perspective

9

Evaluation and evolution: the contribution of the advanced practitioner to cancer care

Ingrid Goodman

Introduction

> The real voyage of discovery consists not in seeing new landscapes, but in having new eyes.
>
> Marcel Proust (1871–1922)

Will you join me on a voyage, help me to explore, to see clearly, to follow the river wherever it goes? I have had freedom to explore my visions and questions during 6 years spent developing a lecturer–practitioner role in oncology nursing in Oxford. My quest now is to find an advanced practitioner role. Thus, in this chapter I will explore two self-generated propositions in relation to the advanced practitioner:

1. The advanced practitioner should develop advanced practice based upon evidence regarding patients' requirements, evaluation of health services, and research
2. The advanced practitioner role should evolve locally and be evaluated within a national strategy.

In exploring these propositions, my aims are to clarify the advanced practitioner role through an examination both of the literature and of personal experience, to explore the contribution of advanced practitioner roles within the cancer nursing setting, and, finally, to consider the potential for a nursing career that incorporates advanced practice.

It is my belief, based on personal experience, that the advanced practitioner should achieve the above propositions by evaluating current practice and identifying service deficits and patients' unmet needs, and should use these creatively to determine the goals of local and national practice development. The advanced practitioner's contribution is particularly important, as it may extend beyond current nursing boundaries, focusing upon meeting patients' needs rather than defining nursing interventions within current definitions of nursing and other disciplines. Of equal importance is the recognition that the multidisciplinary context of advanced practice nursing is critical if proposals are to be realistic and supported by colleagues and politicians.

Meeting the needs of people with cancer and of cancer nurses

Within the context of advanced practice in cancer care, this section explores: the difficulties of meeting the needs of people with cancer; evidence of patients' perceptions of cancer nursing; cancer nurses' stresses, satisfactions, education and skills, and potential developments in cancer care; and the nursing implications.

Professional and political rhetoric and statements of belief frequently refer to the health service being driven by the needs of the population, and recommend patient centred services, for example, the Calman report (Department of Health, 1994). A nationally explicit definition of need seems to be strangely elusive, despite being the apparent key word that defines the focus of national health services. It is difficult then to define how effectively health care and clinical professionals meet the needs of the population and of individual patients. Different definitions of need could therefore influence the focus and nature of practice, including advanced practice (e.g. Maslow, 1970; Bradshaw, 1972; Byrne and Thompson, 1972; Welch et al., 1982; Wingate and Lackey, 1989).

Perhaps this lack of definition contributes towards clinical difficulties. For example, in my experience many nurses aspire to meet all of the needs of their cancer patients, including solving *unsolvable* problems. This, in part, may be due to their lack of knowledge, skills and self-awareness. Nurses and doctors have also been shown to lack assessment skills particularly regarding the assessment of psychological needs and the morbidity of people with cancer (Maguire, 1985; Endall et al., 1993; Tait, 1993).

Patient assessment is a critical skill in the problem solving approach to care and treatment, and forms the basis for the planning and negotiating of treatment and care. Difficulties of assessment that are evident in the literature are currently well recognized by clinical staff. For example, perceptions of the needs of an individual with cancer have been shown to differ between the individual, their relatives, and health care professionals (Hileman and Lackey, 1990), and nurses' ability to assess symptoms and distress have been shown to be inaccurate (Holmes and Eburn, 1989). An aspect of particular weakness appears to be the ability to assess psychological morbidity in cancer patients, which has been shown to be lacking in both doctors and nurses (Maguire, 1985; Endall et al., 1993; Tait, 1993). This poses the question of whether the assessment of need should become a focus for advanced practice to develop, taking the lead for all disciplines involved, or whether there is an alternative approach that would be more effective. Perhaps the key question is: could advanced practitioners achieve more than current practice achieves?

Needs assessment and the planning of priorities in cancer care are becoming increasingly important. Pressure upon resources, shorter in-patient stays, sicker inpatients (Wilkinson, 1995) and a rapid increase in outpatient care, all require highly skilled staff in order to meet individuals' needs within resource limitations. I question whether we are realistic about which needs can and cannot be met, and the reasons for this. Many professionals find this issue distasteful and contrary to their beliefs about patient care. However, it is not only financial resources that limit service capacity. Calman (Department of Health, 1994) states that a cancer centre's essential element is the expertise of the health care professionals within it. If this is so, then the level of expertise and the ability to use it effectively may also limit or expand service capacity. It may be argued that advanced practitioners would expand service capacity and effectiveness.

I would argue that prioritizing patients' needs may be of clinical benefit as well as financial, increasing clarity of purpose and the different contributions to their care. During the times of anxiety (Silverfarb and Greer, 1982), withdrawal, and helplessness (Moorey and Greer, 1989) described by people with cancer, negotiating clear goals of care and specifying contributions towards achieving them (including those of the patients) may promote coping for patients by offering them the control that many seek (Moorey and Greer, 1989; Gammon, 1991). This approach may assist professional staff to focus upon priority needs that have been negotiated with the patient. An advanced practitioner could clarify local staff skill deficits regarding the definition and assessment of patients' needs. Evidence of a mismatch could be used to clarify clinical team aims and skills, and generate topics for staff and patient education.

The advanced practitioner's contribution

In my view, clinical practice should be developed beyond current levels of practice and the advanced practitioner plays a key role in achieving this. He or she, in demonstrating advanced practice, influences and enables others to develop their level of practice and build on existing expertise. The advanced practitioner offers a global and critical perspective, different to that of other nurses, which stems from his or her range of clinical, research, educational and managerial experience and skills. It is this perspective, encompassing many aspects of practice, knowledge and experience, that generates creative questions, ideas and innovations. It exceeds the boundaries of single disciplines by focusing primarily upon patients' needs.

The difficult arena of prioritizing needs, negotiating care, and promoting patient and staff coping, is ripe for tackling by the advancing practitioner. Based upon personal experience and the literature regarding the stresses of oncology professionals (Wilkinson, 1995), I would suggest that clarification of these areas would improve staff coping strategies. An advanced practitioner could explore and evaluate the effectiveness of strategies to support staff and patients, contribute to planning educational initiatives, and evaluate the impact of education and innovation upon patients and practice. These activities could contribute to improving the effectiveness of practice and the use of local expertise. The advanced practitioner might also be involved in measuring these effects and their influence upon service capacity. Perhaps a key factor for advancing practice is freedom for advanced practitioners to take risks and explore their potential across professional boundaries. Such freedom requires authority that is recognized by all professions and patients involved. This issue is explored later.

The caring aspect of nursing should be included as a focus for the advanced practitioner. Central to this focus is the perception of the patient regarding nurses' caring behaviour. I have chosen to focus on two particular studies in which cancer patients' perceptions of nurses' caring behaviours support arguments for prioritizing patients' needs and the consequent nursing interventions with each patient.

In Larsen's study, 57 American patients prioritized nurses' instrumental activities (for example, giving injections) over their affective activities (e.g. comforting activities). Larsen suggests that the primary goal of cancer patients undergoing active treatment is to get better, which includes receiving medications and treatments at the appropriate times. 'Nurses can then move on to the interactions with patients which nurses find meaningful', which she lists as touching, being receptive to patients' needs, and providing individualized care (Larsen, 1995).

Cancer nurses need to ensure that their care really is patient focused and should not fall into the trap of delivering what *they* believe is important. The key point here is that advancing practice using an evidence base requires nurses to challenge their own beliefs, as Larsen suggests. This requires the skills to evaluate and apply appropriate research findings, and the courage to challenge cherished beliefs. Advanced practitioners should demonstrate these skills. This evidence of patients' priorities also suggests that nurses should have a high level of technical competence; this may be of relevance to nurses at all levels of practice, including the advanced practitioner.

The recent National Cancer Alliance (NCA) report (1996) offers useful, detailed descriptions of patients' perceptions of their care and carers in the UK. It offers many suggestions to improve practice. Many of the points raised reflect other research findings, which indicate the need for both technically skilled and knowledgeable practitioners who offer sensitivity and many communication skills. An interesting suggestion is that nurses who have not received a recognized training in counselling should not offer the counselling services that the patients clearly desire.

It is my belief that the advanced practitioner should maintain clinical skills and research the therapeutic aspects of nursing. Evidence of this kind is sorely needed in the current NHS environment in order to justify the need for nurses rather than technicians.

Cancer nurses' stressors, satisfaction, education and skills

Coping with being a cancer nurse in the 1990s is an important aspect of cancer care, towards which the advanced practitioner may contribute. In the UK, the context of rapid and continuous change in health care delivery, technical advances, and rising public expectations, have led to altered causes of stress for oncology nurses (Wilkinson, 1995). A review of three studies carried out from 1986 to 1993 suggests a shift in the sources of stress, with less conflict with medical staff and increased concerns regarding work overload, lack of resources, and staff shortages (Wilkinson, 1995). Nurses continue to have difficulties with patients' deterioration and death.

Evidence from the USA from 38 oncology nurses working at six sites, who examined their rewards and satisfactions (Cohen et al., 1994), also described the pressure of patients having shorter stays and inpatients being sicker than previously. The nature of cancer patients was described as unpredictable and likely to deteriorate rapidly. Emphasis upon the rewards of relationships and comforting activities are contrasted with the resulting difficulties of families venting feelings, and of patients dying and nurses not knowing what to do. Individual learning and development are regarded as rewards, and psychosocial care is singled out as an aspect about which to learn more.

Could an advanced practitioner contribute to improving working relationships, resources, working methods and time management, and assist staff to cope with patient deterioration and death? These are the activities of a team manager. The advanced practitioner's contribution is in the use of his or her skills to identify precisely what the local issues are (for example, the impact of stressors upon staff), and to evaluate the effectiveness of actions taken to minimize stressors and maximize effective coping. In this way, the advanced practitioner could support the local operational manager (that is, the ward sister).

The Calman report (Department of Health, 1994) proposed that care must be planned and led by nurses with postregistration education in oncology and that the nursing service must be structured to ensure patient access to specialist nurses. The need for specialized, educated nurses is also strongly endorsed by the NCA (National Cancer Alliance, 1996). This recognition of expertise is welcome, but is it sufficient? Educational requirements for specific clinical activities are not identified. This gap may generate needs for advanced practitioners, including influencing national policy setting and anticipating the practice implications of development in treatment and services.

The specialized nature of cancer nursing has developed rapidly in the UK since the 1980s. The outcome is a diversity of roles, resulting in inconsistency in nurse activities and education. For example, 'specialist' roles vary from the local nurse with specialized education to international experts. Consequently, it is difficult to define the role of UK nurses caring for people with cancer. Although many work in specialist cancer centres, others are based in medical or surgical units, in specialties such as dermatology, paediatrics, or the community. The level of specialist education within these settings varies enormously.

One example of inconsistent roles and expertise is that of specialist nurses who administer cytotoxic chemotherapy. Currently, many non-specialist clinical units are developing chemotherapy services to meet increasing demand, requiring general nurses to acquire specific skills to administer cytotoxic drugs to outpatients and inpatients. These nurses require focused education in order to be able to fulfil this specific activity. There is a rapidly developing need to educate these nurses and to ensure national consistency of aspects of practice where research identifies boundaries of professional judgement, such as techniques for administration of intravenous therapy. The use of national guidelines to develop standards and policies could be one way of promoting consistent safe practice.

Standards for various aspects of oncology nursing practice have been identified by expert groups, but there is no authority to ensure implementation or evaluation. Perhaps advanced practitioners could contribute to these issues by devising and monitoring a national strategy for identifying and achieving consistency for appropriately specified aspects of practice, for example, evidence based national guidelines for chemotherapy administration. This would include devising evidence based guidelines, leading local implementation, evaluating the impact on practice and patients, and ensuring that nurse education incorporates these initiatives.

Specialist roles

Specialist oncology nursing roles in the UK tend to be either focused on anatomical sites, for example, breast care nurses, or on specific skills, such as those of the chemotherapy nurse. There are also some community liaison and Macmillan roles, which cross hospital/community boundaries. The NCA report (National Cancer Alliance, 1996) on the one hand notes patients' appreciation of specialist nurses, but on the other identifies national inconsistencies regarding roles and patient access.

Specialized nurses are those who have completed a recognized educational programme for cancer nursing and who demonstrate understanding of the common needs, therapies and care in cancer patients. These nurses generally work in clinical teams and are employed across all nursing grades.

There is a need to review current roles and inconsistencies, since many specialist roles have evolved from disease types, medical treatments and institutional boundaries. The current situation begs several questions: is there a need for a different approach to specialized roles; is there a need for both specialist and advanced practitioners; could the advanced practitioners develop from different sources, and also initiate and contribute to national developments? The advanced practitioner could evaluate the contribution of locally based specialized and specialist roles, and I would contend that there is a need for specialized, specialist and advanced practitioners in major cancer centres. This idea is further developed below.

Potential developments in cancer care: nursing implications

Planning for cancer care should incorporate future demands, research and developments that have nursing implications. Service demands and organizational developments identified by Calman (Department of Health, 1994) include a continued increase in outpatients, nursing clinics and satellite clinics, an increasingly elderly population, an increased demand for complementary medicine, and critical pathways. These provide immense scope for practice development, to which advanced practitioners could contribute. It is up to nurses to take the initiative, recognize opportunities, and initiate proactive approaches to practice development. Advanced practitioners have the experience and skills to do this.

Within their educational role, advanced practitioners could help to shape and develop cancer nursing education. By contributing to the development of educational standards for cancer nursing, the quality of nursing care given to patients may be seen to improve. Other areas with potential for development by the advanced practitioner are within the field of technology; for example, the use of virtual reality tools for information giving.

Of equal importance to the educational role of advanced practitioners is their research role. Research in nursing is becoming increasingly important in order to develop and justify new approaches to caring. Advanced practitioners should be involved with research strategies for cancer nursing, perhaps developing cancer nursing fellowships. They should also be concerned with implementing national research and development priorities. There is tremendous potential for research development in cancer nursing. Several areas are listed in Table 9.1.

Table 9.1. Research potential

Treatment developments	Nursing research and interventions
Ambulatory chemotherapy	Rehabilitation and survivorship
Outpatient care	Cancer prevention
Biotherapy	Genetic counselling
Immunotherapy/hormone therapy	Quality of life assessment
High dose radiation therapy	Needs of adolescents
Gene therapy	Innovative symptom relief
Computer prescribing	Nutritional care

The Calman report

A key opportunity for nursing to grasp proactively is the Calman report (Department of Health, 1994). It proposes a structure for cancer services that promotes equal patient access to uniformly high-quality services. The approach claims to be patient focused, with emphasis on evaluation and on specialist staff. An examination of the report reveals many areas with potential for development by advanced practitioners. Key issues within the report are identified in Table 9.2, along with proposals for action. This is an example of how advanced practitioners can grasp the opportunities that could contribute towards addressing many of the issues for cancer nurses. To do this requires a range of managerial and clinical skills, and authority.

Managerial aspects of the advanced practitioner role

The combination of attributes required for advanced practice builds up a profile of combined clinical and managerial expertise. I believe that management is an essential component of the advanced practitioner role. Managerial contribution to the clinical area ensures the authority that this role requires. This necessarily includes budget manipulation in order to develop roles within financial constraints.

An advanced practitioner needs to develop practice in association with the development of the clinical organization and the health service, as the implications of the Calman report (Department of Health, 1994) demonstrate. Clinical developments may require organizational changes, and it is essential that clinical staff should direct organizational development to meet patients' needs. The advanced practitioner incorporates management of clinical services with a recognized contribution to a multidisciplinary management team. This team approach facilitates the advanced practitioner's remit to cross nursing boundaries, and promotes

Table 9.2. Potential opportunities within Calman (Department of Health, 1994)

Key issue	Proposed action
Individuals' perceptions of their needs may differ from those of the professional	Initiate research to explore and evaluate multidisciplinary practice
Good communication between professionals and patients is especially important	Lead other disciplines
The new structure is based upon a network of expertise in cancer care, from primary care to cancer centres	Continue to define professional quality
	Develop educational initiatives (e.g. educating purchasers and community staff)
Emphasis upon integration between professionals in the range of clinical areas that assist cancer patients	Plan national care evaluation strategy
	Clarify and evaluate nurses' roles and contribution
Education, research training and development are emphasized	Negotiate involvement in current requirements to define treatment options for patients and purchasers
	Peer support, sharing, planning
	Collaborate nationally between general, oncology, haematology, community, paediatric nurses
Multidisciplinary consultation and management is essential	Negotiate involvement in multidisciplinary management
Nursing care for inpatients and outpatients should be planned and led by:	Develop and evaluate nurses' consultation contribution, nursing clinics, etc.
1. Cancer units – with nurses who have benefited from postregistration education in oncology nursing	Integrate policies, practices and quality indicators within local clinical areas (community, cancer units, cancer centres)
2. Cancer centres – with nurses with a postregistration cancer qualification	
The nursing service must be structured to ensure access to specialist nurses with site specific expertise and specialist skills	
Moves that improve continuity of care are of particular importance	Develop nurses' roles and contribution creatively
Patients may return to local cancer units for follow-up	Monitor impact of aspects of the Calman report upon patient and family
In cancer centres, the essential element defining it is the expertise of the health care professionals concentrated within it	

sharing and delegation of managerial activities. Consequently, time for clinical activities is possible, and the advanced practitioner's contribution is largely concerned with clinical development, strategic management, and developing evidence for both operational and strategic management.

The discussion so far illustrates aspects of multidisciplinary practice that could be developed by an advanced practitioner. The examples given demonstrate that, to change practice, the role requires clinical, research, educational and managerial skills, and authority. These are combined to evaluate practice and facilitate local and national practice development.

The advanced practitioner's role is varied, but should evolve from local needs, which in one unit may involve teaching and staff supervision, and in another may involve devising and implementing policies for safe practice and management of cancer services. It seems that the advanced practitioner needs to be a professional chameleon, a jack of all trades able to demonstrate expertise in practice, education, management and research. My belief is that the advanced practitioner demonstrates expertise in all spheres and develops particular types of expertise within specific activities. Activities change over time, according to local patient and unit needs and demands. The key to the advanced practitioner role is the ability to combine different types of expertise when needed.

Table 9.3. Analysis of the literature

Topic	Evidence or opinion
Confusion regarding the focus of the advanced practitioner role	*Evidence:* McMillan et al., 1995 *Opinion:* Calkin, 1984; Patterson and Haddad, 1992; Sutton and Smith, 1995
Definitions of expertise, advanced practice, advanced practitioner, specialist practitioner	*Evidence:* Butterworth, 1994; Benner, 1984 *Opinion:* Calkin, 1984; Kapelli, 1993; McGee, 1992; Patterson and Haddad, 1992; Watson, 1995
Emphasis upon the importance of using caring and the uniqueness of nursing	*Evidence:* Benner, 1984; Lewis and Brykcynski, 1994 *Opinion:* Kapelli, 1993; Sutton and Smith, 1995; Watson, 1995
Emphasis upon the need for continual practice and role clarity	*Opinion:* Hamric, 1995; Kapelli, 1993; Sutton and Smith, 1995
Ability to meet extremes of patient need and value uncertainty	*Opinion:* Calkin, 1984; Sutton and Smith, 1995
Importance of vision and extending nursing boundaries	*Evidence:* Butterworth, 1994 *Opinion:* Calkin, 1984; Kapelli, 1993; McGee, 1992; Patterson and Haddad, 1992; Sutton and Smith, 1995; Watson, 1995; Whitely, 1992
Importance of conceptual thinking, ability to articulate own practice and rationale	*Opinion:* Kapelli, 1993; McGee, 1992; Patterson and Haddad, 1992; Sutton and Smith, 1995; Watson, 1995
Importance of a constructive relationship between nursing theory, research, knowledge and practice	*Opinion:* Kapelli, 1993; McGee, 1992; Patterson and Haddad, 1992; Sutton and Smith, 1995; Watson, 1995
Contribution of personal characteristics	*Evidence:* Butterworth, 1994; Davies and Oberle, 1990 *Opinion:* Sutton and Smith, 1995
Level of education and experience needed to achieve advanced practice	*Evidence:* Butterworth, 1994 *Opinion:* Calkin, 1984; Kapelli, 1993; McGee, 1992; Patterson and Haddad, 1992; Watson, 1995
Leadership	*Evidence:* Butterworth, 1994 *Opinion:* Calkin, 1984

The literature and advanced practice

There are numerous definitions of advanced practice and advanced practitioner in the literature, many of which demonstrate some degree of overlap with specialist practice and expertise. In order to generate a hypothesis regarding the advanced practitioner role within the context of cancer nursing, I felt it was first necessary to undertake a personal analysis of the available literature. Several key areas emerged from my review: the concept of advanced practice; the role differentiation, purpose, activities, skills and knowledge of advanced practitioners, clinical nurse specialists and nurse practitioners; individual characteristics of advanced practitioners; education for advanced practice; and the impact and outcomes of advanced practice. Table 9.3 is a summary of this analysis.

From Table 9.3, it is apparent that there is less evidence than opinion in the current literature. Much of the opinion is offered by people with experience of the different roles, and most refer to the literature, frequently to Benner (1984), whose work regarding skill acquisition and the caring aspects of nursing appears to have influenced many authors.

In order to make sense of current thinking, I have also reviewed the recent United Kingdom Central Council for Nursing, Midwifery and Health Visiting (UKCC, 1995a,b) definitions of specialist and advanced practice and practitioners. It is arguable that because they are UK in origin they may be more likely to influence our practice. According to the UKCC (1995a), specialist practice appears to be focused within a specific clinical arena and the practitioner is part of the clinical care team and has managerial responsibilities. Advanced practice is described as 'not another layer to be added to specialist practice', having an apparently more global focus for practice development. Although different, these definitions appear to share some common attributes, including a leadership and development role, and clinical, managerial, educational and research roles. However, both lack specificity.

Having undertaken a review and analysis of the literature, modifying and reforming my own perspective along the way, I was able to develop a personal hypothesis of advanced practice. This hypothesis is now presented and discussed, and proposals are made regarding the skills and working methods needed to establish the advanced practitioner role within a multidisciplinary team in the clinical setting of cancer nursing. In my view, there are clear distinctions between specialist and advanced practitioners.

Personal hypothesis

The advanced practitioner aims to promote the advancement of nursing by using insight and skills based upon experience and knowledge to frame a view or question in a critical and innovative way, thus exploring the nature and scope of nursing. This process of advancing practice is inductive and deductive, requiring conceptual and evaluative skill, and authority to develop and lead innovations. The advanced practitioner enables others to develop their practice as individuals and as a team.

The advanced practitioner evolves within a dynamic process that explores the boundaries of nursing concepts and practice. The process may be started by a response to unmet needs, service deficits or creative problem solving. Consequently, this process requires critical thinking and uses practice to inform theory and vice versa. The process requires clear purpose, but, if a reflective process is adopted, the outcomes may differ from those anticipated (Boud et al., 1987) if inductive ideas are allowed to develop. For example, an evaluation of a specific service problem may raise many associated issues. A recognition of the importance of exploration of these issues may lead to ideas for change that are very different from the original anticipated outcomes. This exploration, leading to a mixture of expected and unexpected outcomes, is the process of evolution. Each step generates the next.

Evaluation and creativity

Creativity may require input from many sources, benefiting from the critical mass of experts within a cancer centre. Within this context, good leadership is essential. Vision and creativity are essential and require the advanced practitioner to challenge cherished beliefs with courage and commitment. Breadth and depth of experience and knowledge are essential in achieving such goals. The analytical skills of observing, questioning and creatively exploring clinical practice critically are key to its success, and may result in generating questions and ideas, following tangents that may lead into the unknown, and the taking of risks. Synthesis, with the application of theory in practice (often developed through reflection) completes the hierarchical thought processes of the advanced practitioner. Thus, the key to a successful advanced practitioner role is evaluation and the use of analytical skills to identify service deficits and unmet needs, synthesizing these creatively to determine the goals of practice development (including the advanced practitioner's own contribution). In this way, analysis and synthesis contribute to the evaluation of practice.

The evaluation of practice, however, involves more than analysis and synthesis. It is also about the identification of useful, critical questions generated from practice, recognition of the importance of evidence, identifying theoretical connections that may generate new perspectives or practices, and acting on opportunities for practice development.

Creativity within the advanced practitioner role combines high levels of analysis with clinical knowledge, experience and skills, particularly those that change actual practice. The unique feature of the advanced practitioner is the synthesis of all of these with vision. Perhaps vision comes from the exploration of the longer term implications of these ideas, combined with managerial insight and experience. Although the attributes of creativity and vision are difficult to define, I am in no doubt that they exist and are fundamental for the advanced practitioner's evaluative contribution to practice development and service delivery.

A key contribution of the advanced practitioner, then, is to develop evaluation methods and to synthesize findings creatively. A less skilled evaluator is more likely to follow rigidly, say, a planned audit, and fail to make connections between issues. The advanced practitioner may work alongside clinical audit colleagues as well as clinicians, contributing to audit design and linking clinical audit, medical audit and research, in a clinically useful way. Evaluation activities will include the development of methods for exploring and measuring specific clinical phenomena. Findings need to be related to the ever-changing clinical context. This could be done by using evaluation methods within an action research process, assisting the advanced practitioner to make ongoing connections between findings and practice, and generating new and clinically relevant ideas.

In addition, an evaluation of the contribution of the advanced practitioner to practice development is important, especially if the role is flexible; the focus may change according to local requirements. This flexibility may be difficult for others, such as purchasers, managers, and some colleagues, to understand. Ongoing evaluation by the advanced practitioner helps to ensure clarity of purpose of the role and demonstration of its effectiveness.

Leadership

The advanced practitioner role is a leadership role. As it evolves, it leads local and national practice, which becomes dynamic, responsive, and evidence based. An advanced practitioner is therefore a visionary leader, who generates, and has the managerial skills to create, an evaluative culture that advances local and national practice and practitioners. The advanced practitioner role is also shaped by managerial, educational and research requirements.

Thus, in order to achieve their goals, advanced practitioners need authority. This may be based upon credibility, level of decision making or sphere of influence (Lathlean, 1995). Currently, NHS authority generally requires a managerial position, and devolved management results in high workloads for clinical staff. My hypothesis requires that the advanced practitioner is able to manage a clinical area, lead a clinical team, and change clinical practice.

The more activities that are required, the less feasible clinical practice becomes, as lecturer–practitioners demonstrated in Lathlean's (1995) study. How can an effective, flexible role with multiple responsibilities be possible with sufficient space for developing clinical practice beyond current boundaries and approaches? My suggestions are methods of working that include multidisciplinary team management, project management and supervision.

Multidisciplinary team management includes delegating day-to-day management to specified team members. The advanced practitioner would maintain strategic managerial activities within a multidisciplinary management team, including doctors and the other relevant disciplines. This team should be seen in the context of the other senior nurses, who should also contribute to practice development, operational management and strategic management. The focus of different senior nurses' roles (for example ward sisters, clinical nurse specialists and advanced practitioners) are different, but they can all contribute, in my experience, to practice and management, using a senior nursing team approach alongside a multidisciplinary management team. The more people who are involved in managerial activities, the easier it is to develop a facilitative style, involving staff and sharing what needs to be done.

Another solution is to plan the advanced practitioner's activities in project management style. Not all activities need to be carried out simultaneously! This approach is supported by my hypothesis that the advanced practitioner will make different contributions at different times due to changing unit needs according to (in my experience) phases of unit development and meeting requirements set by others (for example, achieving national directives).

Education and research

Academic supervision is essential. The advanced practitioner role needs to be developed within a clearly specified contract with a university academic nursing department. The advanced practitioner will benefit from supervision and assistance, which are essential for developing creative approaches to evaluation, and the university will benefit from the advanced practitioner's contribution to departmental research and teaching. The time spent on research and teaching can be planned in phases that are based upon the advanced practitioner's projects. It is important to contract teaching activities and time with an appropriate learner group. Teaching should only be for those who can appreciate the advanced level; the majority of learners' needs can be met by the other senior nurses.

As a result of these three working methods, the advanced practitioner could maintain leadership, strategic management, and responsibility for research. Supervision would enable the development of creative approaches to practice evaluation (research and audit), thus demonstrating the advanced practitioner's impact, and the team's impact, upon patient care. Careful time management using project planning techniques allows for a variety of activities over time, including developing specific aspects of clinical practice.

In my view, there are therefore five key activities of the advanced practitioner role, which should evolve into an integrated meaningful whole: evaluation; creative practice development; managerial activities; research activities; and educational activities.

A supportive setting and an advanced practice culture are crucial for both the advanced practitioner and other team members, and to facilitate team contributions to practice development. In my experience, advancing practice is exciting and contributes towards developing a self-perpetuating culture of questioning practice and generating innovative ideas. Trusting team members with delegated activities within a defined supervision system is a key feature of a supportive setting that advances practice. A facilitative leadership style that enables staff and practice to develop each other is also essential.

My hypothesis extends to supporting the details of the environment for optimum practice, and the expert's requirements identified by Butterworth (1994) as being similar to those that support advanced practitioners. The World Health Organization Delphi study of optimum practice in nursing, midwifery and health visiting (Butterworth, 1994) identified the key characteristics of expert practitioners as innovators, demonstrating leadership and expertise, having key personal qualities including positive communication skills, and being able to work in a multidisciplinary team. It also identified the features within the clinical environment for optimum practice as: a supportive environment; management that respects and supports optimum practice; active involvement in education; active involvement in patient education; the addressing of standards and quality issues; and political awareness. The need to be aware of, and involved in, research activity was also highlighted. The similarity between my hypothesis and Butterworth's findings requires testing. Advanced practitioners could test the findings and contribute further data, thus using practice to inform research.

My hypothesis is summarized below:

- The advanced practice role leads and determines advanced practice, which has clear distinctions from specialist practice. Defining expertise offers a useful contribution to the clarification of levels of practice. However, expertise cannot be defined in isolation from the required supportive environment, and the impact of expertise upon patients requires further investigation.
- The advanced practitioner role is related to multidisciplinary practice that is focused on patients' needs.
- The advanced practitioner role should be flexible and responsive.
- The advanced practitioner should explore approaches to meeting the extremes of patient needs, within the framework of prioritizing patients' needs. Clarifying uncertainties is a key aspect of the advanced practitioner role.
- Having a vision of nursing and the extension of the boundaries of nursing practice are critical aspects of the advanced practitioner role.
- Conceptual thinking and the ability to articulate and rationalize one's own practice are critical aspects of the advanced practitioner role. Both are critical to defining and evaluating the role.
- The advanced practitioner has the potential to offer a unique contribution by synthesizing theory, research, knowledge and practice experience.
- The advanced practitioner requires considerable clinical, managerial, educational and research experience and a minimal academic level of a masters degree.
- The advanced practitioner role requires authority.

A career structure for the advanced practitioner

I would like to propose a clinical career structure in which the advanced practitioner is the pinnacle. Such a structure would need to ensure the development of appropriate knowledge, skills, attitudes and experience. Within the proposed structure (Figure 9.1), the specialist practitioner is seen as a key developmental post, which ensures that the advanced practitioner has developed specialist clinical knowledge and practice. However, global vision, beyond the speciality, of advanced practitioners differentiates them from specialist practitioners. The key skills in which the advanced practitioner exceeds the specialist practitioner are those of global vision and creativity, and the ability to develop these within the wider multi-disciplinary team. To achieve the authority and skills needed to support change, managerial education and experience are necessary. The lack of authority is problematic for many specialist roles.

The proposed career structure reflects the need for a breadth of clinical, managerial and educational experience to achieve the advanced practitioner role. Without advanced practitioners, there is a danger of producing practitioners with a narrow clinical and educational experience and limited managerial experience, which may result in tunnel vision. A career structure for advancing nursing practice should encourage and reward cross-fertilization between clinical nursing, education, research and management. This should widen career pathways and facilitate movement between roles in all areas. It would also recognize the need for nurses to develop expertise to meet patients' needs that do not fit into current service divisions (for example patients in medical wards receiving chemotherapy, or diabetic cancer patients in cancer units). Teaching, supervising others, and being supervised, are implicit in roles at all levels.

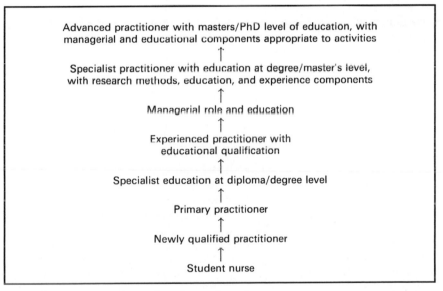

Figure 9.1. A career structure for advanced practice

One difficulty in proposing advanced practitioner roles is the lack of evaluation of the contribution to advanced practice made by the range of current nursing roles. Do advanced practitioner roles already exist in the UK? There are several roles that aim to develop practice, including nurse practitioners, clinical nurse specialists and lecturer–practitioners. I will discuss this latter role from my own experience as a lecturer–practitioner in oncology nursing.

In Oxford, lecturer–practitioners have developed practice within a role mostly encompassing equal time divisions between clinical practice and management (50%) and education (50%). The lecturer–practitioner was described by Fitzgerald (1989) as:

a senior nurse who has mastery of practice, education, management and research. Through demonstrating these collective skills s/he is able to lead a team of nurses delivering a professional service to patients, at the same time developing personal skills and knowledge in him/herself and the nurses working alongside.

The key to the role is to achieve an effective and integrated role, combining clinical practice, leadership and management, with educational activities such as: devising, teaching and developing modules for a range of courses; contributing to departmental development; and developing research awareness and implementing and undertaking research.

There are many similarities between lecturer–practitioners and the advanced practitioner in my proposal. Both are concerned with developing advanced practice and an advanced practice culture. Both require the nurse to apply research findings to practice. Both contribute to service and organizational management and development, and vary in response to local needs. The advanced practitioner differs from the lecturer–practitioner in that he or she has less formal educational activity, is employed clinically with *some* contracted educational time, and (arguably) has more time for clinical practice and research.

Practice developments achieved by lecturer–practitioners in Oxford include: developing patient centred nursing; organizational change; implementing research findings; undertaking research (usually for an MSc course); bridging the theory–practice gap; and educational developments for students and staff (Lathlean, 1995). In my opinion, the main limiting factor of the role is time pressure, which is a view supported by Lathlean's (1995) study of lecturer–practitioners. Her findings clearly demonstrate the difficulties of achieving all the activities of the role. Clinical practice was described by lecturer–practitioners in the study in terms of credibility and practice development, with some meeting service caseload demands. Time and opportunity to develop the nature of nursing or nursing research were very limited within this role, due to an emphasis on the educational commitments and increasing demands of clinical management. Nevertheless, there were many achievements, which are a tribute to the motivation of the lecturer–practitioners, but questions have to be raised about the hours worked to reach these achievements. The most inefficient use of time was supporting junior students, who could have achieved their educational objectives with the assistance of other clinically experienced educators within the clinical team.

Many lecturer–practitioners have the potential to become advanced practitioners, but lack sufficient time to do so. The lecturer–practitioner is required to focus equally on education and practice, whereas the advanced practitioner role, as I see it, should focus on the evaluation of practice. The key element to both roles is the authority to change practice, which Lathlean's study (1995) identified as a crucial element. The advanced practitioner should contribute to education via curriculum planning and teach only those students who are able to benefit from the advanced level, thus freeing more time for research and practice.

My comparison of the advanced practitioner and lecturer–practitioner roles suggests a balance of activities that can be achieved within time management strategies. Comparisons with the numerous specialist and advanced roles in existence should be fully explored before trying to establish new advanced practitioner roles. The disadvantages of proposed roles need to be identified and explored. I have listed some possible disadvantages below, which are based on my personal opinion. However, few, if any, are insurmountable. Table 9.4 compares the potential disadvantages with the arguments in support of the role.

Table 9.4. Potential disadvantages of the advanced practitioner role

Potential disadvantages of the advanced practitioner role	Arguments in support of the advanced practitioner role
Deskilling and frustration of specialist nurses	Advanced practitioner role should support other roles and offer further career progression
Taking over doctors' roles	Should complement changing doctors' roles and be negotiated according to local needs
Expanding awareness of needs for health services that cannot be met within financial constraints	Unmet needs cannot be ignored; this role offers skills to identify unmet needs and to devise and test cost effective strategies for meeting them
Conflict of loyalties between service and individual patients' needs	Same potential as for any other clinical role; ability to propose evidence based and creative suggestions
Too expensive	Likely to demonstrate value for money via benefits generated from evaluation activities

The implications of being without advanced practitioners

A final consideration is that of being without advanced practitioners. Advances in practice have occurred without the contribution of this proposed new role, and so it would be helpful to evaluate how advances have come about and who has undertaken them. Do they explore the potential of nursing or conform to particular definitions? Are these advances confined to improving *current* nursing practices? These questions, although not addressed here, will require further examination in future.

The literature implies that outdated practice may harm patients if demonstrable benefits are not made available to them. For example, the evidence regarding intravenous therapy suggests that practice that is not evidence based is likely to cause longer inpatient stays for immunocompromised cancer patients due to higher rates of infection (Parish, 1982; Goodinson, 1990), and greater patient distress caused by painful cannulas of inappropriate design, size, siting or time left in situ (Speechley, 1978; Doig and Slater, 1988).

My belief is that we need both researchers and advanced practitioners to ensure that research continues. Both groups can develop the evidence base for practice, collaborating with each other; the contribution of the advanced practitioner is the potential to develop research and context together. The advanced practitioner has the unique opportunity of following through from questioning practice to evaluating resulting developments in practice, thus linking research, audit and practice in a clinically meaningful way.

Nursing practice must continue to advance in a manner suited to the future health care context of the UK. That future appears to include devolved management, evidence based practice, closer multidisciplinary teamwork, and multiskilling. In my opinion, this new world will require the advanced practitioner role that I have described, otherwise patients are likely to suffer unnecessarily, difficulties in demonstrating local cost effectiveness are likely to continue, and opportunities for practice development may be missed. The advanced practitioner could make useful contributions in all of these spheres.

Conclusions and action plan

Advanced practice has begun, and roles resembling aspects of the advanced practitioner are developing. This tide of activity and enthusiasm is unlikely to stop; the issue should be to ensure that this activity is directed and evaluated. A national initiative is needed that will define, direct, facilitate and evaluate the evolution of advanced practitioners and lead advanced practice and nursing.

This chapter has explored some evidence and literature regarding examples of practice that require development to meet patients' needs and expectations, and also staff stresses, more effectively. These examples have supported my hypothesis that the advanced practitioner role should be based on evidence regarding patients' requirements and the effectiveness of meeting them. This contributes towards evidence to support the hypothesis that the evaluation of health services should generate the advanced practitioner's activities.

The evaluation of health services requires further exploration to justify or refute my hypothesis. This hypothesis is a belief that I hold, which is based on my experiences. Beliefs, however, have been shown to require testing too; false assumptions can be made despite the best intentions, as Larsen's (1995) study suggests. It is my belief that the development of approaches for evaluating patient care is needed; this is not achieved sufficiently by other roles. Advanced practitioners would identify the focus of their activity within their clinical area and evaluate their impact upon patient care.

An example of government policy, the Calman report (Department of Health, 1994), demonstrates further potential activities for advanced practitioners in cancer care locally, and within a proactive, national initiative. The implications for nursing without advanced practitioners are considered, suggesting a lack of strategic development within cancer care nursing as a specialty and a lack of sufficient developments and evaluation of nursing interventions.

My hypothesis offers a personal perspective, which incorporates most of the issues found within the confusion in the literature. This proposal is devised within the focus of cancer care in the UK, and requires further development for generalist nurses. The advanced practitioner role is identified as the pinnacle of the proposed clinical career structure. The discussion throughout gives examples supporting the hypothesis that the advanced practitioner role should evolve locally and be evaluated within a national strategy.

In summary then, I propose the following hypothesis for further testing: Advanced practice is a dynamic process not a static state. The achievement of advanced practice requires a local advanced practitioner in a leadership role who facilitates the evolution of a supportive culture.

Advanced practice should evolve from the evaluation of local needs and practice, and should be led by an advanced practitioner who follows a creative cycle of evaluation. Consequently, advanced practice and practitioners pass through changing phases of activity, which contribute to health care knowledge and practice. The advanced practitioner is a visionary leader, who evaluates current practice, identifies deficits and unmet needs, and uses these creatively to determine the goals of practice development and the advanced practitioner's own contribution. The role evolves and leads local and national practice, which becomes dynamic, responsive, and evidence based.

Activities are purposeful and flexible and the role generates an evaluative culture, which advances local/national practice, practitioners and leadership. The advanced practitioner focuses on identifying a clear direction for local and national practice, enabling others via facilitation and policy setting, thus developing innovative multidisciplinary clinical practice beyond current nursing perceptions and boundaries. The advanced practitioner contributes to a greater understanding of nursing and patient care, develops and applies knowledge and practice, and tests beliefs and rhetoric.

Advanced practice therefore involves evaluation, vision, creativity, authority and facilitation. These should evolve into an integrated meaningful whole within the advanced practitioner role.

Proposals for action

My proposals for action are listed below:

- Raise funds specifically for the projects listed below;
- Complete a systematic literature review;
- Devise hypotheses for testing, leading to the development of monitoring and evaluation methods regarding the contributions of specialist and advanced practitioners;
- Devise a national register of all specialist and advanced practitioner roles, comparing job descriptions and establishing a national network;
- Compile national data in a national study to identify the processes and outcomes of current and future roles;
- Survey the needs of specialist and advanced practitioners;
- Undertake research to clarify the nature of a supportive environment and culture;
- Develop senior nurse roles into advanced practitioner roles, making use of their managerial authority and budgetary decision making;
- Develop a team of national facilitators to support advanced practitioners, and assist in developing and evaluating their roles and recording data within these processes;
- Establish a clinical career structure encompassing evidence from the

above proposed studies;
- Explore role options for flexible working hours to accommodate the needs of nurses with families and those requiring study leave for doctorates etc.

We are already on a voyage exploring the advanced practitioner's role and advanced practice. Let us set a course and start to follow it, but also follow the courses that emerge.

References

Benner, P. (1984). *From Novice to Expert: Excellence and Power in Clinical Nursing Practice.* Menlo Park, CA: Addison-Wesley.

Boud, D., Keogh, R. and Walker, D. (1987). *Reflection: Turning Experience into Learning,* 2nd ed. London: Kogan Page.

Bradshaw, J. (1972). A taxonomy of social need. In *Problems and Progress in Medical Care: Essays on Current Research,* 7th series (G. McAchlan ed.) Oxford: Oxford University Press.

Butterworth, T. (1994). *A Delphi Survey of Optimum Practice in Nursing, Midwifery and Health Visiting.* Manchester: School of Nursing Studies, The University of Manchester.

Byrne, M. and Thompson, F. (1972). *Key Concepts for the Study and Practice of Nursing.* St Louis, MO: Mosby.

Calkin, J. D. (1984). A model for advanced nursing practice. *J. Nurs. Admin.,* 14(1), 24–30.

Cohen, M. Z., Haberman, M. R., Steeves, R. and Deatrick, J. A. (1994). Rewards and difficulties of oncology nursing. *Oncol. Nurs. Forum,* 21(8), suppl), 9–19.

Davies, B. and Oberle, K. (1990). Dimensions of the supportive role of the nurse in palliative care. *Oncol. Nurs. Forum,* 17(1), 87–94.

Department of Health. (Calman Report, 1994). *Consultative Document: A Policy Framework for Commissioning Cancer Services.* London: DoH.

Doig, J. C. and Slater, S. D. (1988). The misuse of intravenous cannulae. *Scott. Med. J.,* 33, 325.

Endall, M. J., Payne, S., Remington, R. and Royale, G. T. (1993). Detection of anxiety and depression by surgeons and significant others in women attending a breast clinic [poster presentation]. *British Psychosocial Oncology Group Conference,* December 1993, London.

Fitzgerald, M. (1989). *The Lecturer Practitioner: Action Researcher* [thesis]. Cardiff: University of Wales.

Gammon, J. (1991). Coping with cancer: the role of self-care. *Nurs. Pract.,* 4(3), 11–15.

Goodinson, S. M. (1990). Good practice ensures minimum risk factors: complications of peripheral venous cannulation and infusion therapy. *Professional Nurse,* 6(3), 175–177.

Hamric, A. B. (1995). Advanced practice: the future is now. Creating our future: challenges and opportunities for the clinical nurse specialist. *Oncol. Nurs. Forum,* 22, 547–553.

Hileman, J. W. and Lackey, N. R. (1990). Self-identified needs of patients with cancer at home and their home caregivers; a descriptive study. *Oncol. Nurs. Forum,* 17, 907–913.

Holmes, S. and Eburn, E. (1989). Patients' and nurses' perceptions of symptom distress in cancer. *J. Adv. Nurs.,* 14, 840–846.

Kapelli, S. (1993). Advanced clinical practice – how do we promote it? *J. Clin. Nurs.,* 2, 205–210.

Lathlean, J. (1995). *The Implementation and Development of Lecturer Practitioner Roles in Nursing,* [thesis]. Oxford: University of Oxford.

Larsen, P. J. (1995). Important nurse caring behaviours perceived by patients with cancer. *Oncol. Nurs. Forum,* 22, 481–487.

Lewis, P. H. and Brykczynski, K. A. (1994). Practical knowledge and competencies of the healing role of the nurse practitioner. *J. Am. Acad. Nurse Pract.,* 6, 207–213.

MacMillan, S. C., Heusinkveld, K. B. and Spray, J. (1995). Advanced practice in oncology nursing: a role delineation study. *Oncol. Nurs. Forum*, **22**, 41–50.

Maguire, P. (1985). Barriers to psychological care of the dying. *BMJ*, **291**, 1711–1713.

Maslow, A. H. (1970). *Motivation and Personality* (2nd edition). New York: Harper and Row.

McGee, P. (1992). What is an advanced practitioner? *B. J. Nurs.*, **1**, 5–6.

Moorey, S. and Greer, S. (1989). *Psychological Therapy for Patients with Cancer. A New Approach.* Oxford: Heinemann.

National Cancer Alliance. (1996). *Patients centred care. What patients say.* Oxford: NCA.

Parish, P. (1982). Benefits to risks of intravenous therapy: a review of current practices and procedures. *Br. J. Intravenous Ther.*, **11**, 10–19.

Patterson, C. and Haddad, B. (1992). The advanced nurse practitioner: common attributes. *Can. J. Nurs. Admin.*, **5**(4), 18–22.

Silverfarb, P. and Greer, S. (1982). Psychological concomitants of cancer: clinical aspects. *Am. J. Psychother.*, **36**, 470–478.

Speechley, V. (1978). Nursing patients having chemotherapy. In *Oncology for Nurses and Health Care Professionals.* (R. Tiffany, ed.) London: Harper and Row.

Sutton, F. and Smith, C. (1995). Advanced nursing practice: new ideas and new perspectives. *J. Adv. Nurs.*, **21**, 1037–1043.

Tait, A. (1993). Psychosocial care of cancer patients: the nurses' role [poster presentation]. *British Psychosocial Oncology Group Conference*, December 1993, London.

United Kingdom Central Council for Nursing, Midwifery and Health Visiting. (1995a). *Implementation of the UKCC's Standards for Post-Registration Education and Practice (PREP). Fact sheet 6: Specialist Practice.* London: UKCC.

United Kingdom Central Council for Nursing, Midwifery and Health Visiting. (1995b). *Implementation of the UKCC's Standards for Post-Registration Education and Practice (PREP). Fact sheet 7: Advanced Practice.* London: UKCC.

Watson, J. (1995). Advanced nursing practice... and what might be. *Nursing and Health Care: Perspectives on Community.* **16**(2), 78–83.

Welch, D., Follo, J. and Nelson, E. (1982). The development of a specialised nursing assessment tool for cancer patients. *Oncol. Nurs. Forum*, **9**(1), 37–44.

Whitely, M. J. (1992) Characteristics of the expert oncology nurse. *Oncol. Nurs. Forum.* **19**, 1242–1246.

Wilkinson, S. (1995). The changing pressure for cancer nurses 1986–1993. *Eur. J. Cancer Care*, **4**, 69–74.

Wingate, A. and Lackey, N. R. (1989). A description of the needs of noninstitutionalised cancer patients and their primary caregivers. *Cancer Nurs.*, **12**, 216–225.

10

A community hospital perspective on advanced nursing practice

Pat Elliott

Introduction

This chapter attempts to identify how advanced nursing practice was perceived and developed in a community hospital setting. The roles evolved when, in 1993, two advanced nursing practitioners (ANPs) were appointed with the aim of enhancing patient care and developing nursing practice within a large community hospital. The concept at this time was very new and arose from the proposals within the Post-Registration Education and Practice Project (United Kingdom Central Council for Nursing, Midwifery and Health Visiting (UKCC), 1996a). The postholders were given freedom to develop their roles. They evolved in slightly different ways, with one pursuing a research pathway and the other a more clinical focus. Both posts were joint appointments comprising one day a week at a university and four days in practice. It was believed that this would help to bridge the so called 'theory–practice gap' (Castledine, 1980) and advance nursing practice.

The hospital is situated on the banks of a picturesque riverside town. The setting on a summer's day is reminiscent of a sleepy backwater, but not so the hospital; yet, 5 years previously, it was a very different picture, when, along with many other community hospitals, it was fighting for its very survival. For several years there was little evidence of change to meet community need; changes that had been made were of a superficial nature, such as computer terminals on each ward, yet essential facilities that contribute to patient privacy and dignity, such as toilet and washing areas, had been ignored. The management style had been autocratic in nature, with punitive action taken for minor issues. Staff therefore felt inhibited about using their own initiative. The ward sisters tended to follow this autocratic model of managing the wards, and most direct patient care was being delivered by untrained workers. The predominant patient group in the hospital comprised older people, and staff recruitment to this 'Cinderella of nursing' was poor. This negative view of the work did little to enhance the self-esteem of staff. Motivation and morale were also poor. In 1992, a new hospital manager, who had a nursing background, began to change the ethos of the hospital. It was in the midst of this changing environment that she enlisted help in the form of two ANPs to assist in moving nursing forward.

The community hospital is now a thriving, dynamic, progressive establishment, employing 500 staff to service the health care needs of the local community. The emphasis has changed from the general care of older people to specialist areas of rehabilitation, and the hospital now consists of a ward dealing with stroke rehabilitation, one specializing in pulmonary rehabilitation, one in orthopaedic rehabilitation for older people, and one ward that specializes in rehabilitation of people with Parkinson's disease. There is also a day hospital, which initially provided little more than social care but now offers rehabilitation packages for stroke patients and for multiple sclerosis sufferers, in addition to maintenance programmes. The hospital offers a wide range of outpatient facilities, along with a 5-day surgical ward, clinical investigations day unit, and a general practitioner ward, which deals with a wide range of conditions, and to which is attached a palliative care unit. This chapter outlines the perspective of one of the postholders on advanced nursing practice, and also details how the needs of patients led the role development.

Defining the role

At the time of the appointment, there was very little empirical evidence or literature to support the development of the new ANP post. The main source of guidance on the nature of the role came from section 7.6 of PREP (UKCC, 1996a), which stated: 'Advanced Nursing Practice reflects a range of skills which incorporate direct care, education, research and management in health policy making and development of strategies'.

In the UK, it seems there were, and still remain, differences between the terms 'practice nurse', 'nurse practitioner', and 'advanced practitioner'; it is not within the remit of this chapter to clarify all of these roles, but to focus on advanced nursing practice. Many nurses strongly believed that the concept of advanced nursing practice is complex and far reaching. Fulbrook, in a seminar presentation (UKCC, 1996b), argued that the concept was indeed far too complex to define and would therefore be difficult to evaluate. However, as this post was newly created, there would be a call from the trust to evaluate its effectiveness, and before this could be done an attempt had to be made to analyse the concept and define the role.

As there was little empirical evidence or UK literature to support the development of the role, American literature was sought to provide some insight. This confirmed that the advanced practitioner role is indeed complex and has many perspectives. It appeared that 'advanced nursing practitioner' is an umbrella term, which covers a range of practice from the clinical nurse specialist (Hamric and Spross, 1993) to the advanced practice nurse and the physician's assistant (Patterson and Haddard, 1992) (Figure 10.1).

It was believed by the postholder that the role best suited to meet the needs of the community hospital setting most closely resembled the clinical nurse specialist role, which Patterson and Haddard (1992) described as being aimed 'to improve patient care by direct practice and/or role

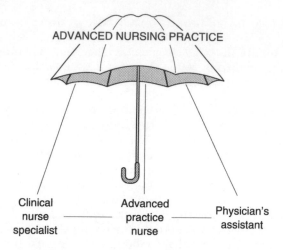

Figure 10.1. Advanced nursing practice continuum

modelling and education of others towards this goal'. It was felt that the most important aspect of the role was focused on direct patient care. Three main dimensions of the role emerged from the literature.

Table 10.1. Nursing practice levels

Practice level	Educational level	Cognitive level	Skill level	Experimental level
Preceptored practice	Diploma (2) Degree (3)	Knowledge comprehension	Novice professional awareness	Exposure participation
Professional practice	Diploma (2) Degree (3)	Application	Competent professional identity	Identification
Specialist practice	Degree (3) Masters (M)	Analysis synthesis	Proficient professional maturity	Internalization
Advanced practice	Masters (M) Doctorate (PhD)	Evaluation	Expert professional mastery	Dissemination

First, the role requires the successful integration of the subroles of clinical practice, education, nursing leadership and support, research, policy influence, and consultant, all of which are aimed at enhancing patient care (Menard, 1987; Hamric and Spross, 1993). Secondly, there is the level of the professional practice of the practitioner. There is an expectation that, with greater experience and knowledge, nurses will function at different levels. Table 10.1 attempts to identify functional criteria within the preceptored, professional practice, specialist practice and advanced nursing practice levels (after Bloom, 1956; Benner, 1984; Sovie et al., 1993; Elliott, 1996; Steinaker and Bell, 1979).

The third dimension is the scope and the influence of the individual's practice. The ANP should demonstrate evidence based 'best practice' within his or her own caseload and assist others in this goal (Bates, 1970) through role modelling, consultation and publishing, and by having political and professional power to influence in a wider arena (Wallace and Gough, 1995).

These three dimensions provided the foundation and framework to aid the postholder in the development of the new role within the community hospital. An exploratory study (Elliott, 1996) later revealed that, in effective advanced nursing practice, a further element was important in addition to the above three dimensions. The study highlighted that the personal qualities and attributes of the ANP were of great importance when attempting to motivate and empower others, and that the creation of a safe environment where there is professional trust and a positive relationship is essential to the free exchange of ideas leading to innovations in practice. As the role developed, it became obvious that flexibility and adaptability were also key elements of advanced nursing practice, in that there was a responsibility for the postholder to be responsive to patients, staff, and the constantly changing professional, political and community needs.

The postholder, having gained a masters degree in advanced nursing practice and having many years of experience in both practice and education, believed that she had attained the level of advanced practitioner (Figure 10.1) and set out to integrate the subroles of education, policy making and researcher into her everyday practice. The underpinning philosophy shared by both the hospital manager and the ANPs was that the key to quality patient care came from the empowerment of staff at all levels. The foundation of empowerment lies in the facilitation of knowledge and skill, through education training and the provision of professional support (Butterworth and Faugier, 1993). Working alongside staff on the ward allowed an analysis of the current state of nursing practice, and, through close involvement, an awareness of the difficulties and the achievements of staff was gained. The analysis of practice outlined pockets of good innovative practice, but also highlighted some major problems:

- High levels of patient dissatisfaction and carer dissatisfaction;
- Poor standard of skill performance;
- Inadequate scope of skills to meet changing patient needs;
- Lack of organization and vision for the future;
- Lack of professional understanding;
- Lack of up to date evidence for practice.

Working in this environment required tact and diplomacy, and also called on nursing intuition. The notion of intuition guiding practice as nurses develop from novice to expert (Benner, 1984), subtly incorporating knowledge into practice, is a feature of advanced practice. In addition, critical thinking skills are also crucial when dealing with problems. Having a solid background nursing knowledge also gives a firm foundation in order to guide practice. Having identified the problems, preliminary objectives were set. These first objectives were aimed at building a foundation for future objectives, as outlined below:

- Develop trust amongst staff;
- Demonstrate clinical credibility;
- Gain professional and personal acceptance in each clinical area;
- Demonstrate effectiveness as a resource person;
- Provide encouragement and support for staff;
- Demonstrate uncompromising professional standards;
- Demonstrate both fast-tracking and strategic programmes of professional education;
- Demonstrate academic credibility, assisting in bridging the theory–practice gap;
- Assist staff to access a rich network of useful resource contacts.

Within 6 months, these objectives were realized: helping staff to discuss their own team values; compiling ward philosophies and mission statements; creating awareness of roles and responsibilities; and redesigning job descriptions and clinical standards. The ANP drew on problem solving skills, change theory, clinical knowledge and intuition in order to develop strategies to help staff within the hospital to develop patient care. Many nurses believe that advanced practice is concerned with undertaking complex technical medically orientated skills, but, within this community hospital setting, the foundations of nursing had to be revisited before staff were ready to develop practice. Helping staff to progress, it was believed, required advanced skills and experience.

A system of primary nursing was developed as a means of facilitating more autonomous and accountable practice, and the nurses were supported by means of clinical supervision (Butterworth and Faugier, 1993) from the ANP. Within 12 months, the situation changed from the sister 'giving orders' to a system where each nurse was working in a more autonomous and accountable manner, being responsible for assessment, planning, implementing and evaluating care for patients from admission to discharge. The use of the nursing process improved, as demonstrated by the results of monthly auditing, and research based practice became evident, as demonstrated by the use of pain charting, wound assessment and mapping, pressure sore risk calculators (Waterlow, 1988), and nutritional assessment. There was a definite move from ritualistic care as reflective techniques (Schön, 1983; Benner, 1984) were employed. Clinical supervision was also structured around a reflective framework (Johns, 1993).

The atmosphere within the hospital appeared to improve, with staff being much more motivated and confident to make changes; there were no patient complaints, and many letters of thanks from patients were received. The ANP believed that the change came about by working alongside clinicians, overtly valuing their contributions, supporting their ideas, giving them freedom to pursue ideas and encouraging them to employ new nursing initiatives. This was aided by her presence on the ward as a role model; the nurses saw her interactions with patients, relatives and other clinicians, solving nursing problems in an holistic manner; she was seen and trusted as a credible practitioner. However, working on the wards highlighted educational issues that required action. Various policy issues also arose, which required change or development of guidelines in order to support practice on the wards. Addressing these issues required the integration of the ANP subroles of educator, policy maker, researcher and clinician in order to facilitate change.

Nevertheless, change was slow. For 12 months change was directed at basic yet essential issues and practices. Subtly, throughout this period, the culture within the hospital changed and there was a readiness to change and develop and an enthusiasm to meet patient needs through role expansion (UKCC, 1993). The time had come to advance practice as a result of changing needs within the local community. All changes were derived from analysis of the needs and problems faced by client groups within the community. New evidence based practice issues also impacted on the need for change. It was ensured that each initiative was undertaken for the appropriate reasons, in that it was believed to be in the 'best interests of the patients' as indicated in the *Code of Professional Practice* (UKCC, 1992).

Clinical developments

Having established a satisfactory foundation for clinical developments, nurses were encouraged to develop specialist areas of practice to meet patient needs in an expert manner, and act as link nurses to support other areas of the hospital. The ethos of empowerment within the hospital allowed the vision of two ward sisters to become reality. One ward changed its focus from general care of the elderly to a progressive 'stroke unit', and another ward developed a focus on pulmonary rehabilitation, being the first inpatient programme in the UK. These developments obviously did not happen overnight and ongoing educational programmes for all the staff on the wards were developed in order to support practice.

A training needs analysis was carried out to support the observations of the ANP, and a planned programme of training was organized and fast-track education made available as clinical issues arose on the wards. A series of updates for nursing auxiliaries was soon under way to encourage them and value their contribution to the ward team, because they had reported feelings of being undervalued. As there were high proportions of unqualified staff, they had a major impact on patient care and it was important that they were equipped with appropriate skills and knowledge and were valued as team members. Professional issue workshops were commenced for qualified staff to create greater awareness of professional accountability, autonomy and legal issues.

As the main focus of the hospital was moving towards expertise in rehabilitation, the ANP collaborated with the local college of higher education to develop two 'credit accumulation and transfer (CAT)-rated modules addressing the concept and practice of rehabilitation. Several nurses who were nearing retirement age joined others on a degree pathway in undertaking and completing successfully the rehabilitation modules. It was particularly exciting to the ANP to see the renewed enthusiasm for nursing that arose in these nurses, who would never have applied to pursue formal further education. Nurses reported that they had previously been made to feel 'past it', but their self-esteem grew, and motivation to put the concepts learned into action flourished. These staff added to the hospital the component of professional maturity (Sovie et al., 1983), combining it with their newly found knowledge in order to make an impact on patient care.

Intravenous drug administration

The need for expansion of the nurses' roles became apparent because the nature of cover in the community hospital often resulted in periods of time where there was medical staff cover only for emergencies. At this time, the nurses did not possess the appropriate skills, nor did they fully understand the implications of the *Scope of Professional Practice,* and were nervous at undertaking expanded roles. This resulted in patients who required intravenous drugs over a weekend period being transferred to the district general hospital, causing avoidable trauma to patients and their relatives, and also fuelling the lack of self-esteem of the nurses. This was obviously not in the best interest of the patients, when nurses could safely develop the skills required to administer intravenous drugs and policy could be adapted to support this need. In response to this problem, a course was developed and run to prepare nurses to administer intravenous drugs in line with the *Scope of Professional Practice* (UKCC, 1993). Skills workshops were held annually, providing a forum where nurses could check their skill, read any new literature on the subject, and reflect on their practice to add to their personal portfolio.

Having successfully introduced nurse administration of intravenous drugs, a further issue of role development arose. If nurses were to follow research based principles in order to reduce intravenous catheter tip sepsis, it is advised that cannulae should be re-sited every 48–72 hours (Elliott, 1990; Peters, 1984). However, if the change time coincided with the week end, when there was only emergency medical cover, the medical staff did not consider routine recannulation within their remit. It was believed that if a bank of nurses could develop and practise cannulation skills, it would be in the best interests of the patients to apply this aspect of research based care. Already having the skills and knowledge allowed the ANP to develop a workshop to prepare nurses for this role and support and supervise them in practice. Again, the subroles were integrated and practice guidelines drawn up to support the initiative.

Resuscitation

A further training issue evolved from the ANP witnessing a shambolic performance by staff during a cardiac arrest, which led to the immediate commencement of resuscitation workshops, policy development, and the commencement of team cardiac arrest simulations (mega-code). The mega-codes involved a simulation of the arrest situation using a manikin, with all members of the team carrying out their specific roles within the hospital resuscitation guidelines, which in turn were based on the European Resuscitation Council guidelines (Evans Medical, 1997). This proved a valuable exercise and included local general practitioner involvement, which also assisted with their own updating. Having refined the cardiac arrest procedure, an audit of all cardiac arrest situations was also implemented in order to monitor practice. Having integrated the subroles of education, policy and guidelines development, research, and clinical supervision, it was found that the most recent cardiac arrests on the wards have been handled extremely well and staff reported feelings of greater confidence. Table 10.2 highlights how the subroles were integrated to effect this change in practice (Elliott, 1996).

Table 10.2. Example of the integration of the advanced nursing practitioner subroles

Subrole	Example in practice
Practitioner	Through involvement in clinical practice, identified deficit in resuscitation procedure and associated practitioner anxiety
Policy influencer	Took forward inadequacies in resuscitation policy; met with staff to develop new policy; presented new policy and guidelines to Nursing Advisory Board for ratification
Educator	Set up resuscitation training sessions; arranged and monitored mega-code simulations
Disseminator of information	Presented new policy and guidelines to meetings and circulated to various staff groups
Researcher	Conducted literature search to gain up-to-date information; auditing of outcomes of performance following training
Clinical supervisor	Discussed with staff anxieties regarding resuscitation, and helped to reflect on 'how to do it better'
Professional leader	Taking forward a clinical problem, arriving at a solution, and motivating staff; effecting a change to a more confident and competent management of a cardiac arrest situation

It is especially important to practice and professional credibility with the general public that, within a community hospital setting where there are no resident medical staff to cover 'out of hours' problems, nurses possess effective up-to-date resuscitation skills.

Aromatherapy

While working with patients in the field of rehabilitation, a situation often arose where it seemed that, medically, there was little more that could be done for patients. It was at this point that the ANP began considering the use of aromatherapy. Having gained the necessary diploma, she developed practice guidelines and standards for conducting aromatherapy, which were ratified by the trust Board. Patients were referred from the wards and the day hospital, and, following thorough assessment, suitable oils were blended and applied through massage. Aromatherapy was seen to have a beneficial effect on postcentral stroke pain, poststroke epilepsy, and muscle spasm. It aided relaxation and encouraged expectoration in those with chronic pulmonary disease, it instilled feelings of wellbeing for patients with multiple sclerosis, and was seen to calm and relax patients who were dying. It was a very useful tool for a suitably qualified nurse to have in her 'tool kit' to complement traditional medicine. In a collaborative venture, one consultant anaesthetist, who ran the pain relief clinic, also began to refer patients for aromatherapy. Such was the demand that again the ANP integrated the subroles to develop and run a foundation course in aromatherapy. This, alongside the development of practice guidelines, assisted in meeting the increasing demands to provide comfort and relief for patients. The interest from nurses was so great that the foundation course continued, and had built into it a progression point leading to a diploma course in aromatherapy, which was also held at the hospital.

Health assessment

One issue that arose from clinical supervision sessions with nurses on the general practitioner ward was that nurses were suffering distress arising from professional disagreements with general practitioners regarding patient care. Community hospitals rely on the goodwill of the doctors and nurses for effective functioning. The doctors often complained that they were requested to visit patients for inappropriate reasons, although the nurses believed that they had valid reasons for the request. On analysing the problem, it appeared that the controversy could be minimized if nurses developed skills in the physical examination of patients and could communicate with medical staff in a more effective manner. Physical examination skills, consisting of inspection, palpation, percussion and auscultation (Jarvis, 1996) have not been traditionally taught in basic nurse education in the UK, yet, in the USA, nurses are prepared for practice with these skills.

In 1995, the West Midlands Region introduced this concept into ANP courses, and American nurses with expertise in physical examination came to the region to conduct workshops. Having attended one of these workshops and spent time in New York practising these skills, the ANP believed that if the hospital nurses were to take the professional lead and develop these skills, there would be many benefits to the hospital. A submission was prepared in order to gain validation of a health assessment course, which would give nurses CAT points at degree level on completion. The course was successful at validation, and the ANP applied her skills in running the course for nurses within the trust, and also supported the practice within the clinical setting. The course not only equipped nurses with physical examination skills, but also allowed reflection on how nursing roles could advance by utilizing these skills. For many, it provided a framework for more effective communication with medical staff. In the day hospital, the skills were utilized to provide full health assessment to be offered to maintenance patients who rarely saw a doctor, and produced an excellent opportunity for health education.

Within the specialist areas such as pulmonary rehabilitation, the skills proved invaluable and prescribing under protocol was made more effective. The skills were later to be utilized by health visitors in a new service development, which was intended to undertake the total care of the 0–5-year age group, and required a complete health assessment of these children to be made. Community nurses and minor injuries nurses also found that, by developing these skills, their practice was enhanced and they believed they had greater confidence because of their increased knowledge base.

The effectiveness of the advanced nursing practitioner role in the community hospital setting

It has been demonstrated through these initiatives developed by the ANP that nursing practice within this community hospital setting has been developed and advanced. Through the postholder's knowledge and experience, and by integrating the subroles of clinician, educator, researcher, policy influencer and staff support, patient care has been improved and staff within the hospital have been given the opportunity to develop themselves and services to meet the needs of the local community. Advanced nursing practice is not just about pursuing individual practice, but is aimed at helping others to develop professionally to give the best possible care to patients. This community hospital perspective of advanced nursing practice has been viewed by the trust as successful in terms of service development and increased patient and staff satisfaction. The model has now been replicated in two other areas of the trust in order to advance practice to meet patient needs. It would appear that, within this community hospital setting, Patterson and Haddard's (1993) perspective on advanced nursing practice achieved its aim to 'improve patient care by direct practice and/or role modelling and education of others towards this goal'.

References

Bates, B. (1970). Doctors and nurses: changing roles and relations. *N. Engl. J. Med.*, **283**, 129–134.

Benner, P. (1984). *From Novice to Expert*. Manlo Park, CA: Addison-Wesley.

Bloom, B. S. (1956). *A Taxonomy of Educational Objectives*. London: Longman

Butterworth, T. and Faugier, J. (1993). *Clinical Supervision and Mentorship in Nursing*. London: Chapman and Hall.

Castledine, G. (1980). Joint service/education appointments. *Nursing*, **2**, 161–168.

Elliott, P. A. (1996). *Celebrating Success and Cascading Confidence: an Exploratory Study Into the Effectiveness of the Advanced Nursing Practitioner Role Through Clinical Supervision* [dissertation]. Birmingham: University of Central England.

Elliott, T. S. J. (1990). *A Guide to Peripheral IV Cannulation for Medical Staff*. Sweden: Vigoo-Spectram.

Evans Medical (1997). *The RTO Resource file: A Guide to the 1997 Resuscitation Guidelines for use in the United Kingdom*. Evans/IMS with the co-operation of the Resuscitation Council of the United Kingdom.

Hamrick, A. and Spross, J. (1993). *The Clinical Nurse Specialist in Theory and Practice*. London: Saunders.

Jarvis, C. (1996). *Physical Examination and Health Assessment*, 2nd ed. London: Saunders.

Johns, C. (1993). Professional supervision. *J. Nurs. Manage.*, **1**, 9–18.

Menard, S. W. (1987). *The Clinical Nurse Specialist: Perspectives on Practice*. New York: Wiley and Sons.

Patterson, C. and Haddad, B. (1993). The advanced nurse practitioner: common attributes. *Can. J. Nurs.*, **16**, 982–986.

Peters, J. L. (1984). Peripheral venous cannulation: reducing the risk. *Br. J. Parenter. Ther.*, **5**, 56–58.

Schön, D. (1983). *The Reflective Practitioner*. London: Temple Smith.

Sovie, M., Bester, J., Young, P. and Dull, S. (1993). Professional development framework, *J. Nurs. Staff Dev.*, **6**, 296–301.

Steinaker, N. W. and Bell, M. R. (1979). *The Experiential Taxonomy*. In *Teaching and Assessing in Nursing Practice*. (N. Penworthy and P. Nicklin, eds.) p. 39. London: Scutari.

United Kingdom Central Council for Nursing, Midwifery and Health Visiting. (1992). *The Code of Professional Conduct*. London: UKCC.

United Kingdom Central Council for Nursing, Midwifery and Health Visiting. (1993). *The Scope of Professional Practice*. London: UKCC.

United Kingdom Central Council for Nursing, Midwifery and Health Visiting. (1994). *Post-Registration Education and Practice*. London: UKCC.

United Kingdom Central Council for Nursing, Midwifery and Health Visiting. (1996a). *PREP – The Nature of Advanced Practice: an Interim Report (Colloquium 1, annex 4)*. London: UKCC.

United Kingdom Central Council for Nursing, Midwifery and Health Visiting. (1996b) *PREP – The Nature of Advanced Practice: an Interim Report*. London: UKCC.

Wallace, M. and Gough, P. (1995). The UKCC criteria for specialist and advanced nursing practice. *Br. J. Nurs.*, **4**(16), 939–944.

Waterlow, J. (1988). Calculating the risk. *Nurs. Times*, **83**(39), 58–60.

11

Advanced nursing practice in a culture of mental health nursing

Dean David Holyoake

Introduction

In August this year, Jo Smith handed in his key to the General Office. Although he was happy to be retiring, it was a sad moment for him. He'd had that key for the last 20 years, and, like all psychiatric nurses, used it every day as a symbol of his authority. Being without a key was like being without the skills necessary in psychiatric nursing. Other nurses had been handing in their keys for the last few months, not because they were retiring, but because the hospital was closing. Services were moving into smaller community units. 'I'm getting out just at the right time', remarked Jo. 'All of this community care stuff will never work.' His sentiments echoed down the long corridors that were once filled with ambling patients begging for cigarettes. The security of the large psychiatric community was disbanding, bringing with it new ideas that were strange to Jo and to patients alike. 'When I first started nursing, there was none of this new fandangled jargon like humanism and holism; it was just common sense that made a good nurse.' The receptionist thanked him for the key. 'I don't see the point to all of this downsizing, clinical specialism stuff, it'll never work. In my day you started as a staff nurse and worked your way up to a charge nurse. You knew where you stood and so did everyone else.'

The change in psychiatric nursing during the 1990s has been dramatic and ruthless. It has brought to the surface a new era in which an emphasis on innovative and daring nursing practice has evolved. Although these conditions at first appear excellent for the advancement of psychiatric nursing practice, there is a reluctance to dispense with the traditional nursing cultures that dominated the care provision of mental health nursing for the last 30 years and ones in which Jo had felt safe.

The title 'advanced nurse practitioner' (ANP) has been part of nursing vocabulary for some time (United Kingdom Central Council for Nursing, Midwifery and Health Visiting (UKCC), 1990), but what is this role? What does an ANP do that other nurses do not? How has this role developed, and what difference will it make as nursing heads towards the millennium? This chapter intends to explore some of the issues connected with the above questions in relation to what it means for mental health nursing. Although there are many more questions to be asked and answered, it would be impossible and unfeasible to attempt an examination of every aspect of advanced nursing practice here. Therefore, it is the intention of this chapter to be a piece of reflective writing of the author's opinions, and thereby further the debate concerning the role. This chapter examines the existing and envisaged roles of the ANP and the history of the role development, and also the difficulties these practitioners are likely to face in their evolution from colleagues within the mental health culture.

The aims of this chapter follow the concepts of 'past', 'present' and 'future'. Within this framework, it will become apparent that the perceptions of mental health nurses belong to a long and traditional culture, which, like most, is suspicious and resistant to change and confused about the nature of the ANP role. The three aims of this chapter are:

1. To provide a historical picture of mental nursing, which emphasizes how mental nursing has braved both psychiatry's domination and general nursing's authority, providing the ideal springboard for the development of the ANP role;
2. To examine and analyse present day thought regarding the ANP role, with emphasis on the ambiguity that the role poses and its relationship to mental health nursing;
3. To provide a framework and draft proposal for future ANP development in mental health.

The past: advancing towards confusion (a specialist culture searching for autonomy)

It seems that the meaning of advanced practice in nursing is unclear and has led to much confusion for mental health nurses (Holyoake, 1995a). This confusion belongs to a long, but settled, tradition within mental health nursing, where, as a first-year RMN student nurse, the highest aspiration would be to gain promotion to a charge nurse post or to become a community psychiatric nurse (CPN). Even with the advent of clinical grading, little changed this respectable climb of personal development within clinical practice. This career pathway provided the framework that allowed most hardworking mental nurses like charge nurse Jo Smith the satisfaction and prospect of improving not only themselves, but the care they provided. According to Chung and Nolan (1994), mental health nurses have historically been discouraged from questioning the nature and development of psychiatric knowledge; hence the cultural development of the large mental hospitals that fostered a territorial feeling that enabled nurses to belong. It also provided them with the mobility to work in all wards without questioning if they had the specialist skills or expertise required for that particular area of care.

However, the days of specialism within mental health nursing were not far off, and, with the break up of these big hospitals, came a dependency on more focused specialisms, such as challenging behaviours, acute care and rehabilitation. Prior to this, boundaries of practice were more often than not set by the long-standing culture of the institution, and adhered to by both nurses and patients. The work of Erving Goffman (1970) provides a testimony to this. The idea that particular nurses should want roles other than those postulated by the culture was, and is, very alien. The visionary, risk taking and perceived leadership role of the ANP would have to conquer the ordered culture of the total institution. Those nurses who were seen by colleagues to be good leaders were described as nurses 'who'd roll up their sleeves and muck in with the rest of us', or someone 'who'd get the job done'. Leadership in mental health nursing was therefore a role (or task) that had never been evaluated and had been medically initiated. Although the picture given here does not praise the good caring practices and massive success mental health nurses have made in humanistic practice, it does begin to suggest the enormous inertia that mental health nurses faced, and continue to face, from the culture to which they belong and have sustained.

Medicine, autonomy and diagnosis

The relationship that Jo Smith had with the consultant psychiatrist was supportive and built upon a mutual respect over 10 years. Jo would often say that Dr Brown was a good man 'but I wouldn't want to cross him'. According to Bowman and Thompson (1995), the relationship between nurses and doctors is generally reported as being poor. The nature of this relationship is based on power and authority, and, although in psychiatry, there is less emphasis on formality, there is no doubt that it exists. This has always had consequences for mental health nurses, in that most interventions (for example, electroconvulsive therapy, rehabilitation programmes, week-end leaves and medication) are medically initiated and led. The need for autonomy, which will be discussed later, seems to be a prerequisite for the ANP role, and one which is at present dependent upon medicine. The more relaxed the relationships within psychiatry, the better the chance of the ANP role to gain autonomy and independence. This is unusual according to Heenan (1991), who noted that in the UK almost half the nurses responding to a survey were not happy with relations between themselves and doctors. Porter (1991) found that, in the absence of the consultant, the nurse's contribution to clinical decision making was considerable, and Brooking (1991) believes that less rigid role demarcation is needed. An earlier analysis of the nurse–doctor relationship by Freidson (1970) utilized the Weberian concept of social closure (the process through which social collectives seek to regulate market conditions in their favour), and argued that medicine had achieved pre-eminence through gaining the patronage of the ruling elite. Mental health nurses can only escape dependence by locating an area of health care work over which they have control. As most areas are nearly always related to medical spheres of influence and share the medical name (for example, psychosis, psychotherapy and dementia), this may never be possible. As noted by Draper (1990), these fields mirror the tradition in which nursing is defined by others rather than by nursing itself in the absence of a common language that might facilitate the description of nursing.

Where does this leave future practice? The answer may involve a role such as that of the ANP, which needs autonomy and a freedom to advance practice from a theoretical base that is nurse-led. Such a move would shift nursing away from what Freidson (1970) regards as a homogeneous paraprofessional group, subordinate to medicine, and engaged periodically in futile attempts to gain autonomy. Supporting this view, Salvage (1988) suggests that, alongside medicine, nursing is said to be a failed profession, and, according to Godin (1996), any minimal autonomy that nurses may achieve is always granted and limited by medicine. As noted by the author (Holyoake, 1996), medicine is still big brother to his little sister nursing, so, when Jo accepted the charge nurse post, he inherited a responsibility that was under the covert management of Dr Brown. Jo would never admit this, and, although he acknowledged that he referred to the ward as 'Dr Brown's ward', he was always quick to mention 'all of the therapy nurses did, including the resource centre'.

Jo was not an autonomous practitioner in the sense in which I refer to the ANP role. He instigated the resource centre because every other ward had one. He relaxed the 'lights out' routine, not because he'd considered the 'patient-led versus institution' debate, or pondered on the ethical under-pinnings of such practice, but because his friend and colleague on Ward 10 had already implemented the practice, after checking with management of course. In fact, the phrase 'patient-led' was considered to be educational jargon by Jo and by many mental health nurses who trained in large institutions. Jo resented the fact that this educational jargon was, and remains, the key to nurse autonomy. Autonomy in practice within mental health nursing culture belongs to a growing dependence upon nurse-led research and theory, of which Jo instigated none. He always took Dr Brown's word for it because 'it was common sense'. The common sense model of nursing is the defender of culture and old order, and not that of the ANP role.

A second facet of the ANP role that has encroached into big brother's backyard is that of nursing diagnosis; diagnosis has always been the prerogative of medicine and nothing to do with nursing. Mental health nurses make skilled decisions every day, based upon their recognition of symptoms, behaviours and interactions of their patients. Unfortunately, they insist on a professional medical diagnosis without question because 'that's the way it is'. Diagnosis is essential to the expert ANP and assists the total team. Melia (1987) suggests that as a result of patriarchal dominance of the medical profession, the expert model of nursing is unobtainable. In today's political climate, professional ambitions must give way to economic reality. It seems that this pessimistic belief predominant in nursing culture promotes the assumption that there is more potential for the philosophies of primary health care (respect for clients, the clients' right to self-determined needs-led care, empowerment, advocacy, holism, equity and autonomy) rather than specialist or advanced practice (risk assessment and manage-ment, liaison, diagnosis, consultation, programme centred administration, collaborative work, research and teaching management) to be the remit of all mental health nursing.

Unfortunately, medically dominated and managerial-led notions of primary care focus on different biomedical models of intervention from those employed by nurses (Ashton and Seymour, 1992). These are therefore medically based and leave no room for nursing diagnosis. As Jo has said in the past: 'A nurse's job is to care, a doctor's job is to diagnose and treat.' In a desperate attempt not to step on Dr Brown's toes, all nurses acknowledge that 'caring' is the concept that distinguishes nursing from all other professional groups, but nursing diagnosis is an indispensable need for modern nursing care.

Mental health nursing versus the general nurse influence

There is a historical difference between mental health nursing and general nursing. The history of general nursing might be described as the history of aristocratic women achieving a first respectability. In contrast, mental health nursing was altogether more masculine and working-class in character (Godin, 1996). Thus, the autonomy given to the early female pioneers of nursing, such as Nightingale, was deemed appropriate for the nurturing attributes of the Victorian feminine character. General nursing is profoundly feminine in make-up, whereas the predominance of males in mental health nursing enables it to present a different culture in which ANP roles may develop. This is an important difference, and, as argued by Godin (1996), the gender-blind tendency of neo-Weberian and Marxist class theory to focus largely upon the social relations of production and distribution of the formal economy in determining the social division of labour, leads to a deficient understanding of nursing. This emphasis on the feminine has led to nurses nearly always being judged as a homogeneous occupational group, best depicted as a busy uniformed general nurse. Gamarnikow's (1978) skilful use of Delphy's (1977) theory of patriarchy, based on social relations in the family and the marriage labour contract, can be used to argue that a male dominated psychiatric culture ultimately has a better chance of equality with medical culture than that of the female dominated general nursing setting. What this emphasizes is that there are many differences between mental health nursing and all other nursing specialties, and therefore the development of ANP roles needs to be situational or regional, and not rigid to the totality of the nursing profession. An awareness of vocation and occupation enterprise of these peripheral members of the nursing community cannot therefore be obtained through writers who implicitly regard nursing's professionalizing interests as being unitary (Witz, 1991; Porter, 1992). In this respect, 'the marginal elements, such as mental health nursing have at best an ambivalent relationship with general nursing' (Godin, 1996).

Summary

1. Psychiatric nursing is currently experiencing a period of rapid change and development, which is challenging the long held traditional culture of the old institutions.
2. This cultural change has involved an increased demand for the specialization of nursing spheres, and has confused traditional career roles.
3. Relationships with medical staff, although not always formal, have highlighted the dependency and need for increased autonomy for a future ANP role.
4. The ANP role could take advantage of such confusion and cultural change in order to develop a common nursing language to initiate nurse-led research and to build the nursing theory necessary for the establishment of ANP roles.
5. Psychiatric nursing is not the same as any other nursing specialty, and has within its domain a number of growing subspecialties, anchored

by the central aim of respect, dignity and non-judgmental acceptance of all patients.

Present: advancing in confusion

This section aims to examine and analyse present-day thought regarding the ANP role, with emphasis on the ambiguity that the role poses and its relationship to mental health nursing.

There seems to exist within the nursing profession a variety of expanded roles, all claiming to be forms of advanced practice. However, the common thread that links the various roles and focuses them on a common goal is not clear (Patterson and Haddad, 1992). The following uncertain words, written in a paper titled 'The advanced nurse practitioner: common attributes' only a few years ago, carry the sentiments of all contemporary definitions of what an ANP role is, should be, and is likely to be. According to McGee (1993), 'the issue that must give cause for concern is not the lack of novel ideas [from nurses about the possibilities for the ANP role] but the lack of clarity with regard to the meaning of these levels of practice in the clinical setting.' Clarification of the situation cannot be sought elsewhere either (Holyoake, 1995b, 1997a,b), and, as McGee (1993) noted, 'it is no use seeking answers in American literature', because there are none. The *role* of the ANP is new (McGee, 1993), but the *concept* of the ANP is not (UKCC, 1990). This mysterious position needs to be explored in an attempt to unravel some of the major themes associated with the role, some of which have already been commented upon, for example, autonomy, increased specialism and diagnosis. It is important to note that very few nursing scholars make reference to mental health nurses; Professor Castledine is one of the few, and it is with his continued support for the role that our analysis of the *present* begins

Recent evolution of the advanced nursing practitioner role

According to Castledine (1991a), there have been four main influences in the move towards advanced nursing practice, and several schools of thought in nursing that have played a part in the development of the role. These four can be summarized as:

- Specialties and specialist hospitals (see below for mental health specialties);
- The Manchester School;
- The Royal College of Nursing;
- Professional influences.

Specialization in mental health nursing includes: research; team co-ordination; discharge planning; psychotherapy; group work; psychoanalysis; behaviourism; cognitive therapy; drama therapy; supervision; bereavement; family therapy; crisis intervention; rehabilitation; substance misuse; the elderly mentally ill; children and adolescence; forensic; community.

Regarding the first influence, the nurse therapist's role evolved at the Bethlem Royal and Maudsley Hospitals in response to developments in adult behavioural psychotherapy. As Castledine (1991a) notes:

Community psychiatric nurses also began to develop specialist skills in more diverse ways than the Maudsley model, although general community nurses have tended to view such specialist developments in the nurse's role with great suspicion.

The second component in the development of advanced nursing practice, the Manchester School research study, showed 'that to become a nurse specialist, a nurse must have practised nursing, must continue to practise and must continue to evolve through practising nursing' (Castledine, 1991a). This demonstrates the importance of continued clinical input and patient contact within the role. Castledine (1991a) argues that 'in many circumstances specialists challenged traditional nursing models by stimulating and taking part in nursing research', thus supporting the argument that increased nurse-led research and theory building is essential for increasing autonomy. Later, Castledine (1993) noted that the nurse practitioner had a role with characteristics, which often included 'a personal caseload, delegated prescribing arrangements, higher decision making'. This indicates a type of autonomy that is, in the case of CPN practice, part of an expanded role; that is, taking on facets of medical roles without direct medical supervision. However, the importance of incorporating such clinical duties, including overdose assessments, needs a sound philosophical base.

Thirdly, almost 10 years ago the Royal College of Nursing (RCN, 1988) published the report of a working party whose remit was to investigate the development of nursing specialties and nurse specialists. As noted by Charlton and Macaulay (1993), the report recognizes and attempts to clarify the confusion that exists between the role of the nurse specialist and that of a nurse working in a specialty area, describing a nursing specialty as:

a component of the whole field of nursing, usually identified by being concerned with an age, sex or popular group (e.g. midwifery or paediatric nursing), a body system (e.g. renal nursing), a health or status situation (e.g. health visiting), a method of investigation (e.g. endoscopy or screening) or another aspect of nursing.

McMurray (1990), however, warns that the categorization of clients by developmental care groups or care settings is artificial, as boundaries between care groups become obscured by practice. Nurses working in a specialty have postbasic education relevant to that area of practice, with a deeper level of knowledge and skill than that obtained through general nurse education. However, the ANP role still remains ambiguous, and, according to Kelly (1996), the term 'specialist' lacks clarity. For many, it conjures up notions of out of the ordinary characteristics, uniqueness and exceptionality. Inherent in the social construction of discourses centred on the term 'specialist' are connotations of expertness; that is, a person who is skilful as a result of practice.

More recently, the PREP report (UKCC, 1994) suggested that specialist nurses will practise within a wide spectrum of specialty areas and will be recognized as providing leadership, support and supervision for nurses and support staff within these specialties. Prior to the PREP report, Castledine (1991b) acknowledged that, although the UKCC (1990) is clear in its intention to recognize advanced practice, the profession is uncertain about what the advanced practitioner really is. He continues to argue that the ANP role should have direct links to clinical practice, noting that 'advanced practice develops out of primary practice and is inextricably linked to it. Developments in many of the practice areas influence the others' (Castledine, 1991b).

In mental health practice, the ANP role remains open wide to interpretation and can be moulded to fit specific needs. Therefore, the primary aim of any budding ANP is to promote acceptance for the role. Such a task will take a long time, and the notion of expertise within an advanced practice role creates an ambiguity between popular acceptance and elitism. When Jo spoke of 'knowing what was what', he was referring to the cultural expectations that mental health nurses have of specific nursing roles. Every nurse would expect charge nurses to be experts in their field, regardless of whether or not they had an English National Board (ENB) certificate to prove it. They would expect a ward manager to have years of experience and know what to do in a crisis, and to have more ward based autonomy than a staff nurse. Even a first-year student nurse at the bottom of this safe hierarchy has an expected remit regarding role, but ask any mental health nurse what the ANP role is, and confusion will be part of the response, followed by a sigh of 'not another type of nurse'. This brings to mind the clarification of role described by Andrews (1989) as 'equal but different'.

When commenting on the PREP report, Castledine (1994) wrote:

Wednesday 23 February 1994 was an historic day for nursing and midwifery in the UK. At long last the council of the UKCC agreed on the final details for the standards for postregistration education ... Three areas of nursing practice which are qualitatively different in nature and non-hierarchical are now recognized: professional, specialist and advanced nursing practice.

Distinct roles for each of the areas (not levels) of nursing were given. The clarification of the advanced nursing role, however, still remains ambiguous, especially for the mental health nurse. Castledine (1994) continues by echoing the proposition put forward by the RCN (1988) that professional nursing practitioners will be seen as the generalists in nursing care provision.

Regarding the specialist area of nursing, the position of the UKCC did not appear over radical, but was, in fact, what one would expect from such a role. Castledine noted:

Specialists will be more restricted to one particular field of nursing care. They will be seen as key clinical managers. They will be someone who is clearly different from a professional practitioner working solely within a specialty. They will be at first degree level.

Much has been written about the clinical nurse specialist role (Hamric and Spross, 1989; Hunsberger et al., 1992; Miller, 1995; Kelly, 1996), but it is important to note that the ambiguity suggested by the line: 'They will be someone who is clearly different from a professional practitioner working solely within a speciality' is only temporarily dismissed by the more concrete consolidation of a first degree. This does not leave much hope for the ANP role, which Castledine does not like to admit when he notes:

> Advanced nursing practice has not been lost, but has been separated from specialist practice as was first proposed in the PREP (UKCC, 1993) consultation document. It is recognized that such key development work is necessary if nursing and midwifery are to progress. The emphasis is on pioneering practitioners, encouraged by management, education and research to innovate and push boundaries forward.

Mental health nurses know that they have to be educated to a minimum of first degree level in order to attain an ANP role. As ambiguous as it seems, the role is not hierarchical and has a direct relationship to clinical practice. The facets of supervision, assessment and diagnosis of particular patients on a referral basis, teaching sessions, and the management of research projects, are just some that would be recognizable to mental health nurses, who would question whether these are skills that are already included in charge nurse/sister roles. In what way would the ANP role push more boundaries? They would also question the difference between a role and a post, and, surely, the strive for expert practice should be sought in preference to any degree.

Boundary pushing, expert superposts and education

The advanced clinical role is bound up with the growing professionalism of nursing, particularly the achievement of autonomy in clinical decision making and developments in education, and the adoption of the 'novice to expert' model (Benner, 1982, 1984). McGee (1993), prior to the PREP report, echoed Castledine's early sentiments by noting that the three areas of practice are termed 'levels'. This suggests a progression through the ranks until a nurse reaches the pinnacle of ANP. For most mental health nurses, as for most nurses practising in other clinical areas, this would appear very alien. A major hurdle later recognized by the UKCC was that of acceptance of the proposed levels/areas of practice by the nursing profession.

McGee (1993) continues by stating that the role of the ANP is a new one; she does not note the evolutionary properties argued by Castledine 2 years earlier (1991a). Thus, for McGee, advanced practice is a new clinical role (UKCC, 1990), based on expert care-giving, but with additional, more formalized roles in teaching, research and clinical leadership. To become an ANP, the nurse must undergo a specified course to a minimum standard of first degree level, which will permit the nurse to practise as an ANP within a specific field. Thus, we have four core facets of the role, all of which are recognizable to mental health nurses in practice. These are teaching, researcher, clinical leadership/expert, and management.

McGee (1993) highlights three major pieces of work on advanced practice, and also points out the scarcity of such work. First, she notes Heffline (1992), who sees the role as 'resting on the nurse who is an expert practitioner. From this base he/she is able to act as a change agent in both theory and practice.' Secondly, Hunsberger et al. (1992):

> based their view of advanced practice on their own survey of neonatal intensive care unit staff in Canadian hospitals. They concluded that the main areas of the

role are as follows: practice that overlaps with the doctor's role in terms of decision making, communication, diagnostic and therapeutic skills.

Thirdly, is Sparacino (1992), who sees the advanced nurse primarily as 'a graduate in nursing who can conduct comprehensive health assessments; he/ she must also have a high level of autonomy and skill in both diagnosis and treatment'. The concepts that are worthy of note here are expert practitioner, change agent, diagnostic skills, autonomy and decision making. It is possible and only right to add to this growing list the attributes of the role proposed by Patterson and Haddad (1992), who acknowledged:

> If one accepts the notion that the goal and purpose of all advanced nurse practitioners is to develop and explore new avenues in a changing health care system, it then follows that flexibility is an essential characteristic of both practitioners and role.

The additional behaviours and attributes of the ANP role now seem to include risk taker, visionary, enquiring, flexible, articulate, change agent, graduate and leadership qualities. To these, it is important to add those of the RCN, whose document *Specialities in Nursing* (RCN, 1988) states that: 'Specialist practice involves a clinical and consultative role, teaching, management, research and the application of relevant nursing research. Only if a nurse is involved in all of these is he or she a specialist.' Arena and Page (1992) also imply expertise in the five subroles of the clinical specialist: educator, consultant, research, clinician and manager.

The major link between all these suggested facets of the ANP role is expert practice. How do we know an expert? Jo would argue that a first year student is not an expert, but that he himself was. It is taken for granted that he is able to fulfil the six criteria proposed by Dreyfus and Dreyfus (1989) as attributes of the clinical expert:

- Problem recognition
- Similarity recognition
- Commonsense understanding
- Skilled knowhow
- A sense of salience
- Deliberate rationality

Once again, the emphasis upon specific education plays an important role within the attainment of an ANP position or area of nursing. The developments in education, whether they are pre- or postregistration, begin primarily in this modern era with the acceptance of the Benner model (1984). McGee (1993) makes reference to Peplau (1965), whom she cites as the first to use the title 'clinical nurse specialist'. The influence of Peplau in psychiatric nursing cannot be underestimated. In a later article, Peplau (1978) wrote:

> The role of the psychiatric nurse also depends upon the length of post-basic nursing education, the scope and depth of knowledge included in it and the clinical modalities for which supervised clinical practice is provided.

What Peplau is quite specific about is the need for clinical supervision within psychiatric nursing. The importance of supervision is apparent to all psychiatric nurses, yet supervision per se is not listed in any of the role facets apart from the UKCC (1994), who link it to the specialist role. The call by educationalists for an upgrading of the profession for a future all-degree level of education seems to be defended by the premise that practice needs to be measurable. As Schön (1988) noted that:

> this distinct specialist contribution must, if it is to be credible, be firmly bounded, scientific and standardized, thereby allowing the distinct possibility of technical rationality to be made explicit or 'fine tuned' to match specific situations.

Although Patterson and Haddad (1992) offer us the visionary and risk taker role, they are unable to provide a useful measurable framework from which mental health nursing can 'technically rationalize' effectiveness. They state that advanced nursing practice:

> ... is about an improvement or moving forward and putting knowledge to actual use. Advanced nurse practitioners engage in activities which contribute to and improve nursing knowledge and practice in response to both the historical and current social demands of the environment. Advanced nurse practitioners define the boundaries of their practice within the philosophical beliefs intrinsic to their profession in order to meet the demands of nursing, patients and society.

Unfortunately, the lack of clarity remains because an individual nurse (whether psychiatric or general trained) who is attempting to fulfil an ANP role should possess, according to Patterson and Haddad (1992), 'certain characteristics and demonstrate behaviours' that might somehow enable them to be 'identified' and 'allow them to contribute to the growth of their profession'. Gatley (1992) suggests that the distinguishing feature of specialist status is an intangible intuitive element, which is not measurable. Calkin (1988) concurs with this view, recognizing that specialist status cannot be achieved without formal educational preparation and experience. The importance of 'expertness' (one of the four core facets) is subject to constraints inherent in the specific nature of the nursing profession and its culture. A comment made by many mental health nurses is 'you don't need a degree to be an expert', but in an emerging culture that is characterized by hierarchical labour markets, a degree represents expertness.

The attempt to iron out the 'skill-mix', and the drive by education to provide a complete graduate professional body, appears to be post-Fordist in presentation, in that the ANP role and the specialist role appear to belong to a defined hierarchy. At present, with the thrust in the UK to review skill-mix, those functions performed by medical and nursing practitioners are constantly under scrutiny. Therefore, the ANP and specialist roles are the new 'super-posts' which rest on top of what Thompson and McHugh (1990) call 'a core work force' with a 'cluster of peripheral employment arrangements characterized by functional numerical and financial flexibility'. Therefore, to answer the earlier question 'what's the difference between a post and a role?', the role is the doing, but the post seems to pay more.

In its defence, the PREP report (UKCC, 1994) recognized the limitations of current preregistration nurse education in meeting the needs of professional practice focused on the delivery of specialist care and case management. According to Kelly (1996):

It is intimated that these 'products' of professional practice require advanced levels of clinical decision making to ensure the delivery of quality care. There is a definite denial of any intention to create a hierarchy within the profession.

The issue at stake is whether the 'specialist nurse' is able to demonstrate advanced levels of knowledge and skills gained from experience (Benner et al., 1992). There are striking similarities between the proposed educational development of the three areas of practice (UKCC, 1994) and Benner's (1984) 'novice to expert model'. In Benner's model, the stages to reach the level of 'expert' are clearly presented, but little note is taken of the fact that stages of progression towards excellence are merely merging points on a continuum, and as such, they impede measurement (Gately, 1992).

When Jo was asked to attend a course relevant to his ward, he was reluctant, but he did. The course on specialized practice was deemed relevant by the school of nursing, but all the nurses who attended it from the hospital complained to each other that it would not work in practice. This nurse specialist concept was alien to the nurses; they preferred teaching sessions about specific tasks in practice. 'I'm an expert in most things that I do, I've been doing it for years', complained Jo to his colleague, who nodded enthusiastically. 'I've worked in acute settings for ten years and I don't need a certificate to prove my skills; ask anyone.' As the course progressed, it seemed to most of the nurses that this idea of specialism was about being an expert, a change agent and an educator. The course facilitator also talked about the dreaded 'R word': research. 'I've always tried to encourage students to do research and I've changed loads of stuff in the ward', remarked Jo to the group. The facilitator had to acknowledge that Jo fulfilled the expectations of his current job description and attempted to get Jo to think about maximizing the potential of his role. 'What more can I do?' questioned Jo. 'I'm an expert, I manage the ward, occasionally I do some teaching and research and now I'm doing this course. If I get a degree, will that make me an advanced practitioner? I understand the subrole stuff about nursing diagnosis, being a change agent, pushing boundaries and being visionary, but will it pay me any more? Will the trust make a post for me, or will I be a free agent, a consultant with an office, from which to flit from ward to ward like one of the old nursing officers?' The session ended with Jo gasping for breath.

His confusion was echoed on the faces of all the nurses in the group. 'If I get my specialist degree I'll be a clinical nurse specialist, but it seems that the boundary pushing, visionary change agent stuff has to be more personal, something that can't be directly measured, so how can it advance nursing practice?' Jo would ponder these questions for months.

Summary

1. At present, the facets of the ANP role are ambiguous to most mental health nurses (see Table 11.1).
2. The promotion of the ANP role would be the primary, and first, task of that role.
3. The implications of higher educational expectations alienate and discourage many mental health nurses from exploring and involving themselves, possibly due to a perception of elitism.
4. Expertness is intrinsically linked to advanced practice and autonomy.
5. A post suggests a definite role; flexibility towards clinical settings is essential for the ANP role.

Table 11.1. Core facets of the ANP role

Vitello-Ciccu, 1984	RCN, 1988	Castledine, 1991b	Patterson and Haddad, 1992
Clinician	Clinical role	Systematic	Flexibility of nurse
Educator	Consultative role	Reflective	Flexibility of role
Researcher	Teaching	Analytic	Risk taker
Consultant	Management	Innovative	Visionary
Administrator	Research	Dynamic	Enquiring
Change agent	Application of	Leadership	Articulate
Advocate	research		Leadership qualities
Sparacino, 1992	Arena and Page, 1992	Calkin, 1992	UKCC, 1993, 1994
Graduate	Educator	Expert	Pioneering practitioners
Assessment	Consultant	Diagnostic	Education
Autonomy	Research	Analyst	Research
Diagnosis	Clinician	Management	Innovator
Treatment	Manager	Knowledge	Push boundaries
		Masters education	

Future confusion (will mental health nursing dress up the old as new?)

It is now consistently assumed that where advanced levels of nursing skill are developed, they are associated with beneficial outcomes. This post-PREP period is a vacuum in mental health nursing. Service development has not been sufficiently established, so the case for the ANP role has not been tested or recognized within a changing culture. According to Lindstrom (1995):

> the aim is not to create a single culture, but to create a single culture which is caring. An important prerequisite for total care is a living caring culture which includes a common pattern of thinking.

A psychiatric culture needs to be different from the general nursing culture template, the latter being 'dependent upon [more] medical generosity' (Lindstrom, 1995). But the need for such generosity is not only medical orientated, as noted by Wilson-Barnett (1995), who contends that 'specialist nursing posts tend to be created by funding through charitable or research soft monies. Once they are well established, such posts become seen as essential.'

Returning to the focus of psychiatric nursing, current philosophy is to place the patient at the centre of all care interventions, regardless of conventional and expected roles. This vogue for humanism is dominant within the mental health nursing arena, regardless of whether or not the practitioner is the team leader, case manager, nurse specialist or ANP. The ambiguity and confusion about the ANP role is, and will continue to be, a contentious vacuity as '[mental health] nurses try to fill their professional vacuum by borrowing philosophies from other disciplines' (Barker, 1990). This is not new, as Barker paints a picture of 'the young, upwardly mobile mental health nurse' who 'talks of promoting mental health within the context of an ecological viable and holistic person-centred conceptual framework.' The use of jargon, eclecticism and quality assurance is in danger of dressing up the old and presenting it as 'the new psychiatric advanced practitioner' whose vernacular language provides the cherry on the top. This 'unideal' role is a real possibility unless mental health nurses examine the need for specific aims regarding the ANP role.

The expanded role

This raises an important issue regarding ANP development, and one that is the subject of current debate, namely, the nature of the extended and expanded roles. Both involve a process of change between two conceptual standpoints, and, for the purpose of this discussion, the definitions of both are taken from the now rather old work of Murphy (1970). Role extension is defined as a unilateral lengthening process, role expansion as a spreading out or a process of diffusion. Both change processes are evolutionary in nature, in that the body of knowledge and the field of practice are constantly emerging. Moreover, both change processes are directed towards the same goal of meeting more adequately the health care needs of our society. The unilateral extension of the nurse's role to incorporate delegated functions might appear to be one answer to the shortage of medical personnel, but for nursing it holds long-range implications, mostly negative, in that nurses will continue to be the handmaidens of medicine.

On the other hand, role expansion, taken literally, implies multi-directional change. Expansion, as a process of role change, is undertaken not only to fill perceived gaps in the health care system, but also to project new and pioneering components or systems of health care (Holyoake, 1997c). Therefore, in order to evaluate whether perceived expanded practice is justifiable within the psychiatric ANP role, questions related to activities of daily living and holism in practice and patient wellbeing are fundamental (Mechanic, 1988). These questions make the link to the professional practice area and contain expansion within the perceived roles of total nursing practice. To push boundaries, the ANP would question: What interventions can my role offer? What are the aims of my role in clinical practice?

Why should mental health nursing be associated with aims? It should be noted that I take it as natural in progressing care that all nurses, including those in mental health, attempt to formulate aims. Aiming is like trying, in that it suggests that there is some predicament entangled in the task, and a very real possibility of falling short or of not succeeding. The development of a psychiatric ANP role is such a task, especially when we consider the difficulty discussed earlier regarding the facets of the role. It is with those facets in mind that a proposed framework will now be discussed, hence tackling the third aim of this chapter, to provide a framework and draft proposal for *future* ANP development in mental health. Such a development has expertise at its core.

The expert practitioner

Jo had recently reflected on a common occurrence in practice regarding a disturbed patient. In the first incident, a patient was angry about not going home at the weekend, and was threatening to punch a window. He was angry and scared. The staff nurse on duty, while talking calmly to the patient, had begun to move closer until he could almost touch the patient, who was hovering by the window with clenched fists. In a split second, the staff nurse pounced, but was too slow to prevent the patient hitting and breaking the window. His injuries, although superficial, required emergency care. A year before this, Jo had been involved in a similar incident, but he knew that rushing in to keep the patient safe would agitate the situation. He remained some distance away and talked calmly until the patient burst into tears and accepted comfort from the big charge nurse. This was not the first time that Jo had encountered such dilemmas in practice, and he recognized the problem as an expert (Dreyfus and Dreyfus, 1989). Jo was an expert, and the nurses who worked with him acknowledged this. Although Jo wanted to push boundaries and develop the subroles of an ANP, he recognized the resistance that such a development would have to face. The fact that many of these facets belonged to all levels of nursing made it hard for himself and others to distinguish between roles.

Most writers assume that the ANP role comprises a number of facets (see Table 11.1). These facets do not clearly belong to primary areas of practice, but may overlap with specialist areas. These facets appear to be not measurable. Most psychiatric practitioners practise to a high level of skill, so what determines their inability to qualify for the ANP role? It seems that the determining factor is first degree level education. In practice, according to Sparacino (1992):

> to acknowledge that there are no gradations between the novice and the expert, some practice settings have instituted clinical ladders, a promotional system which uses both objective criteria and a peer review process to recognize and reward excellent and advanced nursing practice.

The importance of mental health nursing culture, role models, and learning the ropes, is a requisite of becoming an expert. This ritual is more often than not initiated and recognized by other expert colleagues. It is by their say-so that you 'join the exclusive club' and achieve expertise.

This is an issue discussed in the 'Heathrow debate' document (Department of Health, 1994), and the advent of ENB measurability in the form of courses has placed a higher culture upon this extremely suspicious popular culture. The suspicion of such perceived aristocratic intervention by educationalists is made real by the all too common remark 'she's brilliant at the exams, but can't nurse for toffee', thus highlighting the theory–practice gap. This leads us to the conclusion that psychiatric nursing is a highly diffuse and difficult activity in which many earnest nurses engage with great seriousness. It is not a concept that lends itself to picking out any specific activity (as has been hinted at in the list of specialties in mental health nursing already given), but to laying down criteria to which a family of activities must conform in both theory and practice. The central questions worthy of note are: How do we identify an expert nurse in the first place? and, Do all and only those who are identified as experts make use of intuitive judgement in the way that Benner (1984) describes? These questions direct the specific competencies for the psychiatric ANP role; hence the earlier emphasis on aims.

Paley (1996) notes the rift between science and phenomenology in current nursing. Patricia Benner's model of skill acquisition, harnessed to a Heideggerian philosophy (Heidegger, 1962), is one of several currently fashionable theories that highlight the rift between a scientific approach to nursing and its apparent alternative, usually associated with some version of phenomenology. As noted by Rolfe (1997), 'Benner's model suggests that expertise is something that mysteriously develops over time largely outside the control of the nurse.' One component of this mysterious development, which has a profound effect on the ANP role within psychiatry, is the attitudes and practice of colleagues. The implication of a graded and educationally imposed framework for the three areas of nursing practice has the validation of certain competencies at its core (see Table 11.1). This governing enforces an umbrella of imposed responsibility; the individual practitioner has no choice but to comply with the rules, be they appropriate or not. Such a structuralist/Marxist view of the current legislation may seem to be too harsh, but it is important to remember that nurses pride themselves on their commitment and self-improvement, regardless of the rewards offered by governing bodies.

The resistance to such authority can be noted in the reception that the ANP role has received in specific areas, including the type of study days that Jo attended. This resistance is, and will continue to be, prominent in mental health nursing. The individual nurse cannot claim to be a specialist or advanced practitioner without the necessary qualifications, and, although these benchmark courses are justified through their provision of safety, they deny opportunity to many nurses because the role and title are evolving into more than motivated individual excellence; they are also evolving into economically viable posts. The general route to these posts in the UK is currently through postbasic specialist courses run by the national boards. For many psychiatric nurses, there is an acknowledgement that nursing has progressed a long way since the days when a nurse's role was to assist the medical staff, but at the expense of becoming a slave to the postregistration certificate.

This is ironic, since Hamric and Spross (1989) state that clinical nurse specialists are the people to institute the remodelling of the nursing image, stating that they are competent, innovative and willing to shake up the institution with bold new ideas for improved patient care. For many psychiatric nurses, expertise is inextricably linked to credentialling of colleagues rather than through a process of academic accreditation in a specialist area. According to Castledine (1991b), 'It is difficult to give a detailed breakdown of what each of the essential functions of the advanced nurse practitioner role is', but what we do recognize is the importance of continued patient contact within the role, and therefore expert practice which is recognized by colleagues. These are the first requisites of the psychiatric advanced nurse practitioner:

1. *Perceived to be an expert practitioner within a specialty with a post-registration training at degree level;*
2. *Continued clinical practice within at least one specialist area.*

Liaison and consultation

As community care and trust economics progress, it seems that the selling of expertise will become second nature within the contemporary health trade. One aspect of the psychiatric ANP role will involve liaison with other specialties in an interagency consultation capacity. According to Tunmore (1997), liaison mental health nursing has the 'potential to shape the future delivery of nursing care and to identify new and evolving specialisms', such as links with accident and emergency units, health visitors and other non-mental health services. Such a development would require the ANP to conduct assessments and manage a programme centred approach outside of the traditional culture of the mental health setting. The concept of consultation is intrinsically linked to the diagnosis debate already highlighted.

The development of the role cannot avoid the issue because it is very relevant not only in theory, but particularly in practice. I would argue that most expert mental health nurses diagnose continually during every interaction with patients. The need for a nursing diagnostic framework belongs within the ANP role, and it is a need that UK nurses must consider in practice rather than treat as just a concept (Hogston, 1997). It may be that if we do not take nursing diagnosis seriously, a taxonomy like that of the North American Nursing Diagnosis Association will be imposed upon us to fill the void. The need for nursing diagnosis is as important as the need for nursing assessment, and the two are inseparable in theory and practice. By accepting this need, the ANP role accepts the challenge for nursing to take control of its own boundaries. Therefore, when Dr Brown informed Jo that a particular patient had learning disabilities, Jo tried to hint that he felt the patient appeared more depressed. Jo had no diagnostic framework from which to evaluate the responses he received on a day-to-day basis from the patient, but Dr Brown had a specific category into which the patient fitted. Jo could not complain or advocate for the patient. As noted by Hopton (1997) 'psychiatrists require nurses to keep their patients under surveillance in order to confirm their diagnosis and to administer and monitor the treatments they prescribe.' Castledine (1991b) also makes reference to the diagnostic component of the role, and such a facet would surely need to be considered with regard to the psychiatric ANP role.

The ability to diagnose has a direct relationship with being an expert. As Calkin (1984) notes, 'Nurses who excel in analysis and insight when diagnosing and treating human responses are generally known as experts.' Calkin continues by emphasizing my earlier point regarding the influence that the culture and colleagues have on the development of the role: 'Experts by experience generally earn their reputation by having greater or more rapid intervention skills than their colleagues.' Therefore, what makes a psychiatric ANP different from, say, a psychiatric nurse in 'professional practice', is that the ANP would provide a nursing diagnosis and also provide a rationale for choosing diagnostic and treatment processes in a consultancy capacity:

3. *Developing economically viable liaison networks within the wider care trade;*
4. *Leading consultation role;*

5. *Advancing pioneering nursing diagnostic procedures within a specialty.*

Educator

The importance of the educator facet within the ANP role has been highlighted by all nurse scholars (see Table 11.1). This is a justifiable claim, because such a facet is at the core, not only of advancing direct patient care, but also of pushing boundaries and pioneering new approaches to care. The educator facet enables the ANP to role model, mentor, share and assist. The facet incorporates not only clinical based teaching and tertiary education, but more formal classroom teaching and presenting at seminars. If such a role is stripped down to its bare bones, it is primarily about information exchange and the facilitation of such. This is nothing new, and should not propose to be. Nurses of all grades exchange relevant information, be it during a handover or during a break:

6. *Develop relevant teaching within specialties.*

Researcher

The research facet of the ANP role should be at a level that is linked to policy development, evaluation and enforcement. The need to instigate research and co-ordinate projects with other nurses is a skill, and involves an advanced understanding of relevant research methodology, epistemology and ontology. The role demands an in-depth comprehension of identifying research needs within specialties that are nurse-led. As with most nurses, mental health nurses appear to respond more positively to research that is relevant and understandable to them. Such research needs to be of use in practice rather than be dogmatic and left on the shelf to gather dust. The culture of mental health nursing seems only to have made use of second-hand research from other professions and paradigms of scientific enquiry, especially medicine and general nursing. This has not boded well on the whole, and has left it research-impotent and dominated by a seemingly inappropriate body of knowledge that is medicine and psychology-led. It will prove very difficult to revolutionize research in order to give it a pure nursing focus:

7. *Initiate and co-ordinate nurse-led research.*

Management

If afforded a position of autonomy, an ANP could be self-managed. All of the facets of researcher, educator and consultant require management, and the specific time management of such a role would be dependent upon the specialty, the culture and autonomy. The autonomy of such a role suggests self-direction and leadership possibilities to exercise innovative and forward thinking. The inter/intra role conflict engendered by such autonomy is ensured by the need to evaluate and defend the role within the care team; this in itself requires a careful management strategy. The issues of isolation and lack of support in such roles have been noted by Bousfield (1997), who concludes that the challenge is to preserve, protect and promote such specialist roles. This echoes Wilson-Barnett's (1995) earlier sentiments that such specialist posts become essential; however, it is the diversity of the role in the mental health culture that has the potential to create a misunderstanding regarding any management role, because managers are 'supposed to manage in an office' and not 'deal with the patients'.

Mental health nursing and the culture to which it belongs has a need to embrace a new age of consumer groups and contracting, wherein attempts to secure a specialist identity are not futile. It seems that the long-standing trait of accepting all that medicine and general nursing bestows holds no fear for the specialty, due to a history of absorption and an inability to acknowledge a new kind of insight for the future; the engine room for development has always been from outside of the specialty. Management in the past and present has driven on developments in humanist and person centred psychology, which nurses have accepted uncritically; this philosophy of 30 years ago remains with us today, and looks as if it will be predominant for years to come. Thus, the ANP management role, like most, will have to negotiate change not only at a practical level, but also at a philosophical level, although it is difficult to say how this will be achieved. What is clear is that the ANP management role will need to lead the charge against the dominant ideologies that limit the scope of present practice, including medicine, generalism and the existing culture of mental health. I also make the assumption that management is something to do with getting results:

8. Management.

An attempt to provide a number of facets for each of the three areas of nursing can be seen in Table 11.2. These lists cannot be considered definite, and represent the ideas of the author. What they represent is a measured attempt to provide a framework from which nurses can categorize practice within the broad considerations of expertness, management, teaching and research.

Table 11.2. Facets of the three areas of nursing for mental health nurses

Core skills	Specialist	Advanced
Honesty	Exposure	Development of policy
Active listening	Focused knowledge	Enforcement of policy
Problem solving	Accepts uncertainty	Evaluation of policy
Relationship skills	Questions theory	Boundary definition
Care co-ordination	Undertakes research	Research co-ordination
Use of protocol/framework	Expert in a specialism	Initiates and leads change
Acceptance of support	Supports change	Research dissemination
Advanced empathy	Influences policy	Specific knowledge
Assists research	Junior/senior	Supervision and liaison
Team working	Management	Leadership and support
Care planning		Philosophical
		Autonomous
		Diagnosis

Conclusion

This chapter has attempted to widen the debate regarding the ANP role and put forward a position for mental health nursing. The emphasis has focused upon the importance of the psychiatric culture, which has always limited what autonomy and perceptions individual practitioners have had. It has also emphasized the ambiguity regarding the legitimate development of the role, and thus highlighted the need for mental health nurses to take the initiative and seize the opportunity to forge their own role, a role that would attempt not to dress the old up as new, but incorporate core facets that are relevant in practice. This debate will continue to expand along with the role, but, hopefully, as a result of positive reports, rather than from the 'one down' position that this chapter hints that mental health nursing has always occupied.

When I last saw Jo, he said, 'I've been busy doing retirement things.' He was happy with his new life, but he enjoyed talking about nursing. 'You know, I reckon I could have advanced my little bit of nursing a lot more, but I didn't know any better at the time.' He looked at his watch as if he had a ward round to do. 'But hindsight is a wonderful thing isn't it?', he smiled. 'If I could do it all again I'd do that expert diagnosis stuff you keep shouting about.' I guess that Jo, with his years of experience and expertise, was acknowledging that mental health nursing has always been in a two-way relationship with psychiatry, in which the latter had the power. It is an actuality that mental health nursing has never owned its own practice. It has always been bombarded with a composite selection of mental health theory, which has shaped its image from the outside. The ANP role has at its core the facets of expert practice, education, research and management, which it will need in order to pioneer nursing from the inside with a critical new consciousness. There has always been a need to do this, but never greater than now.

References

Andrews, S. (1989). Specialist or generalist nurse? *Primary Health Care*, **6**(2), 8.

Arena, D. and Page, N. (1992). The imposter phenomenon in the CNS role. *Image: J. Nurs. Scholarship*, **24**, 121–125.

Ashton, J. and Seymour, H. (1992). *The New Public Health*. Milton Keynes: Open University Press.

Barker, P. (1990). The philosophy of psychiatric nursing. *Nurs. Stand.*, **5**(12), 28–33.

Benner, P. (1982). From novice to expert. *Am. J. Nurs.*, **82**, 402–407.

Benner, P. (1984). *From Novice to Expert: Excellence and Power in Clinical Nursing Practice*. Menlo Park, CA: Addison-Wesley.

Benner, P., Tanner, C. and Chelsby, C. (1992). From beginner to expert, gaining a differential clinical world in critical nursing care. *Adv. Nurs. Sci.*, **14**(3), 13–18.

Bousfield, C. (1997). A phenomenological investigation into the role of the clinical nurse specialist. *J. Adv. Nurs.*, **25**, 245–256.

Bowman, G. S. and Thompson, D. R. (1995). Strategies for organising care. In *Towards Advanced Nursing Practice*. (J. E. Schober and S. M. Hinchliff, eds.) pp. 222–251. London: Arnold.

Brooking, J. (1991). Doctors and nurses: a personal view. *Nurs. Stand.*, **6**(12), 24–28.

Calkin, J. (1988). Specialization in nursing practice. In *Canadian Nursing Faces the Future*. (A. Baumgort and J. Larson, eds.) pp. 279–296. Toronto: Mosby.

Castledine, G. (1991a). The advanced nurse practitioner: part one. *Nurs. Stand.*, **5**(43), 34–36.

Castledine, G. (1991b). The advanced nurse practitioner: part two. *Nurs. Stand.*, **5**(44), 33–35.

Castledine, G. (1993). Nurse practitioner title: ambiguous and misleading. *Br. J. Nurs.*, **2**, 734–735.

Castledine, G. (1994). UKCC's standards for education and practice. *Br. J. Nurs.*, **3**, 233–234.

Charlton, T. and Macaulay, M. (1993). Good communication heralds successful integration: evaluating the roles of community specialist and general nurses. *Professional Nurse*, **8**(9), 600–602.

Chung, M. C. and Nolan, P. (1994). The influence of positivist thought on nineteenth century asylum nursing. *J. Adv. Nurs.*, **19**, 226–232.

Delphy, C. (1977). *The Main Enemy: A Materialist Analysis of Women's Oppression*. London: Women's Research Centre.

Department of Health. (1994). *The Heathrow Debate: Nursing, Midwifery and Health Visiting Education*. London: HMSO.

Draper, P. (1990). The development of theory in British nursing: current position and future prospects. *J. Adv. Nurs.*, **15**, 12–15. Cited in McGee, P. (1993). Defining nursing practice. *Br. J. Nurs.*, **2**, 1022–1026.

Dreyfus, H. L. and Dreyfus, S. E. (1989). *A Fine Style of the Mental Activities Involved in Skill Acquisition* [unpublished study]. San Francisco, CA: University of California.

Freidson, E. (1970). *Profession of Medicine: a Study of the Sociology of Applied Knowledge*. New York: Harper and Row.

Gamarnikow, E. (1978). Sexual division of labour: the case of nursing. In *Feminism and Materialism*. (A. Kuhn and A. Wolpe, eds.) pp. 96–123. London: Routledge & Kegan Paul.

Gatley, P. (1992). From novice to expert: the use of intuitive knowledge as a basis for district nurse education. *Nurse Educ. Today*, **12**, 81–87.

Godin, P. (1996). The development of community psychiatric nursing: a professional project. *J. Adv. Nurs.*, **23**, 925–934.

Goffman, E. (1970). *Asylums*. Harmondsworth: Penguin.

Hamric, A. B. and Spross, J. A. (1989). *The Clinical Nurse Specialist in Theory and Practice*, 2nd edn. Philadelphia, PA: Saunders.

Heenan, A. (1991). Uneasy partnership. *Nurs. Times*, **87**(10), 25–27.

Heffline, M. (1992). Establishing the role of the CNS in post anaesthesia care. *Post Anaesth. Nurse*, **7**, 305–311.

Heidegger, M. (1962). *Being and Time*. London: SCM Press.

Hogston, R. (1997). Nursing diagnosis and classification systems: a position paper. *J. Adv. Nurs.*, **26**, 496–500.

Holyoake, D. (1995a). *A Study into the Nature of Nurse Interaction with Mentally Ill Young People: How a Nurse Conducts an Examination of Nursing Assumptions in the Advanced Nurse Practitioner Role* [thesis]. Birmingham: University of Central England; London: Steinberg Collection RCN.

Holyoake, D. (1995b). Advancing in confusion. *Nurs. Stand.*, **9**(51), 56.

Holyoake, D. (1996). Medicine is still big brother [letter]. *Nurs. Stand.*, **10**(28), 11.

Holyoake, D. (1997a). Exploring the nature of nurse interaction using an interaction interview schedule: the results. *Psychiatr. Care*, **4**, 83–87.

Holyoake, D. (1997b). A look into the culture club: exploring the perceptions of mentally ill young people about inpatient culture. *Psychiatr. Care*, **4**, 162–167.

Holyoake, D. (1997c). Philosophy of the culture club. *Paediatr. Nurs.*, **9**(8), 16–18.

Hopton, J. (1997). Towards a critical theory of mental health nursing. *J. Adv. Nurs.*, **25**, 492–500.

Hunsberger, M., Mitchell, A., Blatz, S. et al. (1992). Definition of an advanced nursing practice role in the NICU: the clinical nurse specialist/neonatal practitioner. *Clin. Nurse Specialist*, **6**(2), 91–96.

Kelly, A. (1996). The concept of the specialist community nurse. *J. Adv. Nurs.*, **24**, 42–52.

Lindstrom, U. A. (1995). The professional paradigm of qualified psychiatric nurses. *J. Adv. Nurs.*, **22**, 655–662.

McGee, P. (1993). Defining nursing practice. *Br. J. Nurs.*, **2**, 1022–1026.

McMurry, A. (1990). *Community Health Nursing. Primary Health Care in Practice*. Edinburgh:

Churchill Livingstone.

Mechanic, H. F. (1988). Redefining the expanded role. *Nurs. Outlook*, **36**, 280–284.

Melia, K. (1987). *Learning and Working. The Occupational Socialisation of Nursing*. London: Tavistock.

Miller, S. (1995). The clinical nurse specialist: a way forward? *J. Adv. Nurs.*, **22**, 494–501.

Murphy, J. F. (1970). Role expansion or role extension. *Nurs. Forum*, **9**, 380–390.

Paley, J. (1996). Intuition and expertise: comments on the Benner debate. *J. Adv. Nurs.*, **23**, 665–671.

Patterson, C. and Haddad, B. (1992). The advanced nurse practitioner: common attributes. *Can. J. Nurs. Admin.*, **5**(4), 18–20.

Peplau, H. (1965). Specialization in professional nursing. *Nurs. Sci.*, **3**, 268–287. Cited in McGee, P. (1993). Defining nursing practice. *Br. J. Nurs.*, **2**, 1022–1026.

Peplau, H. (1978). Psychiatric nursing: role of nurses and psychiatric nurses. In *Hildegard E. Peplau, Selected Works*. (A. Werner O' Toole and S. R. Welt, eds.) (1994). pp. 120–133. London: Macmillan.

Porter, S. (1991). A participant observation study of power relations between nurses and doctors in a general hospital. *J. Adv. Nurs.*, **16**, 728–735.

Porter, S. (1992). The poverty of professionalization: a critical analysis of strategies for the occupational advancement of nursing. *J. Adv. Nurs.*, **17**, 720–726.

Rolfe, G. (1997). Science, abduction and the fuzzy nurse: an exploration of expertise. *J. Adv. Nurs.*, **25**, 1070–1075.

Royal College of Nursing. (1988). *Specialties in Nursing*. London: RCN.

Salvage, J. (1988). Professionalization or struggle for survival? A consideration of current proposals for the reform of nursing in the UK. *J. Adv. Nurs.*, **13**, 515–519.

Schön, D. A. (1988). From technical rationality to reflection in action. In *Professional Judgement*. (A. Dowie, J. and P. Elstein, eds.) pp. 60–77. Cambridge: Cambridge University Press.

Sparacino, P. (1992). Advanced practice: the clinical nurse specialist. *Nurse Pract.*, **5**(4), 2–4.

Thompson, P. and McHugh, D. (1990). *Work Organisations: a Critical Introduction*. London: Macmillan.

Tunmore, R. (1997). Mental health liaison and consultation. *Nurs. Stand.*, **11**(50), 46–51.

United Kingdom Central Council for Nursing, Midwifery and Health Visiting. (1990). *The Report of the Post-Registration Education and Practice Project*. London: UKCC.

United Kingdom Central Council for Nursing, Midwifery and Health Visiting. (1993). *The Council's Proposed Standards for Post-Registration Education*. London: UKCC.

United Kingdom Central Council for Nursing, Midwifery and Health Visiting. (1994). *The Future of Professional Practice. The Council's Standards for Education and Practice Following Registration*. London: UKCC.

Vitello-Cicciu, J. (1984). Excellence in critical care: educating the clinical specialist. *Crit. Care Q.*, **7**(1), 26–32.

Wilson-Barnett, J. (1995) Specialism in nursing: effectiveness and maximization of benefit. *J. Adv. Nurs.*, **21**, 1–2.

Witz, A. (1991). *Professions and Patriarchy*. London: Routledge.

12

Developing a framework for practice: a clinical perspective

Maureen Coombs and Margaret Holgate

Introduction

The aim of this chapter will be to give a clinically orientated perspective on the advancement of professional practice. It will describe the development of a practice framework in a trust, and the key issues that were raised during its evolution, which were seen to be important in the development and implementation of such a practice framework. These thoughts are distilled at the end of each section as a 'check-list' of practical pointers to be addressed. The final framework is presented towards the end of the chapter, together with indications on how it has been used, lessons to be learned from it, and how the total process has informed and developed the authors' views on the current challenges to professional practice.

As the thoughts and perspectives contained within the chapter are individual to the authors, the authors take full responsibility and ownership for these.

Background

This chapter is set against a backdrop of great change in health care provision. The shift towards a primary care led NHS (Department of Health (DoH), 1990), together with professional (National Health Service Management Executive (NHSME), 1991; United Kingdom Central Council for Nursing, Midwifery and Health Visiting (UKCC), 1992a) and technological progression and increased public expectation, demands that the nursing profession should develop to meet these challenges.

The nursing profession needs to challenge and develop the traditional paradigm of clinical practice to meet the demands of health care provision in the 1990s and beyond. In the current health care climate, all developments must, and should, be scrutinized for their potential benefit to patients, rather than any particular professional group. From this, there must be agreement that the focus of any role change or practice development is the patient (Sutton and Smith, 1995). Nursing must push beyond the known boundaries of the nursing profession in the interests of improved patient care (Ball, 1997). As Chinn (1991) states 'To take charge of our future, we must have the courage to challenge what exists in the present.'

Drivers for change

There have been many influential forces in driving role changes of the nurse over the past decade. The National Health Service and Community Care Act (Department of Health (DoH), 1990) and the new deal on junior doctors' hours (NHSME, 1991) are all key national drivers. This has not only affected the structure and management of the health service, but also the availability and roles of health care personnel. Further forces resulted from professional body reports including the UKCC's *Scope of Professional Practice* (UKCC, 1992a) and PREP, the *Post-Registration Education and Practice Project,* (UKCC, 1990).

Set against these changes, there was also considerable national debate in the professional nursing literature about the nature and function of the many new nursing roles within the health service (Dimond, 1995; Castledine, 1996). The literature has historically referred to nursing role developments as being encompassed within the concepts of expanding or extending practice (DoH, 1994). Role expansion is linked to developments located within nursing as an autonomous, self-determined and discrete service, building on its tradition. Role extension is generally seen as falling beyond the traditional nursing boundaries, towards those of other professional groups, most commonly medicine.

The debate has been further confused through discussion on the nature of specialist and advanced nursing practice. There continues to be a lack of clarity and consensus on the definition of advanced practice, as demonstrated by the current plethora of titles, remits and responsibilities, and grading of these roles (McGee et al., 1996). In addition, the relationship of advanced practice to the concepts of specialist practice has not been fully clarified. Perspectives on advanced nursing practice are reflected through a spectrum of roles, from physician's assistant (medical model) to nurse managed care (nursing model). This situation has recently been further confused by the continuing lack of specific guidance on the nature of advanced practice from the central bodies (Ball, 1997).

The tradition in the John Radcliffe Hospital, and more recently as part of the Oxford Radcliffe Hospital Trust, has been to place few constraints on the scope of nursing practice. This initially developed from the support and vision of nurse leaders at district and local hospital level, and has attracted creative nurses to work in Oxford, allowing innovation and development to be valued. This strategy has enabled Oxford nurses to be among the leaders of nursing practice in this country, supporting such innovations as nursing development units (Pearson, 1983), the role of the ward sister in nursing leadership (Pembrey and Fitzgerald, 1987), primary nursing (Binnie, 1989), and the therapeutic nursing relationship (Ersser, 1991).

Even within this liberated environment, good practice guidelines are required to inform and support any nursing developments. At a time when many clinical units were critically reviewing their services and the contribution that nurses made, or could make, to care delivery, it became apparent that there were several different models of practice development being undertaken. In order to support 'safe practice' without being restrictive, there was a request from the Trust Board that a comprehensive risk management system should be in place, which would address issues that had arisen from such professional role development.

Within the Trust, senior nurse representatives from all the clinical centres met each month to address pertinent operational and strategic issues. This professional practice issue was therefore placed on the agenda as a discussion item for the Nursing and Midwifery Policy Board. In preparation for this, a discussion paper was written, part of which forms the theoretical basis of this chapter. During the ensuing debate, concerns were raised about the multiple practice models being followed within the Trust, from minidoctor to nurse managed care. There were also issues raised about the long-term durability and sustainability of the roles, and the resource availability to support the nurses in these roles.

Due to the national lack of consensus regarding advanced and specialist practice and the role of the nurse within these areas at that time, it was decided not to adopt an approach incorporating a specific level of practice, but to view professional role development per se, and from a perspective that could be easily understandable using the structures and terminology already being employed within the Trust. As a direct result of the debate, it was decided to establish a short-term project group to draw together the relevant issues and concerns, and work them into a usable document for risk management at trust, local clinical area and independent practitioner level to help to guide practice.

The project group comprised four interested senior nurses, which included this chapter's two authors. Each member of the group not only had an active clinical role as a senior nurse in her own clinical area but also carried other unit/trust responsibilities such as management, teaching or corporate project development. The group was charged with establishing a 'framework for practice development' within the Oxford Radcliffe Hospital. The purpose of this framework was to provide a universal algorithm for all nurses to use, which, although allowing freedom for innovation, also ensured the safety of patients and practitioners alike. Although it was primarily devised by nurses for a specific nursing issue, it was felt to be important that the structure was kept sufficiently user-friendly to be utilized by any professional group that was considering professional practice developments.

The framework was devised to provide a flexible structure to take account of practice development within any context of care. The framework would ensure that the nurse undertook roles appropriate to patient need, to an established skill level, and to the level of resourcing. The framework was also seen as a tool that could be used prospectively to direct planning in the establishment of new opportunities for practice development, and could also be used retrospectively to reflect on and audit the practice development. The framework would therefore be useful as a learning tool and a resourcing model, and would provide an evaluation format.

It became clear as the project group met and debated professional practice issues, that a specific decision-guiding framework could be developed, which would focus on specific issues that were felt to be important in informing the arena of professional practice development. These issues are now discussed and later brought together in a distillation of the group's thoughts as the final framework.

The total framework was viewed to encompass corporate, professional, managerial, educational and resourcing issues. The importance of ensuring a corporate and professional 'fit' to meet service, professional and patient needs was seen as paramount in ensuring the success of the practice development. As stated earlier, due to the perspective taken regarding practice development rather than a specified level of practice per se, the framework needed to address all generic facets of practice development and project organization, yet also include specific pointers with regard to individual postholder management. All these areas will now be explored with the resultant implications for practice development management.

Corporate philosophy

Until 1991, the NHS functioned according to a relatively simple model. In a pyramidal structure, policy and control flowed down from the Government via the Department of Health to increasingly smaller geographical and organizational entities, with resource allocation following the same pathway. After 1991, the NHS was restructured to conform more closely to the model of enterprise in the private sector of industry. Health care provision was now provided by trusts and directly managed units for the district and general practitioner fund holders. Services were determined, negotiated, contracted and agreed through contracts (DoH, 1990).

In order to increase the responsibility of the clinicians within the internal market, the large hierarchical hospital organizations were replaced by small semi-autonomous units. This, in effect, devolved the authority and ownership of service delivery to the clinical directorates/units and closer to the point of delivery of care. Placing this into context within the Oxford Radcliffe Hospital Trust, care is managed by smaller multidisciplinary teams called service delivery units (SDUs), functioning at the point of care delivery. This management structure reinforces the devolvement of management and the increased involvement of clinicians in the management and responsibility for service delivery. Although the individual SDUs may plan and manage their local clinical service and need, it is important that this is informed, and indeed can inform, the broader trust corporate philosophy. It is important that, while acknowledging the individuality of each service unit, there is a sharing of common values and aims that are reflected in the philosophy and the annual plans at each level of the organization. This ensures that each constituent part of the organization and the organization as a whole share a common purpose and goals, which can be communicated to patients, staff and purchasers. It is the intention, therefore, that any nursing development is informed by this framework.

In a market orientated work environment, all providers of care are required increasingly to communicate service details to the consumers and purchasers of their service. The ability to communicate and market effectively will contribute to the success of the organization (trust) and its constituent parts (SDUs) in order that it fulfils its responsibility to deliver a high quality service and to enable it to survive financially. The more that purchasers and patients understand about the service delivered and its potential benefits, the more effective will be the use made of that service. A professional practice framework could be used to articulate practice developments to both lay and professional users of the service in order to clarify both the need and the resourcing issues. In this way, the responsibility of the profession to account to the organization for its activities is facilitated through the use of an agreed framework.

Local and national professional frameworks equally have the potential to uphold professional values and standards, and can be used to support more appropriate levels of resourcing in times of increasing service pressures. In this way, a local framework for practice could be used to uphold agreed standards within the organization's business plan.

The framework requires that the nature, resources and outcomes of the activity are described. Using a framework shared with others provides a language and a structure for communication, making it easier to inform those who wish to learn. This framework can also be used to structure supporting arguments in reply to any challenges to the practice development itself. It is important, however, that the framework itself is constantly reviewed and audited so that it does not become stagnant but remains responsive and adaptive to the clinical need. In this manner, the document could be used to provide opportunity for informed risk taking and innovation in practice.

The key questions guiding this section are:

What is the problem or issue involved? Has the problem been identified in past business plans or from user/purchaser feedback? How will be the patient benefit from this change? Is this change consistent with trust philosophy? How will this change help to meet annual plans and service proposals?

Nursing credo

Nursing espouses its own professional values, and therefore local unit and ward philosophies of nursing should be underpinned by the central values associated with caring and nursing. It is important that, at local unit and national level, nursing should be able to articulate its philosophy and its contribution to health care delivery within the current health care service.

Local ward philosophy must also inform, and be informed by, local trust nursing philosophy and strategy. To enable this to happen, it is important that the values and beliefs of the profession at local ward and organization level are reviewed and placed against the needs of patients. Any practice development can then be seen in the light of what is considered to be 'nursing', and can be identified to benefit and enhance the care given to the patient while in the trust hospital.

It is important that, at this point, critical review of the required development occurs to identify whether a suitable 'fit' is made with the nursing philosophy and resources. It may be that, on further examination, the remit of the proposed practice development is not consistent with the nursing philosophy, or that nursing is not the most appropriate health care profession to undertake this activity. If this is the situation, then discussions may need to take place with the health care team to discuss the issue and to identify the most appropriate way forward.

The key questions guiding this section are:

How does this development benefit the patient? Is the change consistent with national nursing philosophy? Is this change consistent with trust and local unit nursing philosophy? Is the nurse the most appropriate person to be involved in this change? What specific skills or attributes can a nurse bring to this development?

Good practice guidelines

The UKCC, as a regulatory body for the profession, requires its members to behave according to the standards and guidelines it lays down, for example, as a code of conduct. In 1992 the UKCC published *The Scope of Professional Practice* (UKCC, 1992a), which repudiated the term 'extended role' and the mandatory certification that occurred with regard to those 'extended' activities. The aim of this document was that practice development would be enhanced and the quality of service provision for the patient improved through innovation. It is important that any practice development is measured against these standards to ensure that 'good practice' is being upheld.

It is also important to consider that both national and local frameworks have potential as documents, to help to mitigate against service pressures. As the code of conduct (UKCC, 1992b) can be used by nurses to protect minimum standards of practice (Hunt, 1994), so a local framework for practice could uphold agreed standards within the organization's business plan. For this reason, it is important that any development is carefully thought through, with benefits to patients and service identified, fully costed, and built into the local business plan. This ensures the profile of the development within the trust and to the purchasers, and agreement in principle to the proposed plan.

The key questions guiding this section are:

Have relevant good practice guidelines and statutory requirements been considered in the light of the proposed development? Are there any issues of concern that need to be addressed in light of this? Has the proposed development been included in the business plan against specific outcomes and resource requirements?

Having considered the professional, national and trust perspectives on practice development, the focus now shifts to influential factors at local practice level. These can be some of the most important issues, as they determine ownership and commitment in sustaining the proposed change. The key factors that were seen to be important were identification of resources, educational provision, and management of the practice development.

Identification of resources

It is vital that a comprehensive review of any resource requirements is undertaken. This includes consideration of the proposed development and the level of staffing required. The level of equipment required, such as a computer, office space, desk, and any travel costs, needs to be obtained. This is important so that the first few months of the postholder's employment is not spent 'wasted' attempting to secure these essential items. If the development is to be audited or requires heavy correspondence with others, then consideration of administrative support is needed, and the buying in of secretarial hours needs to be added into the costing model. It may require creative funding sources to be explored to support the acquisition of this level of resourcing. Flexibility in pay and non-pay budgets, trust funds (as appropriate), or support from industry through sponsorship are possible funding sources.

An important consideration at any of these operational stages is the implementation of an effective support structure to sustain the effectiveness and efficiency of these posts. It is also important so that postholders who are assuming new responsibilities and developing new skills in new territories have support and feedback such that motivation and commitment is maintained.

The key questions guiding this section are:

Is there sufficient staffing to achieve the development? Are there any equipment requirements to enable the staff to fulfil their role? What budget has been identified to offset these costs? Are office, administrative support or computer facilities required? Is the timing of the project realistic? What support structure has been put in place?

Educational provision

The nature of the practice development will determine the level of educational provision that is required. There may be opportunities already available that would support practitioner preparation, or courses may need to be developed. Depending on the skill level required, attendance at a study day or a short course might be sufficient, or, if a major development or change is being proposed, a more formal course might need to be structured and validated. It is important to consider future developments, both educationally and professionally, to determine how these specific educational preparations may fit into the overall plan. This will enable any educational credits gained to be built on in the future.

Depending on the impetus for change locally, it is essential that the curriculum development and strategy are informed by national, professional and local requirements, as raised earlier. This will ensure that the specific nursing focus remains central, and yet takes account of other influencing factors. From this, a more detailed and structured educational programme can be planned. It is important that service and education work together as partners in this area, as only then can education understand service needs and the service side appreciate what is educationally sound and viable.

The assessment strategy for this area of professional practice provision has important issues to be addressed. These focus around the assessment of the developed practice and the question of who is most appropriate to act as mentor and assessor, particularly if new skills are being acquired. These issues are not restricted purely to the acquisition of the new skills/attributes, but must be seen within a continuing framework of clinical supervision, and can be built into a more long-term process including performance review.

This not only maintains quality and standards, but also provides an established support structure, which has been referred to earlier as important for postholders who are assuming new responsibilities and new skills, so that motivation and commitment are maintained.

The key questions guiding this section are:

What assessment strategy has been developed? What opportunity for clinical supervision or performance review has been agreed? What facilities for ongoing education and training have been identified? Is there any budget identified for professional updating? What support structure has been put in place?

Management of the development

The implications of the management of the development must be considered early. Any change can instil great fear and anxiety, not only in those who are undertaking the development, but also amongst those who may be indirectly involved. For this reason, it is important that full consideration is given to any 'knock-on' effects within the service, and appropriate discussions held with relevant people in the organization. This not only serves to inform, but can also be useful in troubleshooting problems early, in raising the profile of the development, and possibly in learning from others who may have similar experiences. The implications for the rest of the team must be examined so that standards of care are raised, and so that team members do not carry extra workload. It is important, to enable all staff to work together, to establish honesty and trust in all communications. It is also important to involve the personnel department and, if appropriate, the staff unions.

It may be that the initiative requires the development of a specific post, and therefore the appointment of a postholder. The preparation of any job description, person specification and salary needs to be thoroughly addressed. It is important, not only for the postholder, but also for the viability of the project, that time is invested at the beginning of the venture in ensuring that all these aspects are rigorously addressed. The use of a definitive job description and specification, and a structured performance review process with outcomes to measure effectiveness, is imperative. These can help to determine the required personal and professional attributes and the necessary skills base to allow the postholder to function at his or her full potential. It is important to address issues relating to requirements for previous experience, and the provision of on-site training facilities.

Provision must also be made for role cover in the event of sickness or annual leave. The total remit of the job needs to be considered, including the identification of specific mandatory or optional aspects of the role. If there is a requirement that the post should be fully operational within a set time, then this also is required to be made explicit, so that both the postholder and the service can have realistic goals and expectations.

The funding for the post, inclusive of any add-on costs, unsocial hours, travel costs, and so on, needs to be clearly identified and secured within the budget. The funding for this post may already exist within the budget or it may be pump primed from an outside source. It is important to make it explicit to all whether the monies are non-recurrent or recurrent in nature; this ensures that there are no false expectations about the longevity of the role.

Finally, in a time of so much planning in a new project, it is easy to forget long-term strategic plans. What of the future of the project and the postholder? What are the career development prospects for the postholder? Where does the postholder progress to in 2, 3 or 5 years time? To maintain future motivation and satisfaction in the role, it is important that consideration is given to future career pathways. Career progression should be structured in advance, and a support mechanism set up to sustain the role, and, more importantly, the postholder.

The key questions guiding this section are:

What 'knock-on' effects can be identified through the system? Has there been open, honest discussion with other members of the health care team? Have the personnel department, and, if appropriate, the staff unions, been consulted for advice? Have the job description, person specification and salary been thoroughly prepared? Where is the funding source for this post? Is the funding pump primed or recurrent? Are unsocial hours and weekends to be covered and financed? What provision has been made for annual leave and sickness cover? Does there need to be previous experience; if not, what training facilities have been made available? Are any of the job activities optional? Is there an agreed time scale for full integration into the post? What are the career development prospects for the postholder? What support structure has been put in place?

Accountability, authority and responsibility

It has been stated as early as the 1960s that one of the weaknesses of nurses as a professional group has been the unfocused nature of their responsibility and authority (Menzies, 1960). By setting boundaries and defining role content within a framework for practice, nurses can be assigned responsibility and authority; clinical decision making will be clear; and practitioners will be accountable for what they do. A framework will also clarify the responsibility of others in the team towards such developments, so that practitioners receive the support they need from their colleagues in terms of respect for their agreed accountability, responsibility and authority.

It is vitally important that all these issues are addressed in an open and direct manner and recorded in writing, particularly to clarify discussions with other health care professionals. If areas of accountability and authority are not agreed, the success of the development cannot be guaranteed. If protocols or guidelines for practice are required, then these need to be agreed and in place at the earliest opportunity, so that there is the scope for the project to develop to its fullest potential.

Within a medicolegal context, a framework that sets levels of competence and service requirements will give support if practice remains located within it. This places responsibility on the practice developers to maintain standards. It also has the potential to save the organization resources that might otherwise have been spent on maintaining a complex system of rules and policing.

Enabling nurses to take role responsibility, rather than task responsibility, ensures that the focus of the nurse is ultimately on delivering total patient care. The use of a framework could liberate practice away from tasks, rituals and routines, and enable the nurse to provide high quality, holistic care.

The key questions guiding this section are:

Have full and open discussions occurred to identify levels of authority and holders of responsibility and accountability at all stages on the framework? Is there full agreement on these issues? Has this been clarified in writing?

The way forward

All the areas discussed above were seen to be of key importance in considering practice role developments. These areas considered national and societal issues, as well as more local influencing factors in determining the appropriateness and success of the development. In bringing these areas together in a systematic way, a framework for practice development was formulated (Figure 12.1). This final framework was discussed and ratified at a meeting of the Nursing and Midwifery Policy Board and then reported on and agreed by the Trust Board. It is now available for use by all clinical areas and by any profession in consideration of any practice development. Although its use is limited, it has been used alongside further research work undertaken at the Oxford Radcliffe Hospitals Trust. Through this, current service roles and needs have been identified in order to inform planning for further educational requirements, so that such developments are supported. Its use is still in its infancy in determining the viability of new practice development roles. Further audit and evaluation is required, not only on the

Considerations in Service Role Developments

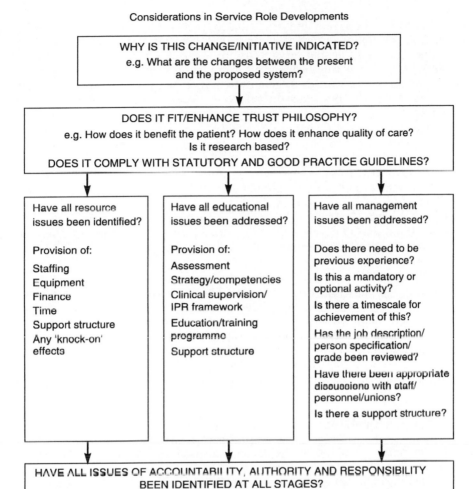

Figure 12.1. A safety net to support professional practice

use of the framework, but also on the value of the framework itself.

Using a framework for practice based on a philosophy that has arisen from professional and managerial theory, an understanding of what nursing is, and an appreciation of what it can achieve, will ensure not only the safety of staff and patients but also enable nursing to advance in ways that will enhance the quality of care delivered by nurses and the rest of the health care team.

Conclusions

A number of themes have arisen from the debate around the purpose and nature of a framework to develop practice. The future of nursing and of new nursing roles depends on the values held by nurses and the vision arising from those values. It is important that nurses do not devalue their belief in holism, continuity and co-ordination in patient focused care in favour of a reductionist, fragmented service culture focusing on tasks; this is not only short-sighted, but will also lead to a reduction in quality patient care. To reverse this trend towards fragmentation, there needs to be critical informed debate among nurses and their fellow professionals in the health care service. There is a real need for a national debate using a common vocabulary about this issue, in collaboration with other members of the health care team and patients. This discussion must be undertaken without professional tribalism, but informed by the discrete professional values each team member can bring.

The focus of any care development must be the delivery of high quality patient focused care. There must be understanding of, and respect for, each individual team member's contribution to the service. It is important to understand that in developing skills in one area, nursing does not threaten the very essence and centrality of that which is nursing unless it replaces that essence.

Having patients as our highest priority does not diminish ourselves as individuals or as a profession. It sets us apart in a powerful way that defines our unique contribution and demonstrates our value to patients, their families, the teams with which we work, and the organizations within which we work. In a culture of lifelong learning, it is vital to be able to see where we have come from and where we are going. It is possible to learn in an orderly and constructive fashion, to have a sense of achievement from the past and not be overwhelmed by the possibilities of the future.

Acknowledgements

The authors wish to acknowledge the contribution of the other members of the project group to the development of the 'Framework for Practice': Nettie Dearman, Lecturer Practitioner, Paediatrics, ORHT; Kim Campbell, Service Delivery Unit Manager, Midwifery Services, ORHT.

References

Ball, C. (1997). Planning for the future: advanced nursing practice in critical care. *Intensive Crit. Care Nurs.*, **13**, 17–25.

Binnie, A. (1989). Primary nursing: where to start? *Nurs. Times*, **85**(24), 42–44.

Castledine, G. (1996). Clarifying and defining nursing role developments. *Br. J. Nurs.*, **5**, 1338.

Chinn, P. L. (1991). Looking in the crystal ball: positioning ourselves for the year 2000. *Nurs. Outlook*, **39**, 251–256.

Department of Health. (1990). *The National Health Service and Community Care Act*. London: HMSO.

Department of Health. (1994). *The Interface Between Doctors and Nurses: a Research Study for the DoH*. London: Greenhalgh.

Dimond, B. (1995). When a nurse wields the scalpel . . . *Br. J. Nurs.*, **4**, 65–66.

Ersser, S. (1991). A search for the therapeutic dimensions of nurse–patient interaction. In *Nursing as Therapy*. (R. McMahon and A. Pearson, eds.) pp. 43–84. London: Chapman and Hall.

Hunt, G. (1994). New professional? New ethics? In *Expanding the Role of the Nurse: the Scope of Professional Practice*. (G. Hunt and P. Wainwright, eds.) pp. 22–38. Oxford: Blackwell Scientific.

McGee, P., Castledine, G. and Brown, R. (1996). A survey of specialist and advanced nursing practice in England. *Br. J. Nurs.*, **5**, 682–686.

Menzies, I. (1960). A case study in the functioning of social systems as a defence against anxiety – a report on a study of the nursing services of a general hospital. *Hum. Relations*, **13**, 95–121.

National Health Service Management Executive. (1991). *Junior Doctors: the New Deal. Making the Best Use of Skills of Nurses and Midwives*. London: NHSME.

Pearson, A. (1983). *The Clinical Nursing Unit*. London: Heinemann.

Pembrey, S. and Fitzgerald, M. (1987). The ward sister: developing the potential of sisters. *Nurs. Times*, **83**(12), 27.

Sutton, F. and Smith, C. (1995). Advanced nursing practice: new ideas and perspectives. *J. Adv. Nurs.*, **21**, 1037–1043.

United Kingdom Central Council for Nursing, Midwifery and Health Visiting. (1990). *Post-Registration Education and Practice Project*. London: UKCC.

United Kingdom Central Council for Nursing, Midwifery and Health Visiting. (1992a). *The Scope of Professional Practice*. London: UKCC.

United Kingdom Central Council for Nursing, Midwifery and Health Visiting. (1992b). *Code of Professional Conduct*. London: UKCC

Commentary: the practice perspective

In Part 3, the perspective shifts once again, this time to focus on practice. This part of the book contains four chapters: the first three present a selection of different perspectives from practitioners themselves, and the final chapter offers a management framework for facilitating practice development roles. It soon becomes apparent on reading this part of the book that advanced practice roles develop in response to both local conditions and the demands of the particular specialism in which they are situated. We might expect, then, that there will be as many advanced practice roles as there are advanced practitioners. This certainly seems to be the case. As Elliott demonstrates in her chapter, even where two new roles are instigated in the same clinical area, they are still likely to develop in different ways. This, incidentally, was the impetus for Coombs and Holgate's practice framework in the final chapter, since 'it became apparent that there were several different models of practice development being undertaken. In order to support "safe practice" without being restrictive, there was a request from the Trust Board that a comprehensive risk management system should be in place, which would address issues that had arisen from such professional role development.'

Clearly, with such a plethora of roles, any selection has to be fairly arbitrary. We have therefore chosen three areas of practice that make very different demands on the role, namely, cancer nursing, the care of elderly people in a community hospital, and mental health nursing. It must be borne in mind, however, that three *different* advanced practitioners writing about the same specialisms would probably produce very different accounts of the roles.

In the first chapter, Goodman gives a personal account of advanced practice from the perspective of a lecturer–practitioner in oncology. In her view, the key activities of the advanced practitioner role are 'evaluation, creative practice development, managerial activities, research activities and educational activities'. However, unlike the roles to be described in later chapters, it tends towards a 'hands-off' approach of strategizing, managing and advising. For example, the practice element of the role is described as monitoring and maintaining standards, multidisciplinary team management, project management and supervision. As Goodman points out: 'The more activities that are required, the less feasible clinical practice becomes.'

Turning to some of the other activities mentioned above, the research role of the advanced practitioner is described by Goodman as being 'involved with research strategies for cancer nursing, perhaps developing cancer nursing fellowships. They should also be concerned with implementing national research and development priorities.' Similarly, 'Within their educational role, advanced practitioners could help to shape and develop cancer nursing education. By contributing to the development of educational standards for cancer nursing, the quality of nursing care given to patients may be seen to improve.' Once again, the emphasis appears to be more on strategizing and prioritizing than on doing research or teaching. Indeed, Goodman adds that one of the ways of fitting all of these activities into a single role is to 'contribute to education via curriculum planning and teach only those students able to benefit from their advanced level'.

For Goodman, then, the primary role of the advanced nurse practitioner is 'to manage a clinical area, lead a clinical team, and change clinical practice'; this role is in stark contrast to the roles described by Fulbrook's advanced practitioners in Part 2, for whom the management role interfered with what they saw as the more important roles of *doing* practice, research and education. Goodman endorses this observation that the advanced practitioner is limited in the number of roles that can be incorporated into her job, but clearly Goodman's priorities lie elsewhere. Perhaps this is to be expected, since she also makes the point that the advanced practitioner role should evolve locally according to specific local needs.

In the second chapter, Elliott gives another, rather different account of the development of a lecturer–practitioner role, this time in a community hospital for the elderly. Unlike many other writers in this book, she sees advanced nursing practice as an umbrella term that covers the clinical nurse specialist and the physician's assistant roles in addition to the more usual advanced practice role. As becomes apparent later, this broad focus is largely in response to the particular demands placed upon the postholder by the community setting and the reduced availability of medical staff, and can therefore be seen as an endorsement of Goodman's call for locally evolved roles.

However, in common with most writers, Elliott sees the advanced nurse practitioner role as being composed of a number of subroles, in her case, those of clinical practice, education, nursing leadership and support, research, policy influence, and consultant, all of which, she emphasizes 'are aimed at enhancing patient care'. However, her emphasis is not on the advanced practitioner's ability to wear a number of different hats and to switch rapidly from one role to another, as many of the North American typologies appear to suggest; rather, as she demonstrates with a number of examples taken from her own practice, she 'set out to integrate the subroles...into her everyday practice'. Thus, a typical practice development might include policy change, educational provision, clinical supervision, consultancy, and evaluation, sometimes all at the same time! Clearly, when Elliott writes of this integration of roles as being aimed at enhancing patient care, she is not merely referring to her own direct clinical intervention, but to the empowerment of her staff. Thus, like Goodman and Barker in previous chapters, Elliott sees the role of the advanced nurse practitioner as essentially one of *advancing* the practice of her colleagues, particularly those who are practising at a lower level.

For Elliott, in contrast to Goodman, probably the most important and effective mechanism for advancing practice is to act as a role model for other staff. Thus: 'The ANP should demonstrate evidence based "best practice" within his or her own caseload and assist others in this goal.' The importance of working alongside other staff cannot be overstated, since it 'allowed an analysis of the current state of nursing practice, and, through close involvement, an awareness of the difficulties and the achievements of staff'. The advanced nurse practitioner role is therefore very much a 'hands-on' approach rooted firmly in clinical practice, and the various subroles relate first and foremost to that practice.

In the following chapter, Holyoake has produced what he describes as 'a piece of reflective writing of the author's opinions' about the nature of advanced mental health nursing practice. Holyoake begins his analysis by noting that mental health nursing has developed in a culture that is both medically led and institutionally situated, and claims that the confusion surrounding new roles in nursing is, at least in the mental health field, a natural result of the attempt to disturb the inertia of institutional practice. His suggestion for dealing with this role confusion is interesting: in order to overcome the institutional inertia that is resisting the clarification and definition of new nursing roles, we need precisely the sort of forceful leadership offered by those very roles. Thus, 'The visionary, risk taking and perceived leadership role of the ANP would have to conquer the ordered culture of the total institution.' In order to define what the role of the advanced mental health nurse practitioner might be, the role must first be established. This suggests an action research approach to role development similar to that described in Part 2 by Manley, in which a provisional role is established and is then evaluated and developed in an action research cycle, and is also reminiscent of Goodman's suggestion of 'using evaluation methods within an action research process, assisting the advanced practitioner to make ongoing connections between findings and practice, and generating new and clinically relevant ideas'.

However, inertia is not the only obstacle to overcome. Mental health nursing, claims Holyoake, is dominated by the medical profession, not only in terms of power relationships and treatments, but also in the language and theoretical models which it employs; in fact, by the whole tradition 'in which nursing is defined by others rather than by nursing itself in the absence of a common language that might facilitate the description of nursing'. The only hope, he suggests, is for mental health nurses to find their own niche away from medical dominance, 'an area of health care work over which they have control'. Holyoake believes that the advanced nurse practitioner role holds the promise of freeing mental health nursing from its subordinate position, and that the key to this is professional autonomy 'to advance practice from a theoretical base that is nurse-led'.

The various subroles of advanced practice, such as researcher, manager and consultant, follow naturally from this emphasis on autonomy, and Holyoake specifically targets the issues of nursing diagnosis and expert practice as being of particular importance to the autonomous practitioner. He claims that nurses are constantly diagnosing, but that, without a nursing diagnostic framework, they are unable to challenge medical diagnoses and act as advocates for their patients. Furthermore, he associates expertise with problem recognition and deliberative rationality, so that 'what makes a psychiatric ANP different from, say, a psychiatric nurse in "professional practice", is that the ANP would provide a nursing diagnosis and also provide a rationale for choosing diagnostic and treatment processes in a consultancy capacity.' Clearly, then, the advanced practitioner must not only make complex professional judgements, but must also be able rationally to justify those judgements and communicate them to other more junior staff.

As with the roles described in the previous chapters, this vision of the advanced nurse practitioner is already looking rather idiosyncratic. This should come as no surprise, however, since Holyoake is at pains to point out that mental health nursing is different from other forms of nursing, coming as it does from an essentially masculine culture, and that furthermore, 'a male dominated psychiatric culture ultimately has a better chance of equality with medical culture than that of the female dominated general nursing setting.' This view is in contrast to Barker's position, expressed in Part 1 of this book, that psychiatric nursing needs to return to its feminine caring roots. Indeed, Holyoake rejects the focus of psychiatric nursing on caring, as an avoidance of having to challenge medical dominance over issues such as diagnosis. Thus: 'As Jo has said in the past. "A nurse's job is to care, a doctor's job is to diagnose and treat." In a desperate attempt not to step on Dr Brown's toes, all nurses acknowledge that "caring" is the concept that distinguishes nursing from all other professional groups.'

Holyoake's emphasis on professional and clinical autonomy naturally leaves him feeling restricted by fixed roles and specific posts with clearly defined job descriptions, particularly since the profession seems to be unable to decide even on a name for the role, let alone a description of what it should entail. He is therefore reluctant to advocate for the establishment of specific advanced practitioner posts, since 'a post suggests a definite role; flexibility towards clinical settings is essential for the ANP role.' He does acknowledge that this is a dilemma for would-be advanced practitioners, however, and in answer to the question of the difference between a post and a role: 'the role is the doing, but the post seems to pay more'.

This dilemma is addressed in the final chapter of Part 3 by Coombs and Holgate, who propose a framework to guide role development without imposing too many management restrictions. Thus, in response to suggestions such as Goodman's that 'perhaps a key factor for advancing practice is freedom for advanced practitioners to take risks and explore their potential across professional boundaries', they point out that: 'The purpose of this framework was to provide a universal algorithm for all nurses to use, which, although allowing freedom for innovation, also ensured the safety of patients and practitioners alike.' This is perhaps as close as Holyoake is likely to come to the autonomy that he sees as being at the heart of advanced practice. Coombs and Holgate continue: 'The framework would ensure that the nurse undertook roles appropriate to patient need, to an established skill level, and to the level of resourcing. The framework was also seen as a tool that could be used prospectively to direct planning in the establishment of new opportunities for practice development, and could also be used retrospectively to reflect on and audit the practice development. The framework would therefore be useful as a learning tool and a resourcing model, and would provide an evaluation format.'

The framework also attempts to address Holyoake's other defining characteristics of the advanced practitioner as being able to make informed clinical decisions, including nursing diagnoses, being able to justify those decisions rationally, and being able to communicate them to others. As Coombs and Holgate point out, their framework 'provides a language and structure for communication, making it easier for those who wish to learn. The framework can also be used to structure supporting arguments in reply to any challenges to the practice development itself.'

Most important of all, the framework represents an acknowledgement that managers, practitioners and educationalists must work together as equal partners in order to overcome the current confusion about advanced practice. The role of the managers and educationalists in this partnership is to impose the boundaries to what can be done, boundaries that are established by the Government, by the professional bodies, by the trusts and by the universities. However, managers and educationalists should also recognize that, within those boundaries, practitioners must be given the autonomy to develop their practice in response to patient need. Thus: 'The future of nursing and of new nursing roles depends on the values held by nurses and the vision arising from those values', and, in order to pursue that vision: 'Nursing must push beyond the known boundaries of the nursing profession in the interests of improved patient care.' This, surely, is at least in part what is meant by advancing nursing practice.

Part 4

Advancing practice: the professional development perspective

13

Advanced practice and the reflective nurse: developing knowledge out of practice

Gary Rolfe

An epistemology of advanced practice

The role of the advanced practitioner is clearly still developing, and there is as yet little agreement on what it is or what it might become. Most writers would agree, however, that it includes a number of subroles, and, while, these vary somewhat, the majority of commentators, including the United Kingdom Central Council for Nursing, Midwifery and Health Visiting (UKCC) and many of the contributors to this book, would include the subroles of clinical expert, consultant and professional leader in their list. The advanced practitioner should therefore be not only an independent clinical decision maker, able to make sophisticated use of clinical knowledge and skill, but also be able to pass on that expertise. Indeed, this notion of an expert practitioner who also facilitates the clinical and professional development of colleagues is arguably the foundation of the role, which should be concerned not only with *advanced* practice but also with *advancing* practice.

Despite a general consensus about the advanced practitioner possessing, using and communicating expert clinical knowledge and skill, little consideration has been given to precisely what this means or how it is to be achieved, that is, to the epistemology of advanced practice. The current trend in the UK at the moment is for evidence based practice (Department of Health, 1989). The evidence on which the nurse is supposed to base his or her practice is usually considered to be a scientific knowledge base derived primarily from research. This scientific, research based knowledge, however, has little to do with the role of the advanced practitioner, and, ironically, those with most knowledge of this kind are not practitioners but academics and researchers, and those most adept at passing it on to others are educationalists. If advanced practice was to be defined by the possession and communication of research based knowledge (and, as the UKCC is suggesting, by a higher degree that proves possession of that knowledge), then most advanced practitioners would not be practising nurses.

Furthermore, as the philosopher Karl Popper pointed out, research based knowledge (what he called 'World 3 knowledge') is freely available to all in books and journals, and yet most knowledge in the public domain is not actually 'known' by anyone. For example, most nursing libraries contain thousands of journals full of research papers, and, although all of them have probably been read by somebody at some time, the details of the vast majority of them are not remembered by anyone, including the authors. Hence, most scientific knowledge is not known by individual nurses, whether they be novices or advanced practitioners. We therefore need to look elsewhere for the clinical knowledge base that is an attribute of advanced practice, and which distinguishes advanced practitioners from their more junior colleagues.

In fact, even a cursory scan of the literature on the nature of knowledge, both in nursing and in related disciplines, will reveal other forms apart from scientific research based knowledge. Benner (1984), for example, following the terminology of the philosopher Gilbert Ryle, distinguished between 'knowing that' and 'knowing how'. For Ryle (1963), 'knowing that' corresponded to traditional theoretical knowledge, for example, knowing *that* bereaved people generally progress through a number of stages of grieving. In contrast, 'knowing how' corresponded to practical knowledge, for example, knowing *how* to counsel a grieving person.

Schön further developed the concept of 'knowing how' with his notion of knowing-in-action, of knowledge embedded in practice, such that:

> I shall use *knowing-in-action* to refer to the sorts of knowledge we reveal in our intelligent action – publicly observable, physical performances like riding a bicycle and private observations like instant analysis of a balance sheet. In both cases, the knowing is *in* the action. We reveal it by our spontaneous, skillful execution of the performance; and we are characteristically unable to make it verbally explicit (Schön, 1987).

It might seem odd to think of practice as a form of knowing, but, as Popper (1979) points out, such knowledge is organismic or located in the body, and as Usher and Bryant (1989) claim, without such knowing-in-action, practice would be random and purposeless. Furthermore, knowing-in-action is expressed not in words, but in the action itself, and has all the qualities of what Polanyi (1962) had some years earlier described as tacit knowledge, personal knowledge that we all possess but find difficult (if not impossible) to put into words.

Benner was particularly interested in this notion of tacit knowledge, which she saw as the hallmark of expert practice. For Benner, the first step towards becoming an expert was to recognize and employ paradigm cases, particular experiences that are powerful enough to stand out as exemplars of practice. These paradigm cases are neither practical knowing how nor theoretical knowing that, but 'a hybrid between naive practical knowledge and unrefined theoretical knowledge'. Furthermore, many of them are too complex to be transmitted to other people, and therefore represent a store of personal experiential knowledge of individual cases and clinical situations that is unique to the nurse from whose experience it is derived.

Although these individual paradigm cases might be useful if the nurse encounters a similar situation, they are more effective when collected together. Thus: 'Expert nurses develop *clusters of paradigm cases around different patient care issues* so that they approach a patient care situation using past concrete situations much as a researcher uses a paradigm' (Benner, 1984, italics added).

For Benner, then, expertise develops as the practitioner begins to accumulate many similar instances of personal clinical experiences about particular care issues and formulates them into a body of experiential knowledge that is generalizable to other situations. Benner (1984) referred to the application of experiential knowledge as 'intuitive grasp', which 'is available only in situations where a deep background understanding of the situation exists'.

As well as scientific knowledge, the expert nurse therefore also possesses at least two other forms of knowledge. First, there is personal knowledge, Benner's paradigm cases concerning individual patients for whom the nurse is caring, and also concerning the nurse as an individual. Secondly, there is experiential knowledge, what Benner referred to as clusters of paradigm cases around specific issues. Therefore, as well as categorizing nursing knowledge according to whether it is practical knowing how or theoretical knowing that, we can also divide it into the three categories of:

- Scientific knowledge, which exists in books and journals, and which is largely the work of researchers and theoreticians;
- Experiential knowledge, which is Benner's 'clusters of paradigm cases' around particular practice issues, built up over time, and which exists largely in the head of the nurse from whose experience it derives;
- Personal knowledge, which is knowledge or experience of unique separate clinical situations with individual patients, or indeed, of the nurse.

By combining these different ways of categorizing knowledge, we can construct a typology with six forms of knowing (Table 13.1).

Table 13.1. A typology of nursing knowledge

	Theoretical knowledge (knowing that)	Practical knowledge (knowing how)
Scientific knowledge	Things that I know, which I discovered from books and journals, through the media or from a lecture	Things that I can do, which I learnt from books, from instructions or for which I follow a set of procedures
Experiential knowledge	Things that I know, which I discovered from my own experience or which I worked out for myself	Things that I can do, which I worked out for myself, based on my own experiences
Personal knowledge	Things that I know, which relate to specific situations or particular people (including myself), which I discovered from my own personal experience or worked out for myself	Things that I can do, which relate to specific situations or particular people (including myself)

Scientific theoretical knowledge includes all the things the practitioner *knows*, which he or she has discovered from books and journals, through other media, or from lectures, and consists of the body of public, accessible, theoretical knowledge of the discipline. Most of what the practitioner reads in academic journals and textbooks is scientific theoretical knowledge, although, as we saw earlier, Popper claimed that theoretical knowledge largely exists independently of the knower.

Scientific practical knowledge includes all the things the practitioner can *do*, which he or she has learnt from books or instructions, or for which a set of procedures is followed, and which, in these days of evidence based practice, is derived mainly from scientific theoretical knowledge. Most nursing guidelines and procedures are currently based on research and are therefore a form of scientific practical knowledge. Indeed, the International Council of Nurses (1996) recommended the writing and publication of 'clinical practice guidelines' as one of the primary means of turning research into practice.

Experiential theoretical knowledge includes all the things the practitioner *knows*, which he or she has discovered from personal experiences or which the practitioner has worked out unaided. This knowledge cannot be described as scientific, since it has not arisen from scientific research, but it is nevertheless generalizable to other similar cases. For example, personal theories about the importance of touch, based on an individual's experiences, constitutes experiential theoretical knowledge.

Experiential practical knowledge includes all the things the practitioner can *do*, which he or she has worked out unaided, based on personal experiences, and which are often difficult to put into words. Again, this knowledge is generalizable to other similar situations, and often comprises what Benner termed 'clusters of paradigm cases'. Experiential practical knowledge can have two sources. It can arise from experiential theoretical knowledge, for example, the way that the practitioner touches patients therapeutically might be based on personal experiential theories of touch. It can also be a 'mutated' form of scientific practical knowledge. For example, the practitioner might start out by basing therapeutic touch on guidelines derived from research, and then modify his or her actions over time until they become unique to that person. Experiential practical knowledge is the defining characteristic of what Benner referred to as 'expertise'.

Personal theoretical knowledge includes all the things the practitioner *knows*, which relate to specific situations or particular individuals which he or she has discovered from personal experience or worked out unaided. This knowledge can be said to be personal in two ways: it is personal to that individual as the knower (that is, known only to that individual); and it is knowledge of particular persons or situations, rather than of generalizable clusters of paradigm cases, including self-knowledge. Much personal theoretical knowledge consists of the things the practitioner knows about individual patients, including their diagnoses, their particular likes and dislikes, and other social, psychological and medical knowledge, and also of things the practitioner knows about himself or herself in relation to the work.

Finally, *personal practical knowledge* includes the things the practitioner can *do*, which relate to specific situations or particular individuals and which are sometimes difficult to put into words, including what Benner referred to as 'individual paradigm cases'. Much personal practical knowledge is derived from the therapeutic relationships that the practitioner has with the patients, and is knowledge of how to respond to them as unique individuals. For example, the practitioner will know that one particular patient will respond positively to touch, whereas another will not; one will prefer to be called by his first name, another will prefer a more formal form of address.

Different writers have stressed the relative importance of various types of knowledge. The Department of Health values scientific theoretical knowledge; Benner argues that experiential practical knowledge is the hallmark of expertise; and Radwin (1995) claims that personal knowledge or 'knowing the patient' is valued most highly by the nursing profession. Many would agree, however, that a combination and synthesis of all these types of knowledge is most desirable (Clarke et al., 1996; Rolfe, 1998), and also that the balance between them shifts, as the nurse becomes more experienced, from an emphasis on theoretical and scientific knowledge as a novice practitioner to a growing reliance on practical and experiential knowledge as an expert (Benner, 1984). It would appear, then, that advanced practice might have a great deal in common with Benner's notion of expertise.

Expertise

Benner described five levels of practice from novice to expert. At one extreme, the novice practises according to explicit rules, 'on abstract principles and formal models and theories' (Benner, 1984). At the other extreme, the expert transcends rules and procedures and practises from an intuitive grasp of particular situations. This intuitive grasp is based not on the context-free rules of the novice, but on concrete paradigm cases drawn from the nurse's own experience, that is, on personal and experiential practical knowledge.

For Benner, expertise is an unconscious act in which the expert practitioner 'matches' a situation with a similar situation from a personal, stored repertoire of paradigm cases (experiential practical knowledge), much as a chess grandmaster 'zeroes in' on the correct move from a mental store of thousands of possibilities. If challenged to rationalize the action, the practitioner is unable to do so; if the practitioner attempts to describe it in terms of rules or algorithms (scientific knowledge), what is described is not expertise, but a lower level of practice. In Polanyi's (1962) words, the expert practitioner 'knows more than [s]he can say' and practises from a largely tacit knowledge base. The practitioner is working intuitively rather than according to an underlying logical process, but, as Benner points out, this intuitive process should not be confused with mysticism. Nevertheless, the expert practitioner is unable to account rationally for the process of intuitive grasp, since it does not follow any explicit, or even implicit, rules; it is 'understanding without a rationale' (Benner and Tanner, 1987), and 'the expert is simply not following any rules! He is ... recognising thousands of special cases' (Dreyfus and Dreyfus, 1986).

If, as Benner claims, expertise is understanding without a rationale, then presumably expert actions cannot be justified by an appeal to logical analysis. As an expert psychiatric nurse cited by Benner put it:

> When I say to a doctor 'the patient is psychotic', I don't always know how to legitimize the statement. But I am never wrong. Because I know psychosis from inside out. And I feel that, and I know it, and I trust it (Benner, 1984).

As the nurse says, she cannot legitimize her statement with a reasoned chain of argument; she simply *feels* that she is right. For Benner, then, expertise is not only an unknown process but an unknowable one; indeed, it is debatable whether she would conceptualize it as a process at all. Although Benner is at pains to distinguish intuitive grasp from mysticism, in practice it is rather difficult to say how they differ.

Benner regards the level of expertise as the highest level of practice, and as we have seen, it is tempting to associate it with advanced practice. However, I have two fundamental objections to this view. First, for reasons that will become apparent, I believe that there are difficulties in attaching the label of 'advanced' to a practice that is, in essence, an unconscious process, or what Langer (1989) calls 'mindless'. Secondly, I disagree with Benner that what she describes as expertise is, in fact, the highest level of achievable practice.

Beyond expertise

The knowledge base from which Benner's expert is practising is largely experiential practical knowledge, with some personal practical knowledge, and, as she rightly points out, this knowledge base is largely tacit and cannot be put into words. This, of course, does not present a particular problem for the expert practitioner in everyday work, since the difficulty with practice based on tacit knowledge lies not in the doing, but in the telling of the doing. However, for the advanced practitioner, part of whose role is a consultant and professional leader charged with the job of 'adjusting the boundaries for the development of future practice, pioneering and developing new roles responsive to changing needs and with advancing clinical practice, research and education in order to enrich professional practice as a whole' (United Kingdom Central Council for Nursing, Midwifery and Health Visiting, 1994), the telling is arguably as important as the doing. If the advanced practitioner is to advance clinical practice through clinical supervision, education and research, then the practitioner needs to be able to gain access to his or her own clinical knowledge base; the practitioner requires an insight into her own *modus operandi*. It is not enough to say, as Benner's psychiatric nurse did, that, although she could not legitimize her clinical decisions, she was nevertheless never wrong since, 'I feel that, and I know it, and I trust it.' Similarly, as Dreyfus and Dreyfus (1986) pointed out (they were writing about how doctors practise, but what they say can equally be applied to nurses):

> In reality, a patient is viewed by the experienced doctor as a unique case and treated on the basis of intuitively perceived similarity with situations previously encountered. *That kind of wisdom, unfortunately, cannot be shared* and thereby made the basis of a doctor's rational decision (italics added).

If the advanced practitioner is to carry out the role suggested by the UKCC and those roles described in this book, then the practitioner's wisdom *must* be shared, and he or she must therefore have personal free and conscious access to it.

Clearly, then, the advanced practitioner needs to be aware of the knowledge base underpinning his or her practice, but the problem, as

Benner (1984) points out, is that 'if experts are made to attend to the particulars or to a formal model or rule, their performance actually deteriorates'. Benner takes this to mean that if the expert is mindful of what he or she is doing while doing it, then performance will suffer. Dreyfus and Dreyfus, from whom Benner borrowed her model of expertise, claim that this can be seen quite clearly from examples such as driving a car or playing the piano. Expert car drivers or pianists are not conscious of their performance; they drive or play without having to pay attention to what they are doing. The expert driver changes up and down through the gears intuitively, and it is only when forced to consciously think about what he or she is doing that mistakes are made, as, for example, when driving an unfamiliar car. Thus:

> Have you ever been driving effortlessly along a city street in a stick-shift car and suddenly found yourself consciously thinking about the gear you are in and whether it's appropriate? Chances are the sudden reflection upon what you were doing and the rules for doing it was accompanied by a severe degradation of performance; perhaps you shifted at the wrong time or into the wrong gear (Dreyfus and Dreyfus, 1986).

The experiential practical knowledge base of the expert is tacit; it cannot be expressed in words. Furthermore, if we attempt to focus on it during practice, our practice deteriorates. As we have seen, the advanced practitioner needs to be able to gain access to, and share the knowledge that underpins that person's clinical practice if the individual is to advance his or her own practice and that of colleagues. For the expert, this presents an enormous problem, since such a person's practice is based almost entirely on practical knowledge or 'knowing how'. What the expert, as Benner describes this person, does not have is experiential or personal *theoretical* knowledge or 'knowing that'. This practitioner can *do*, often to a very impressive standard, but, as Benner's psychiatric nurse demonstrated, is unable to say *why* or *how* he or she can do; the practitioner has the know-how but not the know-that.

Where does this personal and experiential theoretical knowledge come from? Clearly not from books or from scientific research in the way that scientific theoretical knowledge does. In fact, the relationship between experiential theoretical knowledge and experiential practical knowledge is the very opposite of that between scientific theoretical knowledge and scientific practical knowledge. Scientific theoretical knowledge, in the form of research findings or theoretical models, informs and develops scientific practical knowledge in the form of procedures and guidelines. However, experiential theoretical knowledge is informed *by* and arises *from* experiential practical knowledge through the process of reflection-on-action. In the case of scientific knowledge, theory informs practice; in the case of experiential knowledge, practice informs theory.

Thus, experiential (and personal) theoretical knowledge can be developed only by practitioners with a well-founded practical knowledge base on which to reflect. First we learn to do, then we learn, through reflection, to explain how and why we do. Benner's experts never get beyond the doing; they might well be expert at doing nursing, but they cannot articulate the underlying theory. Indeed, they would claim that there *is* no underlying theory, that they are practising intuitively.

However, a theoretical explanation of the process of expert practice has been expounded by a number of writers. Thus, Brook and Champion (1991) reject the notion of irrational intuition and argue that expert practice involves the formulation and testing of hypotheses during the process of practice; Elstein and Bordage (1988) point out that 'it seems practically impossible to reason without hypotheses whenever the data base is as complex as it typically is in clinical problems'; Andrews (1996) claims that so-called intuition is a complex, critical skill, closely related to what Schön refers to as reflection-in-action (not to be confused with reflection-*on*-action, which happens after the event); and, as Schön (1987) notes:

> When the practitioner reflects in action...his experience is at once exploratory, move testing, and hypothesis testing. The three functions are fulfilled by the very same actions. And from this fact follows the distinctive character of experimenting in practice.

It would appear, then, that expert clinical decision making might not be the unknowable and irrational process that Benner imagines it to be, but rather an unconscious form of hypothesis construction and testing. Even Benner herself appears to recognize this when she writes that 'expertise develops when the clinician tests and refines propositions, hypotheses, and principle-based expectations in actual practice situations' (Benner, 1984). If the process is rational and knowable, then it should be possible to elevate it into consciousness, and thereby to transcend Benner's fifth and final level of unconscious expertise with a sixth level of mindful advanced practice.

Knowledge and the advanced practitioner

What is required in order to elevate this tacit 'knowing how' into consciousness, then, is to reflect on it and thereby transform it into propositional 'knowing that'. Benner's expert nurse might be able to say, with a high degree of accuracy, whether a patient is psychotic, but the advanced practitioner, with a body of experiential and personal theoretical knowledge, will be able also to say *how* he or she knows that the patient is psychotic; the advanced practitioner will be able to verbalize her experiential and personal knowledge. When asked to account for her practice, the advanced practitioner will be able to explain exactly how he or she knows what he or she knows and does what he or she does. Unlike Benner's psychiatric nurse, the advanced practitioner would be able to state exactly how to legitimize the statement: 'the patient is psychotic'. The advanced practitioner would do so by reference to textbook and research based knowledge, by citing past case histories of similar patients with whom he or she had worked, and by drawing on specific knowledge about this particular patient and about the therapeutic relationship already built up with that person. The advanced practitioner would, in all probability, come to a decision about the patient in exactly the same way as Benner's expert, but would be able to rationalize and justify that statement, and furthermore, would also be able to pass on this knowledge to others.

I am arguing, then, that different levels of practice can be defined by the different kinds of knowledge employed by the nurse in directing that practice. The novice, straight out of college, has a reasonable scientific theoretical knowledge base from books and lectures, and can apply it in the form of scientific practical knowledge by following rules and procedures (Table 13.2a). As the novice gains experience, experiential and personal practical knowledge bases develop, until the knowledge profile of the expert is acquired (Table 13.2b). However, we have seen that this practical knowledge is tacit; it cannot be explained to others, neither is it recognized by the practitioner, who claims to practise intuitively. Finally, by reflecting on experiential and personal practical knowledge, in clinical supervision or by keeping a reflective journal, the practitioner builds a store of experiential and personal theoretical knowledge (Table 13.2c), which is the hallmark of advanced practice.

Table 13.2. Some knowledge profiles

(a) Novice practitioner		(b) Expert practitioner		(c) Advanced practitioner	
Scientific theoretical knowledge	Scientific practical knowledge	Scientific theoretical knowledge	Scientific practical knowledge	Scientific theoretical knowledge	Scientific practical knowledge
–	–	–	Experimental practical knowledge	Experimental theoretical knowledge	Experimental practical knowledge
–	–	–	Personal practical knowledge	Personal theoretical knowledge	Personal practical knowledge

Thus, whereas Benner's expert lacks the experiential and personal theoretical knowledge base necessary to articulate tacit experiential know-how, the advanced practitioner, through reflection-on-action, has a readily accessible body of personal and experiential knowledge through which to advance personal practice and that of colleagues. Benner's psychiatric nurse might well be an expert, but this nurse is not an advanced practitioner, since all he or she can offer to colleagues is the reassurance that he or she is never wrong. The advanced practitioner is an educator in ways in which the expert can never be. As Schön (1983) points out:

> When people use such terms as 'art' and 'intuition', they usually intend to terminate discussion rather than to open up inquiry. It is as though the practitioner says to his academic colleague, 'While I do not accept *your* view of knowledge, I cannot describe my own.' Sometimes, indeed, the practitioner appears to say, 'My kind of knowledge is indescribable', or even, 'I will not attempt to describe it lest I paralyse myself.' These attitudes have contributed to a widening rift between the universities and the professions, research and practice, thought and action.

The advanced practitioner seeks to narrow the gap between the universities and the professions, research and practice, thought and action, by articulating and synthesizing different knowledge bases, but, more importantly, *advances* practice by not only practising what he or she preaches, but by preaching what he or she practices.

References

Andrews, M. (1996). Using reflection to develop clinical expertise. *Br. J. Nurs.*, **5**, 508–513.
Benner, P. (1984). *From Novice to Expert*. Menlo Park, CA: Addison-Wesley.
Benner, P. and Tanner, C. (1987). Clinical judgement: how expert nurses use intuition. *Am. J. Nurs.*, **87**(1), 23–31.
Brook, V. and Champion, E. (1991). *The Reflective Practitioner*. Tiverton: Fairway Publications.
Clarke, B., James, C. and Kelly, J. (1996). Reflective practice: reviewing the issues and refocusing the debate. *Int. J. Nurs. Stud.*, **33**, 171–180.
Department of Health. (1989). *A Strategy for Nursing: A Report of the Steering Committee*. London: DoH.
Dreyfus, H. L. and Dreyfus, S. E. (1986). *Mind Over Machine*. Oxford: Basil Blackwell.
Elstein, A. S. and Bordage, G. (1988). Psychology of clinical reasoning. In *Professional Judgement*. (J. Dowie and A. Elstein, eds.) pp. 109–129. Cambridge: Cambridge University Press.
International Council of Nurses. (1996). *Better Health Through Nursing Research*. Geneva: ICN.
Langer, E. J. (1989). *Mindfulness*. London: Harper Collins.
Polanyi, M. (1962). *Personal Knowledge: Towards a Post-critical Philosophy*. London: Routledge and Kegan Paul.
Popper, K. (1979) *Objective Knowledge: an Evolutionary Approach*, revised edition. Oxford: Oxford University Press.
Radwin, L. E. (1995). Knowing the patient: a process model for individualized interventions, *Nurs. Res.*, **44**, 364–370.
Rolfe, G. (1998). *Expanding Nursing Knowledge: Understanding and Researching Your Own Practice*. Oxford: Butterworth-Heinemann.
Ryle, G. (1963). *The Concept of Mind*. Harmondsworth: Penguin.
Schön, D. A. (1983). *The Reflective Practitioner*. London: Temple Smith.
Schön, D. A. (1987). *Educating the Reflective Practitioner*. San Francisco, CA: Jossey-Bass.
United Kingdom Central Council for Nursing, Midwifery and Health Visiting. (1994). *The Future of Professional Practice – The Council's Standards for Education and Practice Following Registration*. London: UKCC.
Usher, R. and Bryant, I. (1989). *Adult Education as Theory, Practice and Research*. London: Routledge.

14

Knowing and realizing advanced practice through guided reflection

Chris Johns

This account is of work that has taken place between myself and Helen within guided reflection or clinical supervision.* The two terms are used interchangeably. Clinical supervision has become a focus for attention as a result of *A Vision for the Future* (National Health Service Management Executive, 1993). This document sets out 12 targets for the development of nursing, midwifery and health visiting. Target 10 defines clinical supervision as:

> a term used to describe a formal process of professional support and learning which enables practitioners to develop knowledge and competence, assume responsibility for their own practice and enhance consumer protection and safety of care in complex situations. It is central to the process of learning and to the expansion of the scope of practice and should be seen as a means of encouraging self-assessment and analytical and reflective skills.

From this definition, it can be seen that supervision has a number of intentions. Central to these intentions is the notion of developing and sustaining effective practice.

Helen is a clinical nurse specialist in nutrition in an acute general hospital. This account is structured through our dialogue, which focused around a number of experiences that Helen shared in supervision, and includes my commentary on the meaning of her work in terms of what might be construed as 'advanced practice'. Helen and I have been working together in supervision since January 1995. We aim to meet for 1 hour every 3 weeks. In essence, guided reflection involves my guidance of Helen's learning through her reflection-on-experience, which is a window through which to view herself within the context of her practice. The focus of learning through reflection is to expose, confront, and work towards resolving the contradictions between what is desirable and what is practised. It is the conflict of contradiction and the commitment to achieve desirable work that fuels this process, through the challenge and support of guidance

*My work with Helen was part of a research project funded by a Smith and Nephew Foundation Fellowship. The narrative of Helen's first 12 months in guided reflection is available, along with 13 similar narratives of working with practitioners within guided reflection/clinical supervision, as a model for developing clinical leadership.

(Johns 1994a, 1996). Helen writes accounts of her experiences in a reflective diary structured through her use of the 'model of structured reflection' (Johns, 1995) in order to prepare her for sharing her experiences with me.

Guiding reflection is simply a person being available effectively to challenge and support the practitioner's transformative journey towards new horizons of practice. Guidance acknowledges that reflection alone is an arduous task. Effective supervision is the balance of high support/high challenge to confront contradiction, and high support to sustain the commitment, courage and effort to resolve the contradictions and transform the self as necessary to become effective in achieving desirable work. As I will illustrate throughout this account, achieving desirable work involved Helen 'seeing beyond and confronting herself', to see how she had embodied forces that had limited her ability to achieve this.

From this understanding, learning hinges around achieving and sustaining desirable work. Indeed, a sense of knowing what work is or might be would seem to be the primary notion for understanding 'advanced practice'. Helen does not conceptualize herself as an advanced practitioner. Indeed, when I asked her if she felt she might be an advanced practitioner she just laughed. The concept felt alien.

Speculating what 'advanced' might mean

Perhaps from a research and development perspective, advanced could mean scouting and exploring the territory, rather like the advanced guard of some army of nurses, always looking to expand their territory and needing to know the changing landscapes and horizons. In contrast to expanding the territory, advanced might also mean advancing what is held to be known, in other words, redefining existing landscapes and reshaping known horizons. An advanced practitioner would then be someone who can respond effectively within either of these new or redefined areas of practice. The notion that 'advanced' might distinguish levels of practice is less attractive; it would become an arbitrary concept constituted in terms of artificial criteria. For example, how would advanced be distinguished from basic? What would such a distinction hope to achieve? Perhaps the need for 'advanced nursing' derives from the fact that nurses have not been adequately prepared for the roles they currently undertake. I certainly feel that existing nursing roles have not been well-defined, or have been ill-defined within inappropriate conceptualizations of what constitutes health from a medical model perspective.

Distinctions between levels of expertise have been popularized within the idea of a continuum between novice and expert (Benner, 1984). From this perspective, the notion of advanced could then be seen as *advancing along* this continuum towards expert practice, irrespective of which 'specialty' the nurse works in. The arbitrariness of this distinction will become entwined in what might otherwise be referred to as specialism, a distinction made in conjunction with a specialized field of medicine or health care, and characterized by particular skills and knowledge associated with that specialty that the 'general practitioner' might not possess. The notion of linking 'advanced' to role, in the sense that a nurse 'advances' up a career structure, has usually been associated with increased responsibility, which sharpens the need for certain abilities in order to carry out this responsibility effectively.

At this point I am not going to draw any conclusions to these meandering thoughts. Instead I will invite the reader to gaze at Helen's practice through the rich detailed dialogue of guided reflection, and offer my analysis of this dialogue in terms of reflecting on the central question of what might be construed as characteristic of advanced practice? However, I am going to assume that advanced practice cannot be an accumulation of bits of skills. It can only be a holistic concept, a unitary way of being, and responding effectively to practice in consistent and congruent ways with what the nurse intends to achieve.

Since being in guided reflection, Helen had written a philosophy for her practice (Figure 14.1). Her approach to this work followed the approach of *The Burford NDU Model. Caring in Practice* (Johns, 1994b). Helen also decided to structure her practice using this model because of its reflective nature.

Clinical nurse specialist, nutrition

Philosophy of care
I believe...

- That nursing care offered by the clinical nurse specialist (CNS) in nutrition is centred around the needs of the patient. To this end, the CNS will be available to teach and support patients receiving nutritional support, which will enable them to become partners in their own care. Care is extended to the patient's family and friends as desired.

- That care should be holistic in nature, whether towards recovery through the use of aggressive nutritional support, or towards adaptation with altered health states, including death. At all times, the patient's safety and comfort are paramount. The patient's right to confidentiality and privacy will be respected.

- That when nutritional support is continued after discharge from hospital, the CNS will ensure the provision of seamless care. To this end, patients discharged on nutritional support will have received adequate teaching, and equipment, and will feel supported by the CNS, in association with other health care workers, until they become confident to continue independently.

- That the CNS may act as primary carer or role model and teacher of nurses and other carers. In so doing, the CNS will strive continually to improve patient care by implementing appropriate research findings, and by ongoing evaluation of care. This develops the social value of nursing, and enables others to benefit from the CNS's expertise.

- That in order to be effective, the CNS will need to manage conflict, and so will share her feelings at appropriate times openly. She will support others when needed, reciprocating the caring approach to patients.

Figure 14.1. Helen's philosophy of practice

Framing practice in terms of 'advanced nursing models' is perhaps a significant issue. As Helen's philosophy indicates, her framework for practice involved a belief system that was:

- Focused on holism – that people cannot be reduced to parts or systems without losing their wholeness as human beings;
- Family centred;
- Health focused – in contrast with a health deficit model;
- Based on partnership – that patients' health is their primary responsibility and, hence, they need expert support to enable them to find meaning in the health experience in order to make the best decisions about their future.

Framing practice within such models moves nursing towards being a therapy in its own right and towards complementary and collaborative relationships with other health care workers.

Working with Gerry

In session 21 (26 July, 1996), Helen talked about Gerry, a young man with AIDS: 'I received a telephone call from a staff nurse on a medical ward concerning a patient who had had a "port" inserted 2 weeks ago. They had tried to use it to give drugs but could neither infuse fluids nor withdraw blood. Could I help? The selfish part of me wanted to say "no" because I was busy and this was obviously not a quick fix-it job. The other part of me responded to the staff and patient crisis, so I said I would try to help.

'Gerry, the patient, told me that "everything that can go wrong has gone wrong". He put on what appeared to be an amazing front of cheerfulness; at this stage, I didn't know him well enough to challenge this front. Gerry said he was totally frustrated because this "simple procedure" to insert the port had taken 4 hours instead of 30 minutes. He was unable to use the port so he still had to have drugs peripherally. No one seemed to know what to do next.

'I said I could not promise to solve the problem but that I was there to try. He seemed relieved. My first thought was that the Huber needles were too short, so we agreed to assess the port properly by venogram to look for kinks or thrombi. He agreed, but [the radiotherapist] could not inject radio-opaque dye, so we needed the larger needle to do this.

'Next day, the larger needles arrived and I was able to flush the port out with saline, but the pressure required was still too great to allow a vacuum infusion of Gerry's drugs. I still felt he needed a venogram. The consultant surgeon was asked by the medical consultant to review, as the port had been inserted by her registrar. She asked me to go with her. She then said to Gerry that he needed another venogram with the larger needle and then, if the line would not work, she would remove it and replace it with a Hickman line. Gerry became very agitated and said that he must have a port, he couldn't bear the idea of a Hickman, and that we shouldn't talk of replacement when we didn't yet know what the problem was with the initial port line. This was meant to be for his convenience, not the staff's! I stayed with him and absorbed his anger and frustration. The facade began to slip. I said that to him and Gerry began to cry. We talked of his hopes, his loss, his impending blindness and his frustration. Then, just as quickly as the facade had slipped, he dismissed me. I understood his need for that. I felt very sad for him. I also recalled the identification with my first young cancer patient.

This was my closest confrontation with a young AIDS patient and it was painful. However, the way for me to deal with that was to help Gerry to get what he needed to go on with his treatment, if that was what he wished. I felt immensely angry with the registrar for his arrogance: "I can put the line in."

'On Wednesday morning Gerry had a repeat venogram – it was totally unhelpful. The consultant surgeon phoned me to ask what was happening and offered again to "put something else in". I said that, for Gerry, it had to be a port. She joked that HIV patients were always so demanding; a cancer patient would accept a Hickman. She said: "Well, I could do that. I'm just really embarrassed that this has gone wrong. I've put in lots of ports but my registrar assured me that he could do it. Perhaps we'll have to make sure in future that it is a consultant procedure. After all it's rarely an emergency procedure." I agreed and said that I thought she had been let down. I said that I would discuss the offer with Gerry.

'That afternoon I went to see Gerry. He was having his drugs peripherally. He seemed totally exhausted and close to tears. I told him about this offer. Gerry became angry and said: "She didn't even look at me – she was rude. It's my life not hers! She can go to hell, she's not touching me!" I listened and just stayed with him. Then we looked at alternatives. Gerry sheepishly asked for permission to go to St Michael's as he had his first eye appointment there the next day. I encouraged and supported him with this and confirmed that we would think no less of him. Our door was still open to him but that might be the best option for him. He cried and then dismissed me. On Thursday, Gerry attended St Michael's. Within 30 minutes they had discovered that the port was too small and was kinked. Three days later, they inserted a new one and it's working well.

'Now, on reflection, I feel angry with doctors for attempting things they shouldn't. I feel let down by "experts" who will attempt X-rays they can't interpret. I have channelled this anger by completing a risk management form and discussing it with the Chief Nurse. I am helping (Genito-urinary Medicine) clinic to write a protocol on managing ports, but I have insisted that it must be multidisciplinary and comprehensive to involve such issues as who places the line, what do we order, and who teaches patients, carers and nurses. This experience has confirmed my own practice related knowledge with regard to "ports" and connects with other doctor related incidents with regard to their skills and attitudes. I was able to use the distress I felt to challenge the status quo and to protect future patients. Gerry can have the last word: "Helen – thank you for trying. At least you could see me".'

I challenged Helen with her role responsibility and ethical responsibility within her decision to become involved in this situation. Helen felt managing ports was in her sphere of responsibility, in that total parental nutrition (TPN) could be delivered through this route. From an ethical perspective, Helen felt she was driven by an ethic of care, that here was a patient in some distress who she felt she could help. However, she also acknowledged that she had responded because she wanted to be acknowledged and valued by doctors. This had become a major theme in Helen's work in guided reflection. As this story unfolds, Helen is a powerful player controlling the scenario with consultants who are requesting her advice and help. Helen noted: 'I felt good that the consultant rang me to go to see the patient.'

I challenged Helen about why she felt so sad. She noted that she had a sense of identification with Gerry. He was the same age as her and she felt drawn towards him. She also reacted against the negative attitudes by doctors towards an HIV patient. I termed the phrase 'levels of prejudice'; it was not so bad because he wasn't gay, but worse because 'it' was HIV rather than a more socially accepted cancer. I drew Helen's attention to some literature on nurses' attitudes to patients with AIDS (McHaffie, 1992). I felt Helen had to some extent compensated for the negative attitude of others. She agreed that this might be true. I challenged whether her sense of sadness was pity or compassion. I made the distinction between pity and compassion based on the work by Stephen Levine (1986), that pity was an expression of one's own discomfort rather than genuine concern for another. Helen responded: 'I felt compassion, a genuine reaching out to him in his distress.'

I pointed out to Helen how she had been available to the consultant and supported her, despite her negative attitudes. This was more significant in the light of Helen's residual anger. I challenged her over whether this was a reflection of having absorbed Gerry's distress. Was it healthy for Helen to feel such a sense of moral outrage? Managing her 'feelings' is central to managing her involvement with patients from a holistic perspective. Helen has no choice but to engage her own feelings in responding to another's distress, yet she accepts this. Becoming involved and managing her involvement was another strand of Helen's work within guided reflection, as she strived to embrace her new philosophy of responding to patients and families from this holistic perspective. This work can be seen in contrast to her 'technical problem to solve' perspective when we had commenced working together some 18 months earlier.

Picking up her anger, I affirmed that it was acceptable to be sad for Gerry and outraged at the consultant, because these were human responses to Gerry's distress and to the incompetence of others to respond adequately. Helen demonstrated how she had channelled this negative energy into taking positive action. I reminded her of Lydia Hall's words (1964) that:

> Anxiety over an extended period is stressful to all the organ functions. It prepares the individual to fight or flight. In our culture, however, it is brutal to fight and cowardly to flee, so we stew in our own juices and cook up malfunction. This energy can be put to use in exploration of feelings through participation in the struggle to face and solve problems underlying the state of anxiety.

I also challenged Helen's decision to take a back seat on developing the protocol. I suggested that she needed to lead this endeavour, because she did not trust others to do a good job. This activity would also make her power visible. She agreed.

In Session 22 (15 August, 1996), Helen admitted that she had not picked up Gerry's care with the GUM clinic. Neither had she taken forward the port guidelines. I asked: 'Why not?' Helen retorted: 'Because I'm up to my ears in work!' We agreed on one exclamation mark! Helen had read the McHaffie paper. She said 'It confirmed what we already knew. It was interesting but I was not particularly surprised by what I read.'

Commentary

How might the notion of advanced practice be understood within this text? One assumption is to claim that the essence of advanced practice is the practitioner's ability to be available to work with the 'person' towards achieving 'desirable work'. The claim is not flimsy. I identified 'being available' as the core therapeutic factor in achieving effective work based on realizing *The Burford NDU Model: Caring in Practice* model in practice (Johns, 1996). The extent to which the practitioner can be available is influenced by a number of dimensions (Figure 14.2). Each of these is visible within my dialogue with Helen.

The practitioner is available to work with the patient and family in supporting them to meet their health needs

{
Knowing what is desirable
Concern
Knowing the person
The aesthetic response
Knowing and managing self
Creating and sustaining an environment where being available is possible
}

Figure 14.2. 'Being available' template

Knowing what is desirable

Helen's beliefs about her relationship with Gerry are very visible within the account. She sees and responds to him primarily as a person. His 'problem' with the port is seen within the context of what this experience means to him. From this perspective, she sets out to tune into him in order for them to work together. She creates an opportunity for him to make decisions and acts on his behalf with others as necessary.

Concern

Helen is truly concerned for Gerry. She 'sees' him through the diagnostic label and attitudes of others; being concerned, Gerry matters to her. Her concern sets up possibility (Benner and Wrubel, 1989). My guidance was explicitly intended to nurture and fan this concern.

Knowing the person

Hall (1964) noted that we can only nurse what the patient allows us to see. As such, Helen's skill is to know the person, to penetrate the masks that protect or obscure the other. The existential issue is to see the person within a holistic or unitary perspective (Rogers, 1986). Helen's use of *The Burford NDU model: Caring in Practice* gives her this perspective by tuning her into her beliefs and values within each unfolding clinical moment.

Knowing and managing involvement of self

To respond from a holistic perspective, Helen's 'use of self' is her primary therapeutic tool. To engage another's spirituality and emotions is a spiritual and emotional experience for her. She feels Gerry's sadness. She is outraged at the attitudes of others. She is distressed. As Benner and Wrubel (1989) note: 'whilst caring sets up possibilities it also sets up what counts as vulnerable'. Helen illustrates how she has learnt to understand and manage self, so these feelings or energy can be used positively. Understanding the significance of this work highlights how practitioners like Helen need to be self-aware and have access to support to know and sustain self.

Responding with appropriate and skilled interventions

For Helen, all interventions are viewed within the holistic caring perspective. In this way she juxtaposes her highly specialized technical role with caring. It is significant how consultants consult her for advice and how she becomes Gerry's key worker and advocate. It is Helen who makes the decisions about his care, who gives him permission, who cradles him in his distress, who supports others.

In responding, Helen must grasp and interpret the situation in the moment and be quite clear what she hopes to achieve in negotiation with Gerry. She then responds appropriately. Her work is constantly to increase her repertoire of appropriate interventions. However, it is pertinent to note that her major intervention is 'being there' with Gerry. Helen uses cathartic, catalytic and supportive interventions with him, and confrontational interventions in the face of other health care workers' inappropriate responses (see Heron's 'Six category intervention analysis' (1975), as a framework for considering and rehearsing the therapeutic interventions necessary to respond adequately within any situation).

The 'technical' decisions, and Helen's necessary technical expertise, are relatively straightforward and only complicated in terms of what is best for Gerry. Helen provides this ethical milieu and acts as Gerry's advocate in terms of enabling him to make the best decisions for himself. Gadow (1980) refers to this intervention as 'existential advocacy'. In doing so, Helen inhabits and asserts the powerful moral high ground.

Responding within the clinical situation has been described as the aesthetic response (Carper, 1978; Johns, 1995). How the practitioner responds is influenced by the ethical: 'How should I respond in this situation?'; the personal: acknowledging that who I am is the major factor in the care I give; and the empirical: 'What information is useful to inform my decisions?'

From the empirical perspective, I help Helen to identify relevant theory and research to juxtapose with her knowing-in-practice accessed through reflection. In this way, the theory becomes relevant and is more likely to be assimilated into constructed knowing (Belenky et al., 1986). Perhaps it is only through reflection that research and theory can be meaningfully assimilated into practice. Clearly the 'advanced' practitioner is an informed practitioner, but in ways that are evident through practice rather than merely espoused.

Creating and sustaining an environment where being available is possible

By 'environment' I mean the context of practice and the practitioner's sense of control of her environment in order to be able to respond appropriately. Helen's time is at a premium. She chose to spend her time in this way and indeed felt able to prioritize her work, unimpeded by constraints of others.

Resources are scarce and the use of time is an ethical consideration. Helen's response within the situation reflects a sense of her 'powerful self' and its expression through appropriate assertiveness in working with others. Helen has had to work hard (reflected in her earlier shared experiences) to develop collaborative-type relationships with doctors that facilitate caring. This has been a constant focus for her attention within guided reflection, as she struggled to be valued and acknowledged by doctors, yet she has done this while being true to her beliefs. In doing so, she raises the status of nursing in the eyes of patients and doctors. It is poignant to note how Helen acts to support the consultant while asserting what needs to be done. Helen has learnt to work with traditionally more powerful others, so her expertise is sought and valued.

Working with Emily and her family

Having explicated and illustrated the dimensions of what might be construed as advanced practice, consider the dialogue between myself and Helen in session 23 (9 September, 1996). Helen shared her experience of working with Emily, an 11-month-old girl who had been diagnosed as having a small bowel atresia.

Helen: The mother was offered a termination, but had declined this. On birth, this was very severe, indeed incompatible with life, and shouldn't be treated. However, the mother resisted this. Emily had an operation that increased the gut length 30 cm. A metre was needed to sustain life without TPN. So we were in serious trouble. The doctor's view was that treatment should be withdrawn. The parents are young, unmarried. The grandmother on the mother's side is very powerful. They had met parents of other children who were on home TPN programmes and demanded this for Emily. Emily has had lots of setbacks but she has survived. However, one of her complications is liver failure, so we now have a child who is TPN dependent, with liver damage and gross ascites. She has been referred for consideration for bowel and liver transplant. Then she went off neurologically and needed to be ventilated. A scan showed a large subdural haematoma. The clot was evacuated but this left her with permanent brain damage. She now responds as a 6-week-old baby.

CJ: How was that caused?

Helen: I know, it's curious. As a consequence, she was no longer appropriate for the transplant so she was sent home for terminal care. Then it came to us. I received a phone call asking me to come to a 'professionals'' meeting. My thoughts: 'please don't send her home on TPN!'

On Thursday I went to the ward to read the notes. It was written: 'Go home for terminal care.' I spoke to the ward charge nurse and asked him what were we trying to achieve. She was spending 8 hours between her TPN although she still needed a Hickman line for giving heparin. I returned after lunch to discuss it, expecting to discuss expectations before Emily's parents arrived. But then they arrived. No chance to ask the consultant: 'What are we going to do?'

Emily's grandmother was there: short skirt, dripping in jewellery, aggressive. The health visitor was also there, clearly on the side of the parents.

CJ: Interesting use of words: 'on the side of' – as if a battle was anticipated?

Helen smiled: She challenged me: 'How are you going to get this child home on TPN?!' She pointed out that this child had spent only 2 hours at home since she was born!

CJ: Could you resist this?

Helen: I did. I picked up the issues of the neck line and outlined what it would take to support her at home. I related this to David, another young child who was at home on TPN, and offered to put the parents in touch with his parents. I was challenged by grandmother about taking bloods every day: 'How would this be done?' I resisted this, adding that daily bloods would not be necessary.

CJ: What about this 'terminal' label? What does this mean?

Helen: I know the death cannot be predicted. The health purchaser would have to approve the cost of supporting the child on TPN. They could say 'no'. There was no discussion on other issues, for example, issues such as treating repeated infections. There was no impression that Emily's parents thought that she was going to die.

CJ: There is an issue here about being open and honest and being sensitive, although this may be more accurately put as protecting our own feelings rather than being sensitive to the parents' needs?

Helen: I know. I felt no support from others. It was: 'How are YOU going to do it?' I felt angry about that.

CJ: And still angry?

Helen: No.

CJ: So how has it worked out?

Helen: After the meeting people took their leave. I waited to speak with the grandmother and parents. I said to them: 'It must be hard for you to walk into this meeting, and wondering what was going to be said.' It felt useful, the grandmother was upset.

CJ: Perhaps we need to re-orientate the problem from a technical one to an emotional one?

Helen: That's why I stayed! Lots of anger had gone by the time I left. I thought of alternatives: to take Emily's central line out. She had been to the West Country since she's been at home. She was wide awake and noisy, so much she hasn't slept – she's been so stimulated! They have been very pleased to have this time with her. All they had to worry about was changing her nappy, no drips to do. At the meeting, the grandmother was angry about the size of cot Emily needed because of her ascites. Yet they will have to buy a cot because they can't get one supplied. Small things like that illustrate lack of sensitivity and wind you up!

CJ: Have the professionals paid enough attention to the emotional side?

Helen: No. I have been back to the ward nurses and challenged them: 'What to do, what is right?' It is difficult for them to talk about emotional care. This is a difficult family. The nurses *are* making the effort to put Emily first. There is poor communication between the nurses on the ward and the nurses at this meeting. People are uncertain about what is going on.

(I noted how Helen had rationalized the ward nurses' lack of ability to be with this family, blocked by their own fears and lack of affinity for this family.)

CJ: Why are you left metaphorically 'holding this baby'? Is this your role responsibility? Where are the consultants in all of this?

Helen: I was able to give feedback to the consultant later. I emphasized the need for the professionals' meeting. He is quite ineffectual. He had been incensed at the grandmother's comment that not enough had been done to get Emily home on TPN. He retorted that a million pounds had been spent on her care as it was! He took it personally.

CJ: So you are left taking responsibility. What are you going to do?

Helen: I'm going to get her home on TPN!

We explored the need for Helen to document carefully each decision she made. Helen decided she would write to the consultant and seek feedback on any decisions she made as a way of seeking support and validation. Re-orientating the problem as an emotional one will lead Helen to work with the family, but she could expect a backlash on death. She needed to prepare against this, even though she has established an effective working relationship with this family. There remained lots of unresolved anger likely to come out when Emily eventually died. However, working with the family will offset the 'them–us' tension and bring satisfaction for Helen.

I challenged the concept of the professionals' meeting as a collusive act to determine what we can say or cannot say in front of the parents. Does it go against the idea of open and honest relationships and working with the parents? Why can't we say what we feel and enable others to do so in a supportive way? Is not the professionals' meeting merely a bastion of the medical approach?

I challenged Helen: Link it to your philosophy.

Helen: Yes... so you mean we don't need professionals' meetings? That's food for thought!

A week later I bumped into Helen. She shared her sadness at Emily's death. However, this had been in 'partnership' with the grandmother. Helen needed a hug from me. She needed me to be available to support her as she had supported others. This highlighted the isolation in which she worked, where others were not immediately available to support her with her own sadness. The death of a small child is a tragedy under any circumstance.

In our next scheduled session (7 October, 1996) Helen picked up the idea of the professionals' meeting and exclaimed: 'Yes it is a collusive front – it opened my eyes!' (I noted the turn about.)

Helen: I could see it happening, before my eyes... it was amazing.

CJ: Amazing that we can see the same situation so differently so quickly – as if it had shifted on its axis.

Commentary

Although a very different scenario, the dynamics here are very similar to Gerry's experience.

Knowing the family – knowing self
Helen has to confront herself with her own prejudices against the grandmother and the health visitor and her technical perspective against sending this child home on TPN. Helen is confronted to 'see' the professionals' meeting as a collusive act to assert the professional view and to mute the family's voice. At this meeting, the health visitor acted to support the family's voice, yet Helen heard the distress through the anger and made herself available to work with this family. In doing so, she transformed her negative feelings into genuine concern. As with Gerry, she became the key worker and decision maker, conscious of this responsibility, yet in ways congruent with her holistic caring perspectives. Technology, although significant, is framed within the wider holistic picture.

Annie's experience

Helen linked this point to another recent experience.

Helen: The ward staff had asked me to come to the ward. They said: 'We need your power of persuasion on a lady who needs a nasogastric tube. We thought you could try.'

They were setting me up to fail! I read the notes before I went to see her. I noted that she was deaf. She had had meningitis as a child. When I went to her she was rocking with abdominal pain. She said it was 'terrible'. I talked to her. Her name was Annie. I said we were worried that she was not eating. She said it hurts if she eats. I clarified with her what she thought was happening to her at this time. She said she thought she was dying. She had pointed her hand to heaven to represent death. I said, 'We don't know what's happening, that's why we need to do the investigations.' I asked her if she wanted to die. She said 'yes'.

CJ: How old was she?

Helen: Fifty-three. I thought: 'How can we help her?' I asked her: 'To sort out the pain?' She said 'yes'. I talked to her about how to help her pain. We just sat and I held her hand for about 5 minutes.

CJ: Analgesia?

Helen: Yes . . . why not! I went out to talk to the nurses. I couldn't believe them – they said she had been refusing analgesia. This was 4-hourly IM pethidine. I confronted them: 'Would you accept this?' They saw my point but I could see they were amused that I had not got the tube down. I asserted that was not my priority. I told them that she wanted to die because of the pain.

CJ: Do we know the cause of this?

Helen: She may have secondary deposits from 10 years ago when she had carcinoma of the cervix, plus some radiotherapy complications that meant she had to have a cystectomy and ileal conduit.

CJ: Is there a connection between deaf and daft?

(Helen felt there might be. The patient had a husband and children, although Helen had not met the husband).

Helen: I was intending to turn it around on the ward staff to get them to pay attention to the woman's concern rather than see her as a problem with feeding. It felt like the most important half-hour of the day.

CJ: Does she need the nasogastric tube then? If she doesn't, then why is she staying in hospital?

Helen: Good point. There is the issue about her taking radio dye orally for the CT scan – but I don't know why she can't have an MRI scan. I challenged the nurses – they didn't know.

CJ: You could bypass the nurses and tune into your 'new' relationship with her consultant.

Helen: Yes, I could do that.

CJ: Are you entering into a conflict situation with the ward staff?

Helen: The senior staff nurse is quite receptive and that had an immediate quietening effect on the sniggering health care assistants in the background. It refocused the situation on 'the person of the patient rather than the medical investigations'.

CJ: You helped to do that.

In our next session (28 October, 1996) Helen picked up this woman's care and treatment.

Helen: I went to see this woman's surgeon. He said she couldn't just refuse to have investigations done because the tests done to date did not prove she had cancer. She had to subject herself to investigations. I shifted his perspective – to see her justifiable viewpoint – that he couldn't bludgeon her. He responded by writing up adequate analgesia. He didn't mind at all. Indeed, he found it amusing to be challenged in this way. When I saw her last, she looked as if she was about to die. Her pain was now being adequately controlled. She wasn't being fed, she eats and drinks just a little.

CJ: Will you see her again?

Helen: I will call in and see her from time to time as I'm passing.

CJ: Why?

Helen: Because she knows me and I'm concerned for her. What does it cost me?

CJ: Minutes? Minutes that could be spent with others legitimately?

Helen: Oh well...

CJ: Do you trust the ward staff?

Helen: I do! They had no difficulty in shifting to another focus but they may have difficulty with the fact that we are not feeding her.

CJ: The mystical power of food... that's an intuitive thought.

Helen: Yes... we don't have the 'hospice' mind set.

CJ: Is a hospice an option?

Helen: No, because the cancer has not been proven histologically.

Helen linked this to another woman on a surgical ward who had a large fungating tumour that had broken through the skin; she would not have it biopsied, and because of that, was refused hospice care.

Commentary

Again, Helen sees the person and identifies and responds to her needs. Her concern feels like a moral crusade as she bypasses the ward nurses and junior doctors to confront the consultant. By asserting Annie's perspective, she wins the day. Indeed, she illustrates the force of 'moral argument' and persuades the consultant that the investigations are not in the woman's best interests, based on her knowledge of this woman. The consultant is patronizing, but good humoured. This is a significant point, because, although Helen can achieve collaborative-type relationships with such consultants, this still depends to some extent on their willingness to enter into such collaboration. They have learnt to respect Helen's technical expertise; indeed she knows more about the technical aspects of nutrition than any doctor. She can ride caring perspectives on the back of this technical knowing and shift the perspective from simply a technical perspective to a moral caring perspective.

Realizing the powerful self
Helen's experiences all indicate her realization of her power, yet she must act with tact and assertion, paying due regard to the existing power differentials within practice and the organization. She cannot be influential within adversarial-type relationships, no matter what the extent of her technical expertise. Although she is also powerful in her own right, this power and esteem is brittle and vulnerable, easily 'knocked back'. Yet, through each session, this power becomes increasingly more firm in 'the knowing' through reflection.

Nurses seem to shrink from embracing power, as if a concern for power is antithetical to caring. Perhaps it is also a reflection of how nurses have generally been socialized to perceive themselves as powerless. To claim power is to work actively against power differentials that act to retain the status quo; it is difficult to work with others who may be antagonistic to the idea of the liberated and powerful nurse. Helen has embraced this challenge, yet her vulnerability is evident.

Role framing
An aspect of power is knowing the boundaries of one's legitimate authority to make decisions and act within any situation. Central to this is Helen's sense of autonomy, the extent to which she feels able to make decisions and take action. As Batey and Lewis (1982) have noted, autonomy can be viewed as two types. First, 'structural' autonomy is that which is defined by role, and, secondly, 'discretionary' autonomy is that which the practitioner believes himself or herself to have. To become an effective practitioner requires knowing these boundaries. Helen steps out into new territory

within the scenario with Emily. It is as if she expands her role in accepting responsibility for this family's ongoing care.

Carol's experience

Helen continued: Other things spring to mind. I feel frustrated . . . I get so far and then hold myself back . . . it's hard to break through that.

CJ: Of what?

Helen: Power relations with certain doctors. Although in general I feel I'm more effective, I still get into situations of stress that impact on my sleep, worrying about repercussions. They are usually situations grounded in power, conflict or the infallible self. I am sure, deep down, that this is less than it used to be, but I can't stop it entirely. I feel I'm stewing in my juices! Kicking myself! I am supposed to be able to deal with it. There was this situation the other week-end.

Helen recounted her experience of responding to a woman who had recently been discharged from a London hospital with a gastrostomy tube in situ. The tube had fallen out. The Accident and Emergency department had told her to return the next day, which was a mistake because the gastrostomy hole would close. She contacted the other hospital to find out about this situation and seek advice. The doctors there had been abusive when Helen had suggested a course of action for a woman who needed her gastrostomy tube replaced. They told her to refer her to the doctors. Helen's instinct was to suggest to this woman to return to the other hospital. The woman was happy to wait. Yet she could see that she was right in how she had responded but needed help to deflect her unease at being abused by these doctors. She did refer to the doctors. However, the next day Helen had again become involved, because no one could replace the tube. So Carol had to return to the other hospital anyway, probably for another operation.

Knowing the person

Helen had initially responded to the 'technical' problem, paying minimal attention to who this woman was. On reflection, I challenged Helen to 'see' this person. How did the tube come out? Why was the tube necessary in the first place? Helen noted the woman had a gastric pseudo-obstruction. Perhaps the woman had resisted the logical action of returning to the original hospital because she wanted the attention.

Creating the conditions where Helen could be available

I suggested to Helen that she had taken this situation on board because of the failure of others to respond appropriately. Why had she become involved? Predictably, Helen noted it was because this woman and others needed help. Yet Helen spent many hours attempting to sort this out in the face of abuse and it had left her feeling frustrated. This situation highlights how concern must be managed. It cannot be an unconditional giving, but must be managed within an understanding of her role. The abuse by the doctors reflects the status quo: 'How could a nurse possibly be dealing with this issue?' The doctors assert the status quo through humiliation tactics (Chapman, 1983). Helen knows she should not be flattened by these comments, but she is, reflecting how her sense of subordination is deeply embodied.

Conclusion

Helen's shared experiences within guided reflection make visible the nuances of her practice. It is her journey of self-discovery and transformation. Whether this is advanced practice is a matter of conjecture. I have suggested that the 'being available' template may offer a perspective on what advanced practice might be. The process of guided reflection helped Helen to view her practice from a number of perspectives that would seem essential for knowing advanced practice:

- *Philosophical framing* – clarifying the meaning of desirable nursing practice;
- *Role framing* – clarifying role boundaries, relationships, autonomy, and legitimate authority within practice;
- *Theoretical framing* – assimilating relevant theory and research findings within personal knowing;
- *Reality perspective framing* – enabling the practitioner to see and understand the factors that limit achieving desirable work, while simultaneously enabling the practitioner to become empowered to confront these barriers towards acting in new, more congruent ways.

This account has highlighted the extent to which practitioners such as Helen require significant and *appropriate* support and development to succeed in their roles, particularly if they assert the nature of desirable work in terms of empowerment and caring values rather than the predominant medical model. Guided reflection or clinical supervision enabled Helen to take responsibility to ensure her own practice development and, through review, to monitor her own effectiveness. These are the hallmarks of responsible practice.

References

Batey, M. V. and Lewis, F. M. (1982). Clarifying autonomy and accountability in nursing service: part 1. *J. Nurs. Admin.*, **12**(9), 13–18.

Belenky, M. F., Clinchy, B. M., Goldberger, N. R. and Tarule, J. M. (1986). *Women's Ways of Knowing: The Development of Self, Voice, and Mind.* New York: Basic Books.

Benner, P. (1984). *From Novice to Expert.* Menlo Park, CA: Addison-Wesley.

Benner, P. and Wrubel, J. (1989). *The Primacy of Caring.* Menlo Park, CA: Addison-Wesley.

Carper, B. (1978). Fundamental ways of knowing in nursing. *Adv. Nurs. Sci.*, **1**(1), 13–23.

Chapman, G. E. (1983). Ritual and rational action in hospitals. *Journal of Advanced Nursing*, **8**, 13–20.

Gadow, S. (1980). Existential advocacy. In *Nursing: Images and Ideals.* (S. F. Spicker and S. Gadow, eds.), pp. 79–101. New York: Springer Publishing.

Hall, L. (1964). Nursing – what is it? *Can. Nurse*, **60**, 150–154.

Heron, J. (1975). Six category intervention analysis. *Human Potential Research Project*. Guildford: University of Surrey.

Johns, C. (1994a). Guided reflection. In *Reflective Practice in Nursing: The Growth of the Professional Practitioner*. (A. Palmer, S. Burns and C. Bulman, eds.) pp. 110–130, Oxford: Blackwell Science.

Johns, C. (1994b). Constructing the BNDU model. In *The Burford NDU Model: Caring in Practice*. (C. Johns, ed.) Oxford: Blackwell Science.

Johns, C. (1995). Framing learning through reflection within Carper's fundamental ways of knowing. *J. Adv. Nurs.*, **22**, 226–234.

Johns, C. (1996). Visualising and realising caring in practice through guided reflection. *J. Adv. Nurs.*, **24**, 1135–1143.

Levine, S. (1986). *Who dies? An investigation of conscious living and conscious dying*. Bath: Gateway Books.

McHaffie, H. (1992). Coping: an essential element of nursing. *J. Adv. Nurs.*, **17**, 933–940.

National Health Service Management Executive (1983). *A Vision for the Future. The Nursing, Midwifery and Health Visiting Contribution to Health and Health Care*. London: Department of Health.

Rogers, M. E. (1986). Science of unitary human beings. In *Explorations of Martha Rogers' Science of Unitary Human Beings*. (V. Malinski, ed.) pp. 3–8. Norwalk, CT: Appleton-Century-Crofts.

15

Using portfolios to advance practice

Melanie A. Jasper

If the popular nursing press is to be believed, a professional profile will be a record of a nurse's working history. The content of the profile is anticipated to have come from a portfolio, which provides a current record of all aspects of a nurse's career to date and its anticipated development. Although qualitatively different in actuality, the two terms have passed into common parlance as coterminous, and, for the purposes of this chapter, can be seen to be the same. The purpose of a professional profile is of supporting application to the United Kingdom Central Council for Nursing, Midwifery and Health Visiting (UKCC) for triennial registration. As such, it is supposed to provide evidence that an individual is competent and credible as a practitioner, and has undergone personal and professional development during the previous 3 years.

I have suggested elsewhere (Jasper, 1995a) that this is a short-sighted and simplistic view of the potential that portfolio construction has, both for the individual and for the development of nursing as a practice discipline. In this chapter, I intend to explore the ways in which a portfolio can be developed as a living, dynamic working document that supports advancing practice, rather than the somewhat passive, retrospective record that the professional literature suggests. There are two main ways in which I believe the discipline of creating a portfolio will support the individual practitioner, which are less overt in other developmental strategies, namely, those of critical thinking and writing as learning. These two concepts form the basis of this chapter. However, it is worth taking some time to explore the notion of just what a portfolio is or could be.

The nature of a portfolio

Brown (1992) suggests that a personal portfolio is:

> a private collection of evidence which demonstrates the continuing acquisition of skills, knowledge, attitudes, understanding and achievement. It is both retrospective and prospective, as well as reflecting the current stage of development and activity of the individual.

This view of portfolios as being dynamic and comprising past, current and future professional practice is supported by the myriad of 'how to do your portfolio' articles in the popular press (e.g. Fisher, 1994; Price, 1994), and the variety of commercially produced packages available for purchase (Nursing Times, 1991; Teasdale, 1993). In contrast to this notion of portfolios as facilitating development, are the messages given by the employers, who have largely been silent on the issue of supporting staff in portfolio construction, and the institutes of higher education and the professional bodies for nursing, midwifery and health visiting, who appear to require an 'end-result'. What appears to be happening at present is that nurses are constructing portfolios in order to gain access or advanced standing for courses; for job applications or appraisal, if required to do so by their employer; as part of an assessment strategy for a course; or when (and if) asked to submit for verification for triennial registration by the UKCC.

Thus, at present, two aspects of portfolio construction are evident in practice, as an historical record, and as an educational device, which gives the impression, in direct contrast to the literature, that the portfolio is merely a record rather than a living document. This appears to be the perception of the majority of practitioners who attend portfolio workshops in my university. They have a negative view of portfolios as 'jumping through hoops' and being a paper exercise only. Unfortunately, although the literature does emphasize the rounded view of what a portfolio is, it also tends to focus on fulfilment of the UKCC's criteria (1995), and provides a narrow variety of prescriptive techniques for compiling it. The components of a professional profile, as suggested by the UKCC are:

- Record of factual information;
- Self-appraisal of professional performance;
- Record of goals and action plans;
- Record of formal learning;
- Record of working hours.

This serves only to reinforce the views commonly held about portfolios, and, in some instances, such as the emphasis on critical incident analysis or reflective journals, actively threatens nurses who are unfamiliar with these techniques and are not supported in developing the skills to use them. The emphasis in most of the articles is that the skills are to be developed to support the creation of a portfolio for its own sake, rather than the focus being on practice and individual development. The reason for this appears to be in the way that portfolios have been 'sold' to nurses, suggesting that they have no relevance for the everyday practice of nurses as it occurs. It is no wonder that there is both reluctance and resistance to portfolios per se amongst nurses.

Using a portfolio to advance practice

The situation in which the profession finds itself concerning portfolios is a classic example of the theory–practice gap, which confounds the introduction of many potential developments to nursing practice.

The rationale behind portfolio development suggests that, by using reflective techniques to explore elements of experience, we will develop a new perspective on that element, which will then inform future practice. This is referred to as 'learning'. However, there seems to me to be a missing link here, in that the act of reflection is not of necessity translated into action; just because we see things differently does not necessarily mean that we will act differently. Hence, what is described in most articles as 'reflective practice' is actually reflective process. This may be the reason why reflective practice and portfolios have remained, on the whole, a theoretical concept, rather than being used as the way that nurses learn and develop as practitioners.

How can portfolios be used to aid practitioners rather than imposing an additional burden on their working lives?

The first step, I believe, is that there needs to be a change in the perception of the focus of the portfolio away from career records to arising from and developing practice. If we accept that a portfolio is a collection of evidence that presents us with a picture of (in this case) a practising nurse, then the content of the portfolio has to represent the way in which that nurse practises. It will detail the *process* of practice, rather than simply the aspirations and outcomes of that process.

In documenting the process of nursing in this way, or the way in which nurses learn and advance practice, a body of knowledge will be built up that demonstrates not only individual development but also the way that nursing occurs in practice. For instance, there will be evidence of the thought processes behind the decision making, or the way that alternatives are considered and evaluated before nursing action is taken. In turn, we will have evidence, first hand, of how nurses nurse, rather than how theorists suggest that nurses nurse. This can be seen as practice based knowledge from primary sources, similar in nature to that used by Patricia Benner (1984) when she described the domains of nursing.

If practice based knowledge is accepted as the logical conclusion to a written reflective process, then it opens up exciting and innovative strategies for use within a portfolio, which reflect what a nurse is doing in practice and what nursing actually is from a phenomenological viewpoint, rather than being artificially reduced into preconceived categories such as educational achievements or 'key characteristics'. If the starting point for portfolio development is always clinical practice and the issues or problems that arise from it, then the use of the portfolio as the way that practitioners mediate their development becomes apparent. The portfolio would be a working, dynamic document that a nurse uses creatively to explore issues, define problems, plan action, gather information, create strategies, test alternatives, and evaluate them in practice. Once this point is reached, new issues or ideas will have arisen, which starts the cycle of enquiry again.

Hence, writing for a portfolio can be seen as a cyclical process in which ideas are developed from the recording and analysis of experience, tested out and re-evaluated, and practice is developed. At no time, therefore, can the activity of creating a portfolio be seen as separate from, or irrelevant to, practice. In fact, as a working document, it can be seen as part and parcel of the way that any accountable practitioner would work. Just as practice development arises from practice, the portfolio also needs to be created to serve practice needs as well as individual needs. For instance, an intensive care nurse might have explored the issue of recovery and core body temperature in terms of nursing actions. The outcome of this will be not only revision of nursing procedures, but the anticipation of resource needs, staff education, future developments, and so on, thus developing the issue beyond the limited relevance for the individual. If this can be demonstrated in the way that the portfolio is constructed, then it will, as a matter of course, also fulfil the requirements of the professional bodies, employers and educational establishments.

What, then, makes a practice based portfolio different from those constructed to a prescribed format, such as that created by the English National Board (ENB, 1991) to document acquisition of the 10 key characteristics? The basic requirement is that the portfolio is structured around and about practice, rather than nebulous categories that relate to an individual's attributes and separated from practice. Secondly, the portfolio needs to be a dynamic working document that is regarded as part of practice and as essential to practice, rather than as an added extra. It needs to become the working tool of practitioners who are concerned with advancing practice, and, consequently, with developing themselves. Hence the second step in changing the perception of portfolios for practitioners is in creating a structure that has relevance to both the content and the process of it, maintaining practice issues as a whole, as opposed to reducing them into separate components. This challenges, of course, the reductionist approach to nursing, and acknowledges the complexity of everyday nursing as a totality that is ultimately irreducible in reality.

Structuring a portfolio from practice

Rather than using a variation of the reflective process as identified in much of the nursing literature (Smith, 1995; Andrews, 1996; Teasdale, 1996), which appears to be based around critical incident analysis, I have created a flexible framework, which, I believe, focuses simultaneously on both reflection-in-action and reflection-on-action (Schön, 1983). Hence, the framework incorporates the components of a retrospective analysis, an ongoing log, and an action plan, of the process of developing and advancing elements of practice. These, in fact, are the three staple components and are present in all entries; they are used as a basis for constructing each section and are supplemented with additional categories as appropriate. Examples of additional categories might be progress or process notes, such as ideas to be considered, breakthroughs in thinking, timetabling of a project, and so on. What makes this different from the many published formats for portfolios is that it prescribes neither the content nor the process of constructing the portfolio. The structure itself evolves from the issue, and indeed the starting point for the practitioner is to decide initially on the framework for that issue. This enables the writer to work within a framework that has been created from a specified need, and has evolved from a considered evaluation of that need and a diagnosis of an action strategy. This in itself is part of the reflective and developmental process, and becomes part of the portfolio.

The example given in Figure 15.1 is taken from my portfolio (albeit abbreviated). The framework used for analysis was created specifically to suit the purpose of the problem identified, and is different (although similar) for all of the entries in my portfolio. The idea for this framework, which responds to a specific need and is created from the structure of the experience, was inspired in the first instance by the writing of Tina Koch (1994) in describing the use of a decision trail in a qualitative research project. This excerpt provides a snapshot in time only. The work on this element of my practice is far from complete, and I consider it to be a major challenge to both my own development and to developing a teaching and learning strategy, which, I believe, has as yet unrecognized potential for professional development.

I hope that this example has, in some ways, demonstrated my ideas of how a portfolio can be used to develop practice. However, it would be naive to assume that all practitioners possess the skills to construct a portfolio in such a way. Atkins and Murphy (1993) conclude that, in order to practise reflectively, people need to have developed insight and self-awareness, and be open minded and accepting of criticism. More specifically, however, they suggest that the skills of description, critical analysis, synthesis and evaluation need to be present before a situation can be fully utilized through reflection. This suggests that the successful use of a reflective process in practice is in part dependent on the person having achieved a certain maturational level that incorporates all of those elements. If this is so, and experience with a cross-section of students suggests to me that it is, then it is hardly surprising that both reflective practice and portfolios have received such a hard ride in the profession!

What all of these elements add up to, of course, is the idea that the practitioners have to be critical thinkers in order to be able to advance practice.

Developing critical thinking

In attempting to advance practice, nurses need to be able to think critically about the options that are available to them, select appropriately and justify decision making. Critical thinking can be seen as a transferable skill, which should be developed as a component of any educational programme (Rane-Szostak and Fisher Robertson, 1996). De Bono (1991) suggests that critical thinking is a passive and contemplative activity which involves weighing up, evaluating and deciding on the validity of something, although Yataoka-Yahiro and Saylor (1994, p. 352), in applying this to nursing, propose that critical thinking is 'reflective and reasonable thinking about nursing problems without a single solution and is focused on deciding what to believe and do'.

I like this definition because, for me, it maintains just that 'messiness' or complexity of nursing that I referred to earlier and which is essential to recognize if we are ever to develop a body of nursing practice knowledge. It also draws together the notions that critical thinkers have to have a vast array of skills, knowledge and experience to draw on in order to be able to

---

Figure 15.1. A portfolio extract (opposite)

This section is taken from my own portfolio as a practising teacher, and does, I hope, illustrate the process that enabled me to develop an aspect of my own practice.

Problem identification

Student evaluation at the end of a course highlighted a problem with the integrating mechanism of a learning portfolio used for assessment purposes. The portfolio was used within a shortened common foundation programme for graduates, who had to achieve the same learning outcomes in 6 months as other students achieved over 18. This was our first experience of using a portfolio as a learning and assessment tool, and as such provided significant challenges to us as teachers as well as to the students in developing their skills as independent learners. Teachers identified an additional problem of how the portfolio was to be assessed. The main problems appeared to be related to:

1. Student uncertainty regarding the content and format of the portfolio;
2. Managing the workload of the portfolio;
3. Managing the student–teacher interaction;
4. Achieving consistency in marking.

The challenge to practice

I am convinced, given the experience of the past year, that the strategy of a portfolio is the correct one. The challenges to practice appear to be:

1. To devise a format for the portfolio that will enable the student to feel secure, and yet still maintain the challenge of independent learning and identification of learning needs;
2. Devising marking criteria;
3. Making the tutorial support structure more overt.

Activity log

This activity log ran for 12 pages and details the stages, options and blind alleys that were encountered in the process of meeting the challenges above. It covers approximately 18 months of activity, which included literature searching and review, discussions with colleagues and students, creating and testing strategies and discarding, with justification, the things that were ineffective. What it documents is the process of changing and developing practice which resulted in:

1. A workbook structure for the portfolio (Jasper, 1995b);
2. A set of marking criteria;
3. A flexible student–teacher tutorial system.

Developments to practice

This work on portfolios has convinced me that, contrary to the problems inherent in using such work for assessment purposes, this is an extremely valuable strategy to encourage student based learning. Although the literature on portfolios appears to concentrate, at present, on portfolios as developmental rather than summative, they do appear to provide an integrating mechanism for enabling students to take charge of and control their own learning. In addition, I have learnt so much about the need for student security in terms of structures to facilitate learning and supportive mechanisms that enable students to develop individually. I can also see the value in creating a criterion-referenced marking system for an assessment that is so dependent on the student for content, if not for process. Where do we go from here? There are definitely avenues for development.

Action planning

Personal action My development requires that I find the time to write this up as a journal paper and also present it at conferences (Achieved 1994 and 1995).

Practice consolidation and testing This approach now needs testing with other students on other courses (portfolio as assessment now used for ENB 870 students and incorporated into new Dip. HE curriculum).

Advancing practice This initiative needs further development in terms of moving from a course based educational initiative into portfolio development as a strategy for lifelong professional learning.

And so a new cycle begins!

think their way around nursing problems. This puts critical thinking solidly in the domain of the practitioner who is attempting to advance practice. The American Philosophical Association (APA, 1990) attempted to describe the attributes of a critical thinker, as listed below:

- Habitually inquisitive;
- Trustful of reason;
- Flexible;
- Honest in facing personal biases;
- Willing to reconsider;
- Orderly in complex matters;
- Well informed;
- Open minded;
- Fair minded in evaluation;
- Prudent in making judgements;
- Clear about issues;
- Diligent in seeking relevant information;
- Reasonable in the selection of criteria focused in enquiry;
- Persistent in seeking results that are as precise as the subject and circumstances of enquiry permit.

Although this is, admittedly, a daunting array of features, it suggests that the development of critical thinking is concurrent with, or even dependent upon, maturational processes. A critical thinker appears to need to possess the abilities of assimilation and evaluation that are beyond knowledge and experience; they are about personal development and a capacity to be creative. This creates a link with the suggestion made earlier that the ability to be a reflective practitioner is also dependent upon maturity. Perhaps the two go together as higher level skills that arise not only from knowledge and experience but also from a personal capacity to develop beyond a certain level. The inference here, of course, is that not everyone is capable of becoming a reflective practitioner or of advancing practice. This is not, of course, to suggest that everyone does not have the capacity for development!

Step three in adjusting the practitioner's view of the portfolio is therefore to create the link between critical thinking and advancing practice by seeing the portfolio as a medium for developing critical thinking. Thus, the portfolio becomes a way of mediating the process of developing practice and the acquisition of skills and knowledge to do so.

Looking back again at the APA's list, it is possible to see a link between the characteristics of critical thinking and those used in developing a portfolio using the concepts and structure described in my earlier section. The *process* of examining and developing practice issues through a portfolio will necessarily use and develop skills of critical thinking in the same way. However, a portfolio will provide a documented record of the development of those skills, providing the evidence that an issue has been carefully and logically explored. This highlights the significant difference between portfolio construction as used in this way and many other reflective techniques that might also develop critical thinking, which is the fact that it is recorded in a written format demonstrating the learning, or advances in practice, that have arisen from the thinking processes involved. Allen et al.

(1989) suggest that the connection between writing and thinking has recently been radically reassessed. They claim that, whereas previously, writing was seen as recording thought, the perspective is now taken that writing actually actively develops thinking. It is only a short step from here to making the connection from writing as thinking to writing as learning.

Writing as learning

According to Allen et al. (1989): 'Literacy in the fullest sense is the creating and organising of thoughts, the sorting of assertions and relevant evidence, and the development of and support for reasoned decision making.'

This suggests that writing and thinking go hand in hand in developing critical skills, and supports the explanation given for the infancy of the development of nursing knowledge that, in the past (and largely still to some degree), nursing has been a verbal culture and recruits have limited opportunities to develop critical thinking through writing assignments. Although nursing students demonstrate the development of knowledge and skills through assignments such as writing care plans and developing health promotion packages, they rarely have the opportunity to build on assignments in an incremental way to enable them to reassess their own learning. However, where portfolios are used, even with entry-level students, writing and thinking are developed concurrently as the writer reviews, re-evaluates and reassesses needs for the future.

Allen et al. (1989) describe the assumptions of the *writing to learn* paradigm, in contrast to the traditional *learning to write* paradigm. These are summarized in Figure 15.2.

The writing to learn paradigm appears to support the ideas proposed in this chapter, suggesting that portfolio construction facilitates the development and advancement of practice. In writing portfolio entries, the practitioner develops and expands understanding. For instance, in investigating alternative strategies for wound care with specific clients, a practitioner will not only expand his or her scientific knowledge base, but also make the connections between that and personal specialized experiential knowledge of the client group. In exploring this through writing (assumption 2), the practitioner must also be thinking, because a new perspective on the problem will be developed; there would be little point in merely copying out or repeating knowledge.

The nature of portfolios reflects the nature of nursing: they are messy! Hence, portfolio writing is likely to be cyclical, discursive and dialectical in nature, as the writer tests ideas and discusses them (assumptions 4 and 5). Finally, nursing portfolios will be of limited interest to those from other disciplines. The learning that occurs is personal, and, to some extent, phenomenological. The wider audience arises from colleagues in practice and anyone else who has a stake in the portfolio, such as employers, educationalists and the UKCC.

One of the benefits of written records for practitioners might be that they help us to access the expert's complex thinking mechanisms that are described by Benner (1984) as the 'shift from reliance on analytical rule-based thinking to intuition', and developed by Johns (1995), who suggests

Learning to write	Writing to learn
1. Students can successfully learn content whether or not they can write well	1. Writing is a process through which content is learned or understood (as opposed to memorized or reported)
2. Writing and thinking involve different skills; each can, and perhaps should, be taught separately	2. Writing skills are primarily thinking skills (competence in one is inseparable from competence in the other)
3. Knowing something is logically prior to writing about it	3. Writing is a process of developing an understanding or coming to know something
4. Writing is a sequential, linear activity, which involves the cumulative mastery of components like sentence construction or outlining	4. Writing is a dialectical, recursive process, rather than linear or sequential
5. Communication is the main purpose of writing; written work is a product in which the student reports what he or she already knows	5. Higher order conceptual skills can only evolve through a writing process in which the writer engages in an active, ongoing dialogue with him- or herself and others; learning and discovery are purposes that are as important for writing as communication
6. The student's audience is most often assumed to be the instructor	6. Different disciplines utilize different conceptual processes and thus have different standards for writing; students can best learn writing within their own discipline while writing for real, concrete audiences

Figure 15.2. A comparison of the assumptions of the two paradigms (adapted from Allen et al., 1989)

that reflective practice can 'make explicit the tacit knowledge within experience'. If intuition is seen as part of the working practice knowledge base of expert practitioners (Jasper, 1994), and intuition is the active expression of tacit knowledge as claimed by Johns (1995), then the recording and exploration of an expert's decision-making processes in a portfolio is likely to make these more accessible for developing and advancing practice from an eclectic and practice based knowledge base, and thus for sharing with others. Regarded in this way, the portfolio becomes yet another tool within the nurse's kitbag, which is used to enable better practice.

Step four in our process, then, is to enable practitioners to experience the joy of learning through writing. This is an experience that is highly personal, is usually achieved in isolation, and is a very private achievement. Success tends to act as a motivating force; nurses who can see the benefits for themselves and for their clients tend to build upon that success.

Where to now?

There are a few issues that are beyond the remit of this chapter but which need to be addressed in the future if the portfolio is to move from being more than a fledgling concept. Undoubtedly, the carrot on the end of the stick for most practitioners will be the pragmatic one of a professional profile kept for the UKCC. At present, there is no intention by the UKCC to assess the standard of portfolio work in terms of higher level skills; the criteria for assessment are as yet unannounced and are the subject of a UKCC working party. Using a portfolio for entry to higher levels on a register has been done by at least one other health care profession. The American Dietetic Association (ADA) (Bradley, 1996) uses a portfolio of evidence against six specific criteria (education, experience, professional achievement, professional roles, professional contacts, and approach to practice) for credentialing Fellows of the Association. It has also created both objective and peer evaluation criteria by which the portfolio evidence is assessed. While parallels cannot be drawn with the UKCC at present, it is worthy of note that the criteria for the reregistration of nurses are verified, as is the possible content required in a profile, as set out earlier in this chapter. With the development of specialist sections on the register (although the UKCC is currently ruling out an advanced register), the possibility of stated standards and criteria such as those used by the ADA is not beyond the realms of the imagination.

The second issue that needs to be addressed is an educational one. Clearly, in terms of advancing practice, we are not necessarily talking about learning skills but about the development of alternatives, of new ways of doing things. The teaching and learning strategies used in the education of advanced practitioners need to mirror the processes that they want to develop. Hence, if at the end of a formal course we are hoping for practitioners who are lifelong learners capable of managing and evaluating their learning, then these skills need to be reflected in the process, content and assessment of the course. We also need to create flexible alternatives to the standard, taught, content-driven courses for practitioners who feel that they are working to advance practice but wish to acquire additional skills in such areas as critical thinking, research and writing to learn.

Finally, it seems to me that the portfolio has such potential for the development of nursing practice that we cannot afford to ignore the investment of time, energy and money that a full commitment to it will involve. At present, nurses appear to be using portfolios instrumentally rather than as part of their own development. For this to change, they need to be given the opportunities, from preregistration upwards, to develop the reflective, written and thinking skills needed to turn a portfolio from a record of achievement into a dynamic, living document that reflects the nurse's practice. The benefits of doing this will be advancements in nursing practice.

References

Allen, D. G., Bowers, B. and Diekelmann, N. (1989). Writing to learn: a reconceptualization of thinking and writing in the nursing curriculum. *J. Nurs. Educ.*, **28**, 6–11.
American Philosophical Association. (1990). *Critical Thinking: a Statement of Expert Consensus for Purposes of Educational Assessment and Instruction: The Delphi Report: Research Findings and Recommendations Prepared for the Committee on Pre-college*

Philosophy. Millbrae, CA: American Philosophical Association.

Andrews, M. (1996). Using reflection to develop clinical expertise. *Br. J. Nurs.*, **5**, 508–513.

Atkins, S. and Murphy, K. (1993). Reflection: a review of the literature. *J. Adv. Nurs.*, **18**, 1188–1192.

Benner, P. (1984). *From novice to expert*. Menlo Park, CA: Addison-Wesley.

Bradley, T. R. (1996). Fellow of the American Dietetic Association credentialing program: development and implementation of a portfolio-based assessment. *Journal of the American Dietetic Association*, **96**, 513–517.

Brown, R. (1992). *Portfolio Development and Profiling for Nurses*. Lancaster: Quay.

DeBono, E. (1991). *Teaching Thinking*. Harmondsworth: Penguin.

English National Board. (1991). *Professional Portfolio*. London: ENB.

Fisher, M. (1994). Compiling your portfolio. *Elderly Care*, **6**(5), 15–17.

Jasper, M. (1994). Expert: a discussion of the implications of the concept as used in nursing. *J. Adv. Nurs.*, **20**, 769–776.

Jasper, M. (1995a). The potential of the professional portfolio for nursing. *J. Clin. Nurs.*, **4**, 249–255.

Jasper, M. (1995b). The portfolio workbook as a strategy for student-centred learning. *Nurse Educ. Today*, **15**, 446–451.

Johns, C. (1995). The value of reflective practice for nursing. *J. Clin. Nurs.*, **4**, 23–30.

Koch, T. (1994). Establishing rigour in qualitative research: the decision trail. *J. Adv. Nurs.*, **19**, 976–986.

Nursing Times. (1991). *The Profile Pack*. Open Learning Programme.

Price, A. (1994). Midwifery portfolios: supporting the midwife. *Modern Midwife*, **4**(11), 23–26.

Rane-Szostak, D. and Fisher Robertson, J. (1996). Issues in measuring criteria thinking: meeting the challenge. *J. Nurs. Educ.*, **35**, 5–11.

Schön, D. (1983). *The Reflective Practitioner*. New York: Basic Books.

Smith, C. (1995). Evaluating nursing care: reflection in practice. *Prof. Nurse*, **10**, 723–724.

Teasdale, K. (1993). *Personal Professional Profile*. London: Mosby.

Teasdale, K. (1996). Using personal profiles in reflective practice. *Prof. Nurse*, **11**, 323–325.

United Kingdom Central Council for Nursing, Midwifery and Health Visiting. (1995). *PREP and You: Factsheets 1–8*. London: UKCC.

Yataoka-Yahiro, M. and Saylor, C. (1994). A critical thinking model for nursing. *J. Nurs. Educ.*, **33**, 351–356.

16

Therapeutic use of self: a component of advanced nursing practice

Julie Scholes

Introduction

The domains and competencies of the advanced practitioner role have been described as expert practitioner, leader, researcher, educator, innovator and developmentalist, evaluator, and consultant (Castledine, 1996; Gilliss, 1996; Hixon, 1996; Manley, 1997). In this way the advanced practitioner is seen to have direct and indirect impact on patient care: direct impact through intervention with patients/clients on the advanced practitioner's 'caseload'; and indirect impact through their leadership, educational, developmental and research facilitation roles with other colleagues (Sparacino, 1992; Paniagua, 1995; Castledine, 1996; Manley, 1997). This chapter will focus on the elements of expert practice that are in direct contact with patients and their relatives.

I shall examine the use of self as a therapeutic tool (a construct developed from research conducted in a critical care nursing development unit over a 2-year period) and argue that this is a fundamental component of advanced nursing practice, because, crucial to nurses generating the time, energy and space to work with patients and families in this way, is their mastery of the environment, practical wisdom, expert knowledge base and attention to caring detail. First, I shall locate the notion of expert practice and how this can be realized through the therapeutic use of self within the advanced practitioner's direct caring role.

Benner (1984) described seven domains of expert nursing practice: 'the helping role; the teaching coaching function; the diagnostic-monitoring function; effective management of rapidly changing situations; administration and monitoring therapeutic interventions and regimens; monitoring and ensuring the quality of health care practices; and organizational and work-role competencies'. Brykczynski (1989) identified areas of skilled practice within each of these domains, but of particular interest here are the elements described under the 'helping role' which include:

- Creating a therapeutic environment;
- Presencing or being with a patient;
- Providing comfort;

- Differentiating patient cues of pain and discomfort and using different strategies to resolve these problems (including the use of self);
- Supporting patients' families and friends emotionally and offering appropriate information;
- Guiding and supporting patients through their illness towards wellness tailored to meet their needs and acknowledging their personality.

On face value, one would question how any nurse could practice without incorporating each one of these elements in interactions with either patients or families, but the reality appears to be somewhat different (Rubin, 1996). Benner et al. (1996) suggest that this does not occur until the proficient or expert stage is attained, because it is only at this point in the nurses' professional maturation that they acquire the capacity to tune in to patients and synthesize subtle cues from a vast array of sources, which then influence their 'clinical and ethical comportment'. Put simply, in the earlier stages, nurses have so many fragmented elements to manage in order to achieve competency that this occludes their capacity to achieve the whole. What differentiates experts from the rest is their fluid practice and capacity to harness each one of Brykczynski's skills without knowing they have done so. How they do this is the subject of this chapter. It is argued that the capacity to presence, connect with the deeply unconscious patient, and draw upon a vast repertoire of interventions tailored to meet the individual needs of the patient is the essence of the art of critical care nursing, and, as such, the very notion of advanced nursing practice (Tanner et al., 1993). Before addressing this, it is important to identify how we gathered the data to illuminate these findings.

Approach

As this study was being undertaken on a nursing development unit, the aim was to engage the participants in as much deliberative reflection upon their role as possible. In this way the research served as an educative opportunity (Elliott, 1991), because, through the process of data collection both the researcher and the participants gained insight into the work and practice of critical care nurses and ways in which this could be enhanced. Therefore, reflection and reciprocity were central tenets of the approach. At first, we started by gathering data through participant observation. Field notes were recorded and shortly after the observational period the nurses were engaged in a reflective dialogue (Scholes and Freeman, 1994) about the events that had occurred during the observational period. There were two problems with this. First, the speed with which the nurses interacted meant that detailed recording became problematic, and, while writing field notes, a series of important events took place, which went unrecorded but were central to the overall intervention sequence. The second problem was that many of the nurses found it difficult to articulate the sequence of events in detail because much of their interaction was so integral to their caring repertoire that it defied explanation without further prompt.

It became evident that video-recording the interactions would serve as a useful means of gathering all the elements of an interaction (Botorff and

Morse, 1994; Botorff and Varcoe, 1995). Later, the nurses were interviewed in front of their video recording and asked to describe their interactions and sources of knowing that underpinned their decision making and repertoire of caring interventions. In this way, they had the chance to 'look, look again and hopefully see' (Gepp, 1996) the elements of practice that formed the whole of the interaction.

The use of video in the critical care setting is loaded with ethical concerns. Although the camera was primarily aimed at the nurse, the patient inevitably came into shot. Gaining informed consent from the patient was invariably an impossibility due to the condition that had initiated their admission to the unit. We therefore developed an elaborate protocol by which we would gain vicarious consent from relatives to proceed with the video. (The staff and research team primarily developed the protocol, which was subsequently sanctioned by the local Ethics Committee on behalf of the Trust.) Because we strictly observed this protocol, it necessarily restricted the amount of footage we were able to record (total 28 hours), as there were many instances when the situation was deemed inappropriate to proceed. However, when we did film, we found the video footage and the content of the reflective interviews illuminated rich detail about the nurses' interactions with patients. This also served as a potent learning exercise for the nurses who engaged in this process, serving both to celebrate good practice and to identify ways in which practice could be enhanced, and subsequently shared, with more junior colleagues. This data then informed progressive focusing (Parlett and Hamilton, 1972) and purposive sampling (Erlandson et al., 1993) of subsequent observations and interviews.

All the concepts generated through constant comparative analysis of the data (Glaser and Strauss, 1967) were subject to participant validation through focus groups (Janiesick, 1994), and scrutiny and comment on draft reports (Simmons, 1987; Stake, 1994). The data that this approach elicited will now be presented and compared with formal theories from the literature. First, how the nurses became established at the beginning of each shift is detailed in order to illuminate how they gained mastery of their environment, a necessary activity that pre-empted therapeutic engagement with the patient. The elements of presencing and therapeutic engagement are then examined. After the exploration of the therapeutic use of self, the ways in which advanced practitioners drew upon some of these skills to interact effectively with the relatives is discussed.

Getting in the know and getting organized

When nurses first came on duty, we noticed that they went through an elaborate process of information exchange, organization and checks. Information was conveyed in three distinct episodes: through a general overview of all the patients on the unit; at a bedside handover; and then directly through comprehensive patient assessment. At each episode, the information became more detailed and intimate. When the nurse 'took over' the patient, they would introduce themselves then run a series of checks on the equipment, handling and relocating the equipment and changing the parameters of alarms. Most importantly, nurses were seen subtly to shift the location of visual displays to a position of personal preference. As each piece of technology was handled, this too was subtly relocated before moving on to the next. We noticed that the more experienced nurses were in critical care, the more likely they were to alter the layout of the environment and create their own preferred practice territory (Scholes and Moore, 1997). The process of 'getting organized' and 'getting in the know' served important purposes because it built a picture of the patient located in the environment, which then informed subsequent decision making and interventions (Tanner et al., 1993).

In both observational and video recordings, we captured experienced nurses interacting with patients in a pattern that was repeated throughout the shift. Because of the repetition we called this a 'flight path'. As they proceeded through their flight path, we noticed that they would scan the visual displays from any location in their practice territory. Just as an experienced driver scans the rear view mirror at regular intervals, the nurses scanned the visual displays, but were unaware of the regularity of this activity until watching themselves on the video. In the process of scanning the visual displays, they could ascertain if there were any changes to the readouts and intervene immediately to check if this was an anomaly or a cue to the patient's changing condition. When an altered cue was detected, the nurses were aware that they had gathered this information from the visual displays, but assumed that this had happened by chance or intuition, rather than acknowledging that this information was gathered through their regular scanning process.

The activities at the beginning of the shift were far from routine. Creating a practice territory enabled nurses to create the space through which they could run their flight path. More importantly, the relocation of equipment and visual displays meant that visual access to this information was maintained from whatever position in the practice territory. The equipment was lined up against the patient so that the objective data from the readouts was in direct proximity to correlate with the qualitative visual assessment of the patient.

Although all the practitioners on the unit learnt to do this series of activities (through in-service training and preceptorship), the way in which it was done and the meaning attributed to the activities differed according to the practitioner's experience. For the novice to critical care, this activity was a routine cumbersome process, but for the experienced and expert practitioner, organization and getting in the know enabled them subsequently to practice with rhythm and fluidity, but, why did the experienced practitioners have such a highly stylized pattern of working?

First, creating a practice territory allowed nurses visual access to all salient information from any vantage point, to enable them to formulate decisions. Secondly, this created the space through which they could practice their own rhythmic and systematic care, tailored (through knowing the patient) to individual need. Most importantly, this pattern allowed experienced nurses to free their conscious attention to tune in to patients and engage with them in a meaningful way. The process of covering information repeatedly at the beginning of the shift drove into the nurses' memory the baseline information against which they could judge subsequent changes. The more established critical care nurses were able to read chunks of information and formulate a judgement (Carter et al., 1987), whilst the experienced nurses were able to scan all the available material and notice an altered cue. They could then immediately intervene or hold back, according to the significance that the nurse placed upon that cue relative to the overall picture presented by the patient (Schraeder and Fischer, 1987). This demonstrates how expert practitioners use their perceptual awareness to single out the relevant cue, rather than deliberate and analyse all the available material to formulate a judgement and then consider what action to take (Benner and Wrubel, 1989).

The ways in which the nurses uncovered information about the patients as people were crucial to this process; this came from the longitudinal relationship with them and their relatives. Knowing the patient (May, 1991; Tanner et al., 1993; Radwin, 1995) came from various sources, primarily from the relatives' descriptions of the individual when in good health. Careful observation of the relatives' interaction gave the nurses some important clues, as did photographs and any background information from other practitioners involved with the patient throughout the illness (Tanner et al., 1993; Scholes and Moore, 1997). This information enabled the nurses to make judgements about how they would interact with the person, the degree to which the individual was tactile, formal or relaxed. The patients' responses to various interventions and their changing condition throughout their episode in the critical care unit strengthened this understanding and helped the nurses to detect more subtle cues and responses (Schraeder and Fischer, 1987; Tanner et al., 1993; Macleod, 1994).

All this took time, and, therefore, mastery of the environment, a sound knowledge base and practical wisdom against which accurate decisions could be formulated, and an array of interventions that could be used, were crucial. The expert practitioner could draw upon a vast array of possibilities and use the most appropriate in an apparently seamless and fluid sequence. This has been described by Chinn and Kramer (1991) as 'aesthetic knowing'. These practitioners therefore had the technical and practical know-how, which could be reflectively operationalized without conscious deliberation, based upon the direct 'feeling' of an experience and 'subjective acquaintance' with the patient (Carper, 1975). This knowledge meant that they could manage complex situations and incorporate multiple activities into one apparent action or minor deviation, thus creating the time and space to manage the unpredictable (Carter et al., 1987) and to practice the therapeutic use of self.

There were various elements and skills that underpinned the holistic manifestation of therapeutic engagement. For the purposes of clarity, they will be described individually, but the reader should remember that, in the process of segmenting and describing the parts of the interaction, this belies the fluid and rhythmic behaviours it seeks to describe. However, the description is put forward to illustrate the elements and skills that underpin apparently basic caring qualities that resurface in the practised art of the expert or advanced practitioner (Johnson, 1994; Macleod, 1994).

Presencing: being there

The nurses working in critical care were constantly aware of the need to convey to a deeply unconscious patient, who was surrounded by invasive equipment and technology, that they were alive and valued, and that there was hope. To do this, they needed to reach the patient and make that person aware of their presence and communicate their concern and care (Walters, 1995; Benner et al., 1996). However, the nurses were also acutely aware of the patient's distorted reality brought about by the equipment and sedation (Hudak et al., 1986), and had an implicit desire to prevent the patient from being jolted into this 'technical nightmare' by their actions. Certain interventions were recognized as having the potential to do this, but every endeavour was made to minimalize their impact and swiftly restore a peaceful resting state for the patient, free from discomfort and pain. Balancing the two meant that they established a complex process of gently alerting the patient to their presence, explaining their actions, and confirming therapeutic meaning whilst undertaking an intervention. Much of this was achieved through touch and talk, but also in the way that they handled the patient and dextrously manoeuvred equipment so that it did not cause additional discomfort. Macleod (1994) located this capacity to pay attention to detail and convey care through everyday acts as the essence of expert practice. How these nurses gained the unconscious patient's 'attention' prior to any caring action is described to illuminate the detail involved in the basics of everyday interactions.

Engaging with the patient

When patients were approached, this was invariably from the side, with nurses alerting patients to their presence by calling their name and simultaneously touching their hand or shoulder (the engaging hand). The nurses would then locate themselves into patients' apparent visual field, dictated by the location of their head upon the pillow. As the nurses spoke, they would gently increase the pressure of touch and remain quite still, allowing patients to accommodate to their proximity. The nurses read whether or not patients had engaged with them through subtle cues like changes in the pupil indicating some focusing, a blink or some other facial expression. Once the nurses had connected with the patients in this way, they became quite still, fully concentrating on the interaction.

When explaining a procedure, they would maintain the engaging hand but use the other to locate or zone the area that was about to receive attention. For example, if patients were to have endotracheal suction, nurses would lightly touch the end of the tube; if they were to have chest physiotherapy, they would lay a flattened hand upon the chest. Each movement was slow and precise, punctuated by stillness to gauge if the patient had understood what was said, and offering the chance for feedback.

Emphasis was conveyed through a flattened hand or a stroke, which was depressed in rhythm to the nurse's voice pattern. Stroking was often the interaction of choice to encourage a response, although touching the face with the back of the hand was the interaction most often associated with assurance over an activity (Scholes, 1996). If a patient became highly agitated, and the nurse had ensured that the patient did not require a positional change or medication, the nurse would place a flattened hand on either the arm or the knee and remain quite still, using a soothing explanation to orientate the patient. If, during this time, an alarm went off, the nurse would maintain the engaging hand but turn slowly to mute the alarm and scan the visual displays. What is important is that the nurse did not break contact with the patient once connection had been made with that person. If the clinical decision necessitated, then the nurse would slightly increase the pressure of the touch and move away to respond. However, on return, the process of re-engaging would be observed prior to any subsequent intervention.

Closure

Just as engaging and making their presence known was skilfully deployed to prevent 'jolting', so too, was closure. The nurse would draw back slowly from the patient's visual field and gently increase the pressure of the touch as a parting gesture, and next stand quite still for a moment to assess if this had disturbed the patient from a restful state. If there was no further response, the nurse would then turn and carry out other indirect patient care activities (Scholes, 1996).

The maintaining hand throughout the interaction and the increased departing pressure are both therapeutic touch strategies of Shiatsu and massage (Beresford Cooke, 1996). However, the nurses were unaware of what they did (until witnessing this on the video and then checking this out in their own observation of colleagues), nor did they have any formal theory or training that could have informed this action. Yet, consistently, this pattern of therapeutic interaction was witnessed in nurses acknowledged by their peers as being expert critical care practitioners; but the source of knowing that informed these interactions remains elusive.

Differentiating the genuine from simulated action

Experienced nurses had two distinct paces: one slow and deliberate when in direct contact with the patient; and the other swift and darting around the unit. Once engaged with a patient, stillness and concentration demonstrated 'emotional presence' (Swanson, 1991) and authenticity (Parse, 1992). Connecting with the patient in this way enabled nurses to convey their care and willingness to dialogue, and created the opportunity by which they could detect feedback that the patient was orientated to the moment. Gadow (1989) argues that it is through establishing meaningful connections that the art of nursing is realized, but this is not part of the caring repertoire for all experienced nurses (Rubin, 1996).

Authentic and simulated interactions are discernible from each other. Attentiveness, proximity and receptivity differentiate the genuine from the simulated posture. The genuine connection is made for the good of the patient rather than seeking personal merit for the nurse (Bishop and Scudder, 1990), while the simulated connection is a castaway gesture, divorced from other action and performed to impress an observer (Scholes, 1996). The authentic connection is made through a concern to care (Benner at al., 1996), and is marked by concentration and attention to detail (Macleod, 1994) and noticing the difference the contribution makes (Benner and Wrubel, 1989). Therefore, the capacity to realize such art requires a level of proficiency and willingness to generate such a moment, and an understanding to make sense of the interaction. Because of this, genuine presencing is firmly located in the domain of the expert or advanced practitioner (Johnson, 1994; Macleod, 1994; Benner et al., 1996).

Tuning in: reading the cues

Knowing the patient (Tanner et al., 1993; Benner et al., 1996) was crucial to understanding the subtle cues and, more importantly, their significance. This emerged over a period of working with patients and their relatives, assimilating small pieces of information and entering into a deliberative detection process to uncover more about them as people, for example, their vulnerability or stoicism, reactions to pain and stressful encounters (Tanner et al., 1993; Morse, 1996). Ultimately, this led to nurses being able to distinguish between patients' cues of discomfort and pain, as well as fatigue and changes in mood. Just as this information helped to frame the act of caring, it also enabled the nurses to recognize patterns of response against which judgements about progress or decline could be gauged (Benner et al., 1996). If the patient was on the unit for a prolonged period, the nurses were able to make judgements about the life force of the patient and they articulated issues surrounding the patient's capacity to 'pull through' or that they had 'given up'. Benner et al. (1996) identified this ability to read the patient amongst practitioners who they defined as either proficient or expert, although those nurses, like the ones in the research study described here, did not necessarily connect with all the patients and their families. To a certain extent this was based upon individual chemistry and a capacity to engage with patients and their families. However, certain predisposing skills and professional attributes did exist to make this more likely, especially when combined with a prolonged episode with, or intense understanding of, the patient as person (Tanner et al., 1993).

Knowing a patient's personality helped to inform the nurses' actions and how they could respond to greatest effect. Having insight into a patient's hobbies gave nurses a hook on which to build lighter conversation. Traditionally, critical care nurses have encouraged relatives to bring in favoured tape recordings of music or messages from the family alongside family photographs (Tanner et al., 1993). All of this builds a picture of the patient's personality and how to connect appropriately with him or her.

Therapeutic use of self

Through the process of connecting with patients and responding to their subtle cues, nurses used themselves as therapeutic tools to calm, orientate and return patients to a peaceful rested state. In addition, nurses used self to alleviate respiratory distress, build patients' confidence and trust in their interventions, bring hope, and lighten their mood. To do this, the nurses needed:

- Comprehensive knowledge of the specialty and their own therapeutic potential to inform when and how to act;
- Specific communication skills through which they could dialogue and

understand the responses of unconscious patients and intervene proactively;
- Confidence in the appropriateness of their actions;
- A willingness to take informed risks to offer alternative therapeutic responses to suit a patient's personality;
- Feedback in terms of positive outcomes for the patient (Benner et al., 1996).

The therapeutic use of self was linked to self-knowledge, self-growth, practical wisdom and a wealth of applicable scientific knowledge (Uys, 1980). Thus, science and art became one in terms of the caring act (Leininger, 1984; Orem, 1991; Johnson, 1994) and an expression of the nurses' emotions and feelings (Watson, 1988); but the therapeutic use of self had a dynamic feedback loop: the more it was used, the greater was the confidence to act in this way and the greater was the practical wisdom and range of alternatives that could be applied to any given situation (Scholes, 1996).

The ways in which some of these skills were transferred across to the care of relatives of a critically ill patient will now be addressed. (The term 'relative' is used here to describe any significant other who held a deep rooted emotional bond with the patient.)

Guiding patient's families and friends emotionally and offering them appropriate information

'When a patient is admitted for critical care, they are in physiological crisis, but their relatives enter the department in psychological crisis' (Roberts, 1986). How nurses responded to the needs of family and friends during this sudden life event transition was crucial to the subsequent relationship between the staff and the family. This implies that, although nurses had time to establish themselves with the patient, to frame their act of caring, the initial impact with the relatives established the template against which all other actions were subsequently judged. The sequence of events or crises that the relatives had to face could be broadly categorized into the following:

- Waiting for information and confirmation about the patient's condition and chances of survival;
- Coming to terms with the reality of both the situation and the strange technical environment;
- Overcoming the reality shock and gaining some security from the strangeness of the technology and environment, which confirms that all that could be done was being done;
- Making sense of events and seeking to understand the situation and implications of the treatments;
- Gathering sufficient information about the situation and context to enable the relatives to reclaim the person from the critically ill patient, engage with the person and participate in his or her care;
- Feeling that they were making a contribution to the well-being of their relative (the patient), to bring comfort to them (Zainal and Scholes, 1997).

The way in which the nurses enabled the relatives, through their transition from being outsiders in an alien environment to participants in care, was built over time and grounded in a relationship of trust and rapport. Making immediate connections with relatives who are in a heightened state of distress and anxiety came from experience that informed professional wisdom and empathic engagement. Handling such complex situations is a sphere of excellence that can be located within the advanced practitioner's direct caring role. Four key characteristics could be identified: establishing trust; professional wisdom; empathic engagement; and therapeutic use of self. Each one of these characteristics and their application to the context of enabling relatives through their crisis will be examined.

Trust, argues Meize-Grochowski (1984), is the foundation of a therapeutic relationship and implies confidence in the actions of the trusted. Adequate information that could be trusted as realistic was the relatives' chief concern, which was second only to their primary wish that the patient would fully recover. Trust came from the way in which the nurses interacted with them and the patient. Watching, attentiveness and 'emotional presencing' (Swanson, 1991) did much to confirm in the relatives' minds that the patient was in the best place and receiving all that technology and care could provide. However, the relatives had to cope with the contradiction that, although the patient was receiving such treatment, the outcome could not be predicted. This placed them in a context of uncertainty, which influenced their capacity to adapt to the situation and negotiate their own transition (Mischel, 1990). Helping the relatives to cope with the uncertainty of the patient's condition and enabling them to have a realistic perspective of the survival chances were important; but the nurses were also aware of the need to present a realistic picture without extinguishing hope, hope being the sustaining emotion with which to handle uncertainty (Morse, 1996).

The impact of a relative's sudden admission for critical care leaves family and friends in a state of bewilderment, anxiety and confusion. The physical environment of the critical care unit and the location of invasive technology and equipment to the patient, alongside pathology or trauma, distort the features of critically ill patients and do much to make them unrecognizable. The patient becomes a stranger, and the emotional impact this has on the relatives is to increase their loneliness, anxiety and uncertainty. Connecting with an alienated lonely relative through expressions of care and compassion are ways to reach those who are suffering; to make such connections, there is a need for wisdom and a self-awareness of one's own fragility (Younger, 1995). Therefore, the presence of a wise practitioner, whose connections with the individual is based upon a sense of need and humanity, is the way to help the relatives through their crisis (Morse et al., 1994). The refined skills to achieve this in practice are grounded in experience and expertise.

This picture is one of complexity, through which certain core caring skills can reduce the turmoil for the relatives and enhance their opportunity to participate in care. However, elements of expert practice were evident in the ways in which not only 'complicated' or 'problematic' family situations were handled but also throughout the everyday encounters (for the expert nurse) with relatives of patients admitted to the unit. Connecting with the relatives and being deemed trustworthy, honest and genuine have been shown to be hallmarks of the qualities that relatives identify as excellence in critical care nurses (Zainal and Scholes, 1997). Most importantly, one of the key factors that enables relatives to feel that they can trust the nurse originates from their appraisal of the nurse interacting with their relative (as a patient). The capacity to presence and engage therapeutically with the patient, although not articulated in this language, has been identified as excellence in caring and inspired trust, even if the patient does not survive, because relatives gain great comfort from the nurse's skill to keep the patient pain free and rested (Zainal and Scholes, 1997).

Relatives value highly a nurse's interest in both them and their family, and can include the nurse as part of an extended family picture or as a 'friend' who made things more tolerable. Finding the right balance between enabling the relatives to be stoic and to release their anxiety through periods of emotional fragility have been shown to be crucial to the expert practitioner's capacity to work effectively with relatives in a meaningful and therapeutic way (Morse, 1996).

Discussion

The therapeutic use of self seems, at face value, to be essentially a way of presencing and knowing the patient and relatives that does not require any specialist or advanced skill. Read out of context, this could be viewed as a basic human caring quality grounded in common sense, but Macleod (1994) argues that such qualities demand 'uncommonly common sense' and an altruistic investment of self within the professional role that has matured into genuine practical wisdom (Hixon, 1996). While on the journey towards professional maturity and proficiency, the practitioner acquires fragmented blocks of learning and competence, which have to be deliberated over before they are operationalized and used to effect (Carter et al., 1987; Benner et al., 1996). Such deliberation consumes the energy and attention of the less experienced practitioner, leaving little residual capacity to give self to the everyday act of caring. The therapeutic use of self is seen as the holistic return to basics, which only emerges once practitioners have a solid command of their specialty, practical wisdom, and a profound knowledge that can be applied to the real world context of complexity and upheaval.

Authenticity, presence and connectedness are the hallmarks of the way in which expert practitioners were seen to reach the deeply unconscious patient and use themselves as a therapeutic tool. This raises an important issue. Expert practitioners are unable to articulate their capacity to practice in this way because it has become so integral to their repertoire of caring (Benner et al., 1996). Perhaps one of the features of advanced practitioners is their capacity to find innovative approaches to transfer these skills to others and to find ways to articulate the epistemology of practice in a meaningful and understandable language to their colleagues. We should remember, however, that, if we take the practitioner away from the direct caring context, the skills become muted (Fox-Young, 1995). Therefore, one of the greatest celebrations of the advanced practitioner role is the notion that these practitioners will retain their direct caring role with the subroles of educator, researcher, leader, strategist and evaluator (Manley, 1997). If the balance between the roles cannot be sustained, the consequences for these practitioners and the excellence they espouse might well become eroded, so that they become a jack of all trades and master of none. Perhaps one of the greatest features of advanced practitioners will be their capacity to integrate successfully all these roles, without compromising any one. In this way, we shall see advanced nurse practitioners making a significant difference in the lives of their patients, their relatives and their colleagues.

References

Benner, P. (1984). *From Novice to Expert: Excellence and Power in Clinical Nursing Practice*. Menlo Park, CA: Addison-Wesley.

Benner, P. and Wrubel, J. (1989). *The Primacy of Caring: Stress and Coping in Health and Illness*. Menlo Park, CA: Addison-Wesley.

Benner, P., Tanner, C. and Chesla, C. (1996). *Expertise in Nursing Practice: Caring, Clinical Judgement and Ethics*. New York: Springer Publishing.

Beresford Cooke, C. (1996). *Shiatsu Theory and Practice*. New York: Churchill Livingstone.

Bishop, A. and Scudder, J. (1990). *The Practical, Moral and Personal Sense of Nursing: a Phenomenological Philosophy of Practice*. Albany, NY: State University of New York Press.

Botorff, J. and Morse, J. (1994). Identifying types of attending: patterns of nurses' work. *Image J. Nurs. Schol.*, **26**, 53–59.

Botorff, J. and Varcoe, C. (1995). Transitions in nurse–patient interactions: a qualitative ethology. *Qual. Health Res.*, **5**, 315–331.

Brykczynski, K. (1989). An interpretive study describing the clinical judgement of nurse practitioners. *Schol. Inquiry Nurs. Pract.*, **3**, 90–91.

Carper, B. (1975). *Fundamental Patterns of Knowing in Nursing*. New York: Teachers College, Columbia University.

Carter, K., Sabers, D., Cushing, K. et al. (1987). Processing and using information about students: a study of novice and expert postulant teachers. *Teaching Teacher Educ.*, **3**, 147–157.

Castledine, G. (1996). Clarifying and defining nursing role developments. *Br. J. Nurs.*, **5**, 1338.

Chinn, P. and Kramer, M. (1991). *Theory and Nursing: a Systematic Approach*, 3rd ed. St Louis, MO: Mosby-Yearbook.

Elliott, J. (1991). *Action Research for Educational Change: Developing Teachers and Teaching*. Buckingham: Open University Press.

Erlandson, D., Harris, E., Skipper, B. and Allen, S. (1993). *Doing Naturalistic Inquiry: a Guide to Methods*. Newbury Park, CA: Sage.

Fox-Young, S. (1995). Issues in the assessment of expert nurses: purposes standards and methods. *Nurse Educ. Today*, **15**, 96–100.

Gadow, S. (1989). Clinical subjectivity: advocacy with silent patients. *Nurs. Clin. North Am.*, **24**, 535–541.

Gepp, D. (1996). *The Shoot*. (BBC 2, 3 October.) London: British Broadcasting Corporation.

Gilliss, C. (1996). Education for advanced practice nursing. In *Advanced Practice Nursing: Changing Roles and Clinical Applications*. (J. Hickey, ed.), pp. 22–32. Philadelphia, PA: Lippincott–Raven.

Glaser, B. and Strauss, A. (1967). *The Discovery of Grounded Theory*. Chicago, IL: Aldine.

Hixon, M. (1996). Professional development: socialisation in advanced practice nursing'. In *Advanced Practice Nursing: Changing Roles and Clinical Applications*. (J. Hickey, ed.), pp. 33–53. Philadelphia, PA: Lippincott–Raven.

Hudak, C., Gallo, B. and Lohr, T. (1986). *Critical Care Nursing: a Holistic Approach*, 4th ed. Philadelphia, PA: Lippincott.

Janiesick, V. (1994). The dance of qualitative design, metaphor, methodolatry and meaning. In *Handbook of Qualitative Research*. (N. Denzin and Y. Lincoln, eds.), pp. 209–19. Newbury Park, CA: Sage.

Johnson, J. (1994). A dialectical examination of nursing art. *Adv. Nurs. Sci.*, **17**(1), 1–14.

Leininger, M. (1984). Caring: a central focus of nursing health care services. In *Care: the Essence of Nursing and Health*. (M. Leininger, ed.), pp. 45–59, Thorofare, NJ: Slack.

Macleod, M. (1994). It's the little things that count: the hidden complexity of everyday clinical nursing practice. *J. Clin. Nurs.*, **3**, 361–368.

Manley, K. (1997). A conceptual framework for advanced practice: An action research project operationalising an advanced practitioner/consultant nurse role. *J. Clin. Nurs.*, **6**(3), 179–190

May, C. (1991). Affective neutrality and involvement in nurse–patient relationships: perceptions of appropriate behaviour among nurses in acute medical and surgical wards. *J. Adv. Nurs.*, **16**, 552–558.

Meize-Grochowski, R. (1984). An analysis of the concept of trust. *J. Adv. Nurs.*, **9**, 563–572.

Mischel, M. (1990). Re-conceptualisation of the uncertainty of illness theory. *Image: J. Nurs. Schol.*, **22**, 265–262.

Morse, J. (1996). *Comforting: Enabling Enduring and Facilitating Suffering*. (Mebius Kramer Lecture, Utrecht, 26 April 1996.) Edinburgh: Campion Press.

Morse, J., Miles, M., Clark, D. and Doberneck, B. (1994). Sensing patient needs: exploring concepts of nursing insight and receptivity used in nursing assessment. *Schol. Inquiry Nurs. Pract.*, **8**, 234–261.

Orem, D. (1991). *Nursing: Concepts of Practice*, 4th ed. St Louis, MO: Mosby-Yearbook.

Paniagua, H. (1995). The scope of advanced practice: action potential for practice nurses. *Br. J. Nurs.*, **4**, 269–274.

Parlett, M. and Hamilton, D. (1972). Evaluation as Illumination: a new approach to the study of innovatory programmes. Occasional Paper no. 9, Centre for Research in the Educational Sciences, Edinburgh: Reprinted in *Evaluating Education: Issues and Methods: an Open University Reader*. (R. Murphy and H. Torrance) pp. 57–73. London: Harper and Row

Parse, R. (1992). Human becoming: Parse's theory of nursing. *Nurs. Sci. Q.*, **5**, 35–42.

Radwin, L. (1995). Knowing the patient: a process model for individualised interventions. *Nurs. Res.*, **44**, 364–370.

Roberts, S. (1986). *Behavioural concepts of the critically ill*, 2nd ed. Norwalk, CT: Appleton-Century-Crofts.

Rubin, J. (1996). Impediments to the development of clinical knowledge and ethical judgement in critical care nursing. In *Expertise in Nursing Practice: Caring, Clinical Judgement and Ethics*. (P. Benner, C. Tanner and C. Chesla, eds.), pp. 170–192. New York: Springer Publishing.

Scholes, J. (1996). Therapeutic use of self: how the critical care nurse uses self to the patient's therapeutic benefit. *Nurs. Crit. Care*, **1**(2), 60–65.

Scholes, J. and Freeman, M. (1994). The reflective dialogue and repertory grid: a research approach to identify the unique contribution of nursing, midwifery or health visiting to the therapeutic milieu. *J. Adv. Nurs.*, **20**, 885–893.

Scholes, J. and Moore, M. (1997). Making a difference: the way in which the nurse interacts with the critical care environment and uses herself as a therapeutic tool. *ITU NDU Occasional Paper Series no. 2*. University of Brighton.

Schraeder, B. and Fischer, D. (1987). Using intuitive knowledge in the neonatal intensive care nursery. *Holistic Nurs. Pract.*, **1**(3), 45–51.

Simmons, H. (1987). *Getting to Know Schools in a Democracy: the Politics and Process of Evaluation*. London: Falmer Press.

Sparacino, P. (1992). Advanced practice; the clinical nurse specialist. *Nurse Pract.*, **5**(4), 2–4.

Stake, R. (1994). Case Studies. In *Handbook of Qualitative Research*. (N. Denzin and Y. Lincoln, eds.), pp. 236–247. Newbury Park, CA: Sage.

Swanson, K. (1991). Empirical developments of a middle range theory of caring. *Nurs. Res.*, **40**, 175–180.

Tanner, C., Benner, P., Chesla, C. and Gordon, D. (1993). The phenomenology of knowing the patient. *Image: J. Nurs. Schol.*, **25**, 273–280.

Uys, L. (1980). Towards the development of an operational definition of the concept 'therapeutic use of self'. *Int. J. Nurs. Stud.*, **17**, 175–180.

Walters, A. (1995). A Heideggerian hermeneutic study of the practice of critical care nurses. *J. Adv. Nurs.*, **21**, 492–497.

Watson, J. (1988). *Nursing: Human Science, Human Care: a Theory of Nursing*. New York: National League for Nursing.

Younger, J. (1995). The alienation of the sufferer. *Adv. Nurs. Sci.*, **17**(4), 53–72.

Zainal, G. and Scholes, J. (1997). Adapting to crisis: the relatives' experience of intensive care and the nurses' therapeutic role with the family. *ITU NDU Occasional Paper Series no. 3*. University of Brighton.

Education for the advanced practitioner

Gary Rolfe

Part 4 of this book has explored the notion of advanced practice as mindful expertise, and has focused on the development and exploration of personal and experiential 'knowing how' and 'knowing that', and on a number of methods for uncovering such knowledge and bringing it into consciousness. In this final chapter, I will explore some of the issues to be considered when establishing an educational course for advanced practitioners.

Educational needs of the advanced practitioner

There are a growing number of courses, usually at masters level, that offer a diverse range of approaches to advanced practitioner education; indeed, this diversity is to be expected, given the lack of consensus over what constitutes advanced practice. Some of those courses are skills based, some provide advanced theoretical knowledge in particular specialisms such as critical care or mental health nursing, and some offer a combination of skills and knowledge in some or all of the subroles of advanced practice identified by the American Nurses' Association (McLoughlin, 1992), namely research, education, management, leadership and consultancy. All of the above would meet the criteria of one or more definitions of advanced practice in current usage, and each is designed to appeal to a particular type of practitioner with particular learning needs.

The debate around the educational needs of the advanced practitioner has become the focus of a wider dispute about the nature of the role, and has polarized educationalists into two opposing camps. This dichotomy of views can be seen clearly in the report of the listening exercise conducted by the United Kingdom Central Council for Nursing, Midwifery and Health Visiting (UKCC, 1996). On the one hand, some educationalists have advocated a model in which 'the pathways to advanced practice needed to be fuelled by many different experiences, structured reflection and individually tailored study', with a portfolio and 'expert peer' panel approach to assessment. In contrast, others 'stressed the importance of a competency based framework for postregistration education' with a more formalized means of assessment based around the demonstration of specific clinical knowledge and skills.

Clearly, these two educational models reflect different perspectives on the nature of advanced practice, which was summarized by the UKCC (1996) as follows:

There was a split regarding understanding of advanced practice. Some participants saw advanced practice as a list of extended tasks and occupational competencies gained through a structured period of study at masters level and supervised clinical practice; others understood it as a broader way of looking at and developing nursing gained through a portfolio of experience, structured reflection and individually tailored study. Broadly, the first group saw advanced practitioners within a doctor substitution model and thought therefore that advanced practice required a high level knowledge base founded predominantly in the biological sciences, physical health assessment skills, evidence based and supported by assertiveness and communication skills training. Focused education was seen as essential in preparing nurses to take on new roles in primary and secondary health care settings, but the development of nurses and nursing appeared unimportant. In the second group, the knowledge base suggested was eclectic and more process oriented. The ability to constantly question practice, high motivation, commitment to *nursing* development, confidence and self awareness, underpinned and informed by structured critical reflection were seen as crucial. Advanced practitioners in the second group were expected to be grounded in practice but to have research, education and consultancy functions as well. Advanced practice was seen to be very much about advancing the practice of others.

Consensus amongst the respondents largely favoured the second group, and 'the nurse practitioner model of doctor substitution either in acute or primary care was not felt to meet the criteria for advanced practice' (UKCC, 1996).

However, although the two camps appear to have set themselves in opposition to one another, they are in fact responding to the educational needs of two different groups of practitioners, each of which complements the other. Before discussing an educational programme for the advanced practitioner, it is therefore necessary to distinguish the role from what we might, following the terminology of the UKCC, refer to as the clinical nurse specialist (CNS).

The UKCC originally conceived a hierarchical relationship between the advanced nurse practitioner and the CNS, in which nurses could progress from nurse practitioner to specialist practitioner to advanced practitioner. However, this view was later modified, so that 'advanced practice is not an additional layer of practice to be added to specialist practice' (UKCC, 1995). Nevertheless, the suggestion of a hierarchy continues, with specialist practitioner educational programmes being 'no lower than first-degree level' while advanced practitioners would be 'undertaking studies which are likely to be at masters and PhD level' (UKCC, 1995). It is rather difficult to untangle the precise relationship between the two, and the latest pronouncement from the UKCC does little to help the confusion in stating: 'It does not...make sense to label a particular activity as advanced. The UKCC is keen that specialist practice should embrace as many practitioners as possible rather than be exclusive (UKCC, 1997).

For the purposes of this chapter, it might be useful to polarize the roles of the specialist practitioner and the advanced practitioner, since this will help to clarify the very different educational needs of the two groups. This dichotomy is not intended to suggest a hierarchical relationship, nor an exclusivity of function. There is clearly some overlap between the two roles, and it is right that there should be. The differences between them are outlined in Table 17.1.

Table 17.1. The specialist and advanced practitioner roles

Specialist practitioner	Advanced practitioner
The specialist practitioner is concerned with content, with *what* he or she practices, for example, the application of specialist knowledge.	The advanced practitioner is concerned with process, with *how* he or she practices, for example, the use of clinical judgement.
The role of the specialist practitioner is a mixture of practice, teaching, research and education in varying proportions to suit local needs	The role of the advanced practitioner is grounded in clinical practice, although it might include other subroles from time to time, such as teaching, research and consultancy.
The specialist practitioner is primarily a technical role.	The advanced practitioner is primarily a therapeutic role.
The knowledge base of the specialist practitioner is primarily scientific knowledge. If this knowledge base is to be maintained, the specialist practitioner must continually update his or her specialist knowledge through academic study. It is therefore possible for the specialist practitioner to have a role that includes only a small practice component.	The knowledge base of the advanced practitioner is predominantly practical and experiential knowledge. If this knowledge base is to be maintained, the advanced practitioner must remain in practice. By definition, it is not possible to have an advanced practitioner whose role is primarily managerial or educational.
The specialist practitioner reflects on the *content* of nursing, that is, on what he or she does.	The advanced practitioner reflects on the *process* of nursing, that is, on how he or she nurses.
Supervision focuses on caseload management and specific clinical issues.	Supervision focuses on the process of clinical practice. It employs specific issues to explore process.
Because the knowledge base of specialist practice is scientific, it can be developed through taught courses at all levels, focusing on the teaching of relevant clinical content and learning how to access and critically appraise that content.	Because the knowledge base of advanced practice is experiential and personal, it cannot be developed through formal taught courses, but through reflection on the process of nursing. It is inappropriate to expect nurses to register on courses (at whatever level) to learn how to become advanced practitioners.

Educational implications of the role

Clearly, this view of advanced practice has a number of fairly explicit educational implications, which run counter to most traditional approaches to both specialist and advanced nurse education. Most significantly, it suggests that the student will enter an advanced practice course with a well-developed knowledge and skills base, although, of course, he or she might not be able to articulate it. The educational model most appropriate for advanced practice courses is therefore *not* of a more skilled, more knowledgeable practitioner imparting clinical wisdom to a less-expert, less-knowledgable student (the so-called 'mug and jug' model), but rather of a partnership of equals, of an expert educationalist (but not necessarily an expert clinician) helping an expert nurse to explore his or her own practice, to generate knowledge from that practice, and to disseminate it to others. This is the model advocated by Rogers (1983) of the educationalist as a facilitator rather than as a teacher.

The practitioner might need to learn new skills to enable him or her to generate, explore and disseminate the practice based knowledge; research skills, teaching skills or supervision skills might be required, but these are not the *necessary* skills of an advanced practitioner. They are merely tools to facilitate the role. A course comprised predominantly of those elements would not constitute a course in advanced practice as it is understood here. In fact, an advanced practice course of the kind being advocated here would not primarily be aimed at developing practical skills of any kind, or with imparting specific clinical knowledge. Rather, it would be concerned with the interface between knowing and doing, with how knowledge is translated into practice and with how knowledge is generated and extracted *from* practice.

Clearly, such a course would not be content laden, and the aim would not be (as we have already seen) to disseminate content based knowledge, but to develop transferable process skills, the skills of learning how to learn, of critical and self-critical appraisal, and of building knowledge and theory from practice through reflection-on-action. Core content would therefore be restricted to the knowledge and skills associated with critical reflection, and, in particular, of clinical supervision and reflective writing. If individual students required specific content in the course of their studies, then the role of the educationalist would be to facilitate them to identify what knowledge they needed and how to find it, either by accessing taught courses or through private study. Because each student would have individual and unique learning needs, programmes of learning would have to be student centred and individually tailored, perhaps through the use of a learning contract. This approach is in keeping with the UKCC (1996) recommendation that courses for advanced practitioners should be concerned with 'structured reflection and individually tailored study'.

Furthermore, because such a course would focus on the processes of practice rather than on the content, and because content is individually negotiated and pursued, it could very easily be multidisciplinary, not just across the different nursing disciplines but across the helping professions generally. The ultimate aim would therefore be to develop flexible, reflective and reflexive lifelong learners in a fast-changing professional environment where specific content based knowledge has a limited life.

It should be apparent by now that advanced practice as it is described here cannot be taught; it is a body of personal and experiential knowledge and skills that accumulates over time through doing and then reflecting on that doing. A course for advanced practitioners should be precisely that, a course for practitioners who are already practising at an expert or advanced level, and as such it would not 'produce' advanced practitioners but rather enable advanced practitioners to articulate and learn from what they do and also accredit them educationally for what they already are. This approach is largely in keeping with the findings from the UKCC (1996) listening exercise that 'we can only facilitate the emergence of advanced practitioners rather than being able to create them'.

We have already established that the focus of the work of the advanced practitioner is on practice rather than on research, education or management (although these elements might or might not constitute a small component of the role). The focus of a course for advanced practitioners should therefore also be on practice, and could, for example, be structured around practice based projects in the student's own clinical area, and the generation of personal and experiential knowledge from those projects through guided reflection and reflective writing. Furthermore, the notion of a dissertation by research is clearly inappropriate, since it emphasizes the importance of scientific knowledge at the expense of experiential and personal knowledge.

If courses for advanced practitioners are to focus on practice and the generation of experiential and personal knowledge rather than on theory and the dissemination of scientific knowledge, then we are faced with a number of problems around the issue of how to assess and evaluate practice at an advanced level. These problems are both practical and epistemological, and are compounded by the numerous rules and regulations about levels, philosophies and methods of assessment imposed by academic institutions.

The practical problems revolve around the difficulty in determining who would be qualified to assess practice at advanced level, since, by definition, the practitioners undertaking such a course would be at the forefront of their professions and already pushing at the limits of expertise. Educationalists might have the skills of assessment, but would lack the clinical expertise to make informed evaluations of advanced practice.

The epistemological problems are more intractable, and are concerned with the nature of advanced practice and the ways in which it manifests itself. We have already seen that the knowledge base of advanced practice is complex, unique to each practitioner, and not easily expressed in words, and that the behavioural component is slippery and avoids simple categorization. Advanced practice does not manifest itself in simple, observable measurable behaviours or in generalizable propositional knowledge, and so we cannot adopt a 'tick box' approach to its evaluation. As the UKCC (1996) points out: 'advanced practice is not directly related to a list of tasks to be performed or occupational competencies', but is concerned with 'structured reflection and individually tailored study'.

One way of resolving this problem is to make a distinction between evaluation and assessment. Evaluation is the act of making a value judgement, of determining the quality of something, whereas assessment (as the term is used here) is an educational undertaking employed as part of a mechanism of academic accreditation. Evaluation is concerned with making judgements about clinical quality, assessment with making judgements about academic worth.

Once this distinction has been made, our task becomes easier. All students need to be assessed for the award of academic credit for their study. Academic assessment requires educational skill and expertise, and is usually undertaken by an educationalist. In theory based courses designed to transmit propositional knowledge, the process of academic assessment is relatively unproblematic, since the educationalist would usually have a well-developed knowledge base in the subject being assessed, and would therefore also be in a position to make an evaluation of the extent to which the student had mastered that knowledge base.

However, in a course for advanced practitioners, where the knowledge base is experiential and practical, the educationalist is usually not equipped to make such an evaluation, although he or she would still be required to carry out an assessment. Fortunately, we have seen that one of the core characteristics of an advanced practitioner is the ability to be reflectively self-critical, through clinical supervision, through reflective writing and through other reflective techniques. Thus, the problem of who assesses and evaluates advanced practice can be resolved by requiring the advanced practitioner to evaluate his or her own practice critically, and for the educationalist to assess that critical evaluation. Students on a course for advanced practitioners would, in effect, be required to produce a reflective critique of their own practice in the form of a course assignment; that assignment would then be assessed by a course tutor in much the same way as a critique of, say, a research report, that is, in terms of the high-level cognitive skills of evaluation, synthesis and analysis. Of course, the task of self-evaluation is made more difficult by its subjective, reflexive nature; it is easier to evaluate the work of someone you do not know, rather than your own work. However, we have seen that this ability to be reflectively self-critical is precisely the cognitive skill that distinguishes advanced practitioners from those practising at a more basic level; advanced practitioners can access, explore and learn from their own experiential and personal knowledge.

Finally, it is worth considering the academic level of courses for advanced practitioners. The UKCC, as we have seen, originally set the level at masters or PhD, but part of the reason for that decision is probably related to the hierarchical nature of the various roles. Thus, if specialist practitioner programmes were to be at degree level, then advanced practitioner courses would have to be at least at masters level. However, most of the participants who took part in the UKCC's listening exercise (UKCC, 1996) reinforced this decision, with only the representatives of medical organizations dissenting, the conclusion being that nurses educated to masters level 'may be construed as threatening to the medics' (UKCC, 1996).

Part of this threat might be related to the finding from the listening exercise that the medical representatives believed that 'everyone "belonged" to a doctor', and that, since doctors themselves are not usually educated to masters level, it would be difficult for them if some of the workers 'belonging' to them were more educated than they were. Nevertheless, from a purely educational perspective, it is clear that the reflective and reflexive nature of the educational experience associated with the academic needs of advanced practitioners can be provided only at such a level.

MA in advanced professional practice: an example of a course for advanced practitioners

I will now briefly describe a course for advanced practitioners that is being offered at the University of Portsmouth. (Readers who are interested in courses for specialist practitioners, are directed to the account by Gibbon and Luker (1995) of the masters programme offered by the University of Liverpool.) It was designed according to the model of advanced practice outlined in Part 4 of this book, and has the following features:

- It is an interdisciplinary/multiprofessional course for advanced practitioners in any area of health care. Applications have been received from practitioners in a range of disciplines including nursing and midwifery, the medical profession, and the professions allied to medicine.
- It strives towards a student centred partnership between practitioner and educationalist, in which each is acknowledged as an expert in his or her own field of practice. The content is brought to the course by the participants themselves, based on the reflective philosophy that learning about practice means learning *from* practice.
- It is process driven rather than content laden, with a focus on the processes of practice that are common to all health care practitioners, providing an opportunity for nurses, therapists and doctors to work together and share knowledge and experiences in a truly interdisciplinary way.
- It is practice based and project focused, and is constructed around work being undertaken by the course participants in their own practice areas as part of their everyday activities.
- It encourages a flexible approach to learning in which course content and learning methods are negotiated through individual learning contracts.
- It provides the opportunity for interdisciplinary group supervision on a regular monthly basis.

I am not claiming that this is the best way, or the only way, to design a course for advanced practitioners; it is merely *one* way. It is therefore being offered as an example rather than as an exemplar, as a slice of experiential knowing how and knowing that, from which the reader can take as appropriate to individual needs.

The course structure

The course includes six compulsory core units:

- Learning contract and portfolio (2 units);
- Practice development through supervision;
- Critical reflection;
- Project proposal;
- Project report.

Within the 'Learning contract and portfolio' unit, students will negotiate the balance of credits required for the award of Master of Arts. These remaining units may be selected from a wide range of electives from across the spectrum of University courses, although the students must be able to justify their selection in relation to their personal and professional development, as well as to the overall coherence of their personal programme of study. Additionally, some core units may be taken again, this time as options, and students may also elect to take an option written especially for this course, entitled 'Critical review of a previous project'.

Learning contract and portfolio (core)

These units act as the unifying mechanism for the course, and, as such, run throughout the time that the student is registered for the award. The first unit is intended to facilitate the student's progression through the core units of the programme up to postgraduate diploma level. The second unit builds on the first, and focuses on the options and electives that complete the programme to masters level. There is no formal syllabus content to these units. The learning contract is guided by the focus of the students' own professional practice and by the individual skills and knowledge that they wish to acquire. Within the learning contract, the students will identify the combination of units that will enable them to meet those learning needs. This will be reviewed each semester and renegotiated as appropriate. The review of progress is achieved through the collection of evidence of learning in the portfolio.

Each semester, the portfolio will act as a reflective review in which the students will evaluate the evidence collected against their learning contract and assess their own progress. This in turn feeds back into a review and reassessment of the learning contract as new needs are identified and plans are made to fulfil these. In the final semester, the reflective review will provide a commentary on the whole course, demonstrating how the learning outcomes stated in the learning contract have been achieved. Thus, the portfolio acts as the cohesive mechanism for the course, where units are brought together and reflected upon as a whole. In addition, students will assess the process of their learning and how it contributes to the attributes of a practitioner who is committed to advancing practice.

Practice development through supervision (core)

This unit provides ongoing peer support through regular monthly meetings of the student group. The focus of the group is on the clinical supervision of practice through a range of formal and informal structures, as this is thought to offer the most appropriate framework for reflecting on personal and experiential knowledge from practice. The unit also aims to provide a forum for the sharing of ideas, educational and emotional support, the discussion of project work and other course work, and an exploration of the experience of course participation. Thus, although the content of the unit focuses on the development of the knowledge and skills of the clinical supervision of practice, the means to achieve that end include a range of models of clinical and educational support, including mentoring, preceptorship and 'buddy' systems.

These learning methods will also be set in the context of a dynamic, functioning group, and a number of models of group processes and dynamics will be explored through discussions and reflection on the ongoing learning group. Regular attendance and peer support will therefore be stressed as the key elements to a successful learning experience. The assessment of this unit will be through two short-case presentations and a written reflective account of the student's contribution to the supervision group.

Critical reflection (core)
This taught, content based unit runs throughout the first semester, and provides the students with a range of theory and knowledge necessary to undertake the project based units and the 'Practice development through supervision' unit. It is therefore a key unit and provides the theoretical underpinning that informs the whole Advanced Professional Practice programme. It is assessed through a written critique and a seminar presentation of a critical incident.

Project proposal (core and option)
Following a short taught component, this unit is structured around a programme of individual tutorials, during which the students will be expected to develop a proposal to undertake a practice based project in their own work area. The unit has two sets of learning outcomes: process outcomes related to the design and writing of a project proposal, which are common to all students taking the unit; and content outcomes, which relate to the specific proposal being undertaken, and which are individually negotiated with each student. The unit assignment will be a written project proposal following the guidelines specified in the taught component, and will assess both process and content learning outcomes.

Project report (core and option)
In this practitioner based enquiry, the students will implement the project outlined in the 'Project proposal' unit, which is a prerequisite for this unit. The project will usually be based in the students' own work area, and will typically include a practice innovation and an evaluation phase. The students will be responsible for their own learning and assignment work, calling on the support of the tutor and named specialists in practice areas as appropriate. With tutorial guidance, they will identify key and relevant syllabus content and texts to support the implementation and evaluation of their project. The project could be of any size, from a planned change to individual practice to a large-scale project involving an entire practice area. The unit has two sets of learning outcomes: process outcomes related to project design and report writing, which are common to all students taking the unit; and content outcomes, which relate to the specific project being undertaken, and which are individually negotiated with each student. The unit will be assessed by a written formal report with a particular focus on discussion and evaluation of the project.

Critical review of a previous project (option)
Students may elect to take up to two critical reviews of projects that they have previously undertaken before joining the course. The projects should be practice based and can be of any size. The unit has two sets of learning outcomes: process outcomes related to project evaluation and report

writing, which are common to all students taking the unit; and content outcomes, which relate to the specific project being undertaken, and which are individually negotiated with each student. The unit is structured around a programme of individual tutorials and group seminar presentations, and, in keeping with the course philosophy, credits will be awarded for a critical evaluation of the project rather than for its successful outcome.

Conclusion

The content, structure and academic level of a course for advanced practitioners must clearly reflect the needs of the practitioners themselves. This raises difficulties with courses for advanced practitioners, since there is, as yet, no clear and widely accepted agreement on what advanced practice is. The view of advanced practice taken in this chapter is congruent with that expressed in my earlier chapter, and sees it as practice based, as concerned primarily with personal and experiential knowledge, and as focusing on the processes of professional judgement rather than on skills and propositional knowledge.

This perspective has a number of explicit educational implications, which have been discussed in some detail, and has resulted in the design of a practice based course at master's level, which seeks to accredit clinical work by requiring the practitioner to carry our reflective evaluations of his or her own practice. However, it is also acknowledged that other definitions of advanced practice will result in other models of course design, and that we should not be narrowing the focus of the educational experiences on offer to practitioners at any level.

References

Gibbon, B. and Luker, K. A. (1995). Uncharted territory: masters preparation as a foundation for nurse clinicians. *Nurse Educ. Today*, **15**, 164–169.
McLoughlin, S. (1992). Congress on nursing practice meets. *Am. Nurse*, **24**, 23.
Rogers, C. R. (1983). *Freedom to Learn for the 80s*. Ohio: Merrill.
United Kingdom Central Council for Nursing, Midwifery and Health Visiting. (1995). *Implementation of the UKCC's Standards for Post-Registration Education and Practice (PREP)*. London: UKCC.
United Kingdom Central Council for Nursing, Midwifery and Health Visiting. (1996). *PREP – The Nature of Advanced Practice: an Interim Report*. London: UKCC.
United Kingdom Central Council for Nursing, Midwifery and Health Visiting. (1997). Advancing professional practice. *Register*, **19**, 5.

Commentary: the professional development perspective

Part 4 returned to the two fundamental questions posed by Albarran and Fulbrook in the opening chapter of the book: 'What is advanced practice?' and 'What is an advanced practitioner?' However, in the intervening chapters, the answers to these questions have developed into two themes, with some writers focusing on *advanced* practice and others on *advancing* practice. The difference, as we have seen, is more than semantic. The label 'advanced practice' suggests that some practice is not so advanced, and therefore places it in a hierarchy. This is the view expressed by Fulbrook's respondents, which he summarized as: 'Advanced practice is expert clinical practice, which is at a higher level than that delivered by non-advanced practitioners', and by Goodman's assertion that 'the advanced practitioner role is defined as the pinnacle of the proposed clinical career structure', but, whereas 'advanced' is an adjective that describes a particular level of practice, 'advancing' is a verb that describes an activity. Advancing practice is therefore not a state but an action. As Johns pointed out, advanced practice might mean 'advancing what is held to be known', and, for him, 'the notion that "advanced" might distinguish levels of practice is less attractive; it would become an arbitrary concept constituted in terms of artificial criteria.'

Similarly, Barker suggested in Part 1 that: 'The critical aspect of the role of [advanced practitioners] might be to advance practice, acting as a role model to all those defined, implicitly, as *basic* practitioners.' However, unlike Johns, Barker appears to be happy with the idea that the term 'advanced' distinguishes a higher level of practice from that of 'basic' practitioners. Similarly, Holyoake suggested three levels of 'core', 'specialist' and 'advanced'; Elliott offered four levels of 'preceptored', 'professional', 'specialist' and 'advanced'; and Goodman proposed seven levels from 'newly qualified' to 'advanced'. What they all appear to be suggesting is that in order to be *advancing* practice, whether it is his or her own or that of colleagues, the nurse must first attain a higher level, which we might call *advanced* practice. In this final part of the book, an attempt is made to develop the notion of the nurse achieving a level of *advanced* practice from which she is then able to *advance* practice.

In the first of the five chapters of Part 4, Rolfe explores this issue by outlining a typology of nursing knowledge, which includes not only generalizable knowledge from scientific research, but also experiential and personal knowledge: not only theoretical 'knowing that', but also practical 'knowing how'. Although this typology is derived from the work of theorists, it is supported by the views of advanced practitioners themselves. Fulbrook illustrated this in an earlier chapter, where his sample of advanced practitioners claimed to use 'personal knowledge' and 'knowledge from clinical experience rather than knowledge from formal education' to make clinical decisions. Similarly, Elliott identified the use of 'nursing intuition' in her own practice, and Holyoake linked advanced practice firmly to Benner's notion of intuitive expertise. Advanced practice would therefore appear to transcend the application of scientific knowledge. As Stilwell observed, 'protocols of care cannot account for every situation', and nurses must employ a range of knowledge and skills that take them far beyond scientific, research based knowledge; and, as Barker added, although knowledge gained from scientific theory and research has its place, 'it may not bring nursing closer to a clarification either of the *basic* or fundamental role and functions of the ... nurse, or the possibilities for *advanced practice.*'

These latter views would seem to suggest that advanced practice might be no more or less than Benner's concept of expertise. However, Rolfe argues that Benner's experts practice from an incomplete knowledge base, which omits experiential and personal theoretical knowledge, and that they are therefore unable to articulate the theory underpinning their practice. By reflecting on their practical knowledge, advanced practitioners are able to build theory out of practice, and thereby make conscious the so-called intuitive practice of the expert. For Rolfe, the conscious awareness of their own knowledge base is the most important aspect of the advanced practitioners' work. If they are to advance the practice of others, then they must be able to articulate the knowledge underpinning their own practice in order to share it with their colleagues. As Holyoake pointed out earlier: 'The educator facet enables the ANP [advanced nusc practitioner] to role model, mentor, share and assist. ... If such a role is stripped down to its bare bones, it is primarily about information exchange and the facilitation of such.'

Rolfe's suggestion that advanced practice goes beyond Benner's 'understanding without a rationale' towards a model of analytical decision making is also supported by Fulbrook's advanced practitioners. As Fulbrook pointed out: 'Although intuition and heurism were considered part of advanced practice, informants did not reject analytical ability. In fact, on the contrary, it was frequently mentioned as an important factor that was necessary for advanced practice.' Thus: 'When advanced practitioners make decisions, they do so having acknowledged all the factors that impinge on a particular situation and having weighed up the possible consequences of a variety of possible interventions.'

Advanced practice is therefore seen as mindful expertise, and, unlike Benner's expert, advanced practitioners are able to articulate the underlying rationale of their clinical decisions, to 'preach what they practice', and thereby advance the practice of their colleagues not only by example but by explanation. This, perhaps, is what Barker meant earlier by the advanced practitioner developing conceptual maps that 'will provide the provisional knowledge that will help so-called novice nurses find themselves within the caring relationship'.

This notion of advanced practice as being distinguished by the generation of a body of experiential and personal *theoretical* knowledge that informs practical 'know how' is implicitly or explicitly stated in most of the definitions, check-lists and discussions from earlier chapters. Frost, for example, stated that: 'It is my view that advancing practice is about developing the way in which nurses understand how they make decisions, analyse the consequences of what they do, and adapt nursing to improve the health outcomes for the people they serve.' Similarly, Stilwell pointed out that 'the nurse must become an expert problem-solver, using a range of knowledge and skills to identify and respond to health need, while helping patients to choose and achieve their individual health goals.' Likewise, Read produced a check-list of 10 attributes of the advanced practitioner, which she gathered from the literature, before offering an observation from a group of advanced practitioners themselves that 'the crucial factor is the level of decision making and responsibility for a caseload rather than the nature of the tasks undertaken.' This practitioner's perspective was reinforced by Fulbrook, who noted from his findings that 'the excellence of care that [advanced practitioners] give is not measured in relation to their ability to perform tasks but in their ability to assimilate a wide range of knowledge and understanding, which they apply to their practice'; by Elliott, who claimed that critical thinking skills were crucial to her own advanced practice; and by Goodman, who added that: 'Conceptual thinking and the ability to articulate and rationalize one's own practice are crucial aspects of the advanced practitioner's role.'

This view of the advanced practitioner as the possessor and transmitter of a body of experiential and personal knowledge has an extremely important implication: by definition, the advanced practitioner *has* to have a practice. That is not to say that advanced nurse practitioners must do nothing but hands on nursing. They might well be researchers, educators and/or managers as well, but first and foremost they are practitioners, and it is the knowledge that they generate from their practice that informs and supports their other roles.

Again, this notion is supported by most of the writers in this book, and, whereas some appear to take the practice focus of the role for granted (for example, most of the contributors to Part 4), others are more explicit about the predominance of the practice role. Thus, Manley advocated four subroles of expert practitioner, educator, researcher and consultant, but concluded that 'all four subroles are *practice based*, requiring both practical and theoretical knowledge' (our emphasis). Similarly, Fulbrook's advanced practitioners saw the essence of advanced practice as being clinical, but with subroles that included change agent, consultant, educator and researcher, but not manager, and Elliott described the integration of her subroles in the practice setting. Only Goodman questioned this emphasis on hands-on clinical work, suggesting that the advanced practitioner plays more of a strategic and managerial role in relation to practice.

Clearly, then, educationalists and managers cannot be advanced practitioners in nursing (although they might achieve advanced status in the practice of teaching or management), and this, as later chapters demonstrate, has implications for the education and supervision of advanced nurse practitioners. In particular, it challenges the traditional models of education and practice development as the transmission of knowledge and skills from non-practising lecturers or managers to novice practitioners. Educationalists and managers cannot, by definition, be advanced practitioners, so their credibility as experts in advanced practice, and thus their ability to teach, manage and assess advanced practice, is called into question.

If educationalists cannot teach advanced practice, managers cannot manage it, and neither group can assess it, then who can? One answer to this question, which is explored in the last four chapters, is that it is, in fact, the *wrong* question; we should not be asking who can teach, manage and assess advanced practitioners, but how they can be facilitated to teach, manage and assess themselves. According to this view, advanced practitioners should be autonomous and self-regulating, and their relationship with managers and educationalists should be a relationship of peers, each acknowledging the skills and expertise of the other in their respective fields of practice, a view expressed by Holyoake earlier in the book.

As Johns pointed out, the advanced practitioner must be enabled 'to take responsibility to ensure her [Helen's] own practice development and, through review, to monitor her own effectiveness. These are the hallmarks of responsible practice.' Similarly, Goodman stressed the importance of advanced practitioners being able to evaluate their own practice. This view is embraced wholeheartedly by Rolfe in the final chapter on education for the advanced practitioner, and is also supported in the earlier chapter by Coombs and Holgate (who, writing from a managerial perspective, were understandably more cautious), in which they proposed an organizational framework for advanced practice. They argued that limits and boundaries to responsibility, authority and accountability have to be set, but that: 'By setting boundaries and defining role content within a framework for practice, nurses can be assigned responsibility and authority; clinical decision making will be clear, and practitioners will be accountable for what they do.' Similarly, Frost advocated an autonomous role, but pointed out that, in order for this to happen, 'employers, statutory and professional bodies, and policy makers in a number of professions have to work together in ways that cross conventional boundaries.'

Following on from Rolfe's argument that the hallmark of advanced, autonomous practice is the generation by the nurse of her own body of clinical knowledge through reflection-on-action, the following chapters explored three such ways that this might be attempted. Thus, Johns maps out a model of clinical supervision based on guided reflection, in which a skilled educator enables skilled practitioners to make sense of their clinical experiences. Clearly, the role of the educator in guided reflection is rather different from the traditional role, and, as Johns points out, it entails exposing, confronting and resolving contradictions between what is practised and what is desirable.

Similarly, Jasper advocates the use of reflective writing as a means of exploring and developing knowledge from practice. Like Johns, she sees reflection as an educational process, claiming that, 'by using reflective techniques to explore elements of experience, we will develop a new perspective on that element, which will then inform future practice. This is referred to as "learning".' Like Johns, she is concerned not just with generating knowledge out of practice, but with ensuring that this knowledge is then employed to *improve* practice.

Clinical supervision and reflective writing are engaged in at all levels of practice, but it is argued here that, for the advanced practitioner, they transcend what is normally referred to as reflection or reflective practice. For nurses who are not at this mindful level of practice, the processes of guided reflection and reflective portfolio-writing are largely descriptive; these nurses are able to give an account of their experiences but have difficulty in justifying or rationalizing them, in uncovering the underlying processes. Like Benner's psychiatric nurse quoted earlier by Rolfe, they can reflect on the fact that they made a clinical judgement but they cannot say *why* they made that judgement rather than a different one.

Of course, this has implications for the application of experience in practice. As Jasper points out, what is usually described as reflective *practice* is most often merely reflective *process*; it is one thing to reflect on experience, but it is quite another to use that experience to improve practice. If, as Benner asserts, expert practice is practice with no underlying rationale, then no amount of reflection will enable nurses to move beyond a descriptive account of what they did. They will therefore not be able to generalize their learning from one particular experience to other situations; they will not be learning from their mistakes (or, indeed, from their successes).

Although the process of reflection is, for most practitioners, descriptive, at the level of mindful advanced practice it becomes an analytical process; because they have access to their decision making strategies, reflection for advanced practitioners is not merely a question of 'what happened?', but also of 'why did it happen?' Thus, despite her protestations, Johns' supervisee, Helen, is clearly practising at an advanced level, at least as it is described in this book. However, the similarities between guided reflection and reflective writing end there; a closer examination of the two chapters will reveal that Johns' clinical supervision and Jasper's reflective portfolios are not simply two ways of facilitating the same process; they are different processes, which produce different kinds of knowledge.

Guided reflection is a verbal process, but it is also an interpersonal one. It is concerned with exploring thoughts and feelings with another person and is best suited to uncovering personal knowledge, particularly knowledge about nurses themselves and about their personal therapeutic relationships with their patients. For Johns, then, 'the essence of advanced practice is the practitioner's ability to be available to work with the "person" [patient]' (what Stilwell described in an earlier chapter as making a 'meaningful connection' with the patient), in order to achieve what Barker calls the 'proper focus' of nursing, understanding the person who experiences the illness. As Johns demonstrates so graphically, this personal knowledge is often of an intimate and sensitive nature, and the process of uncovering it can be very painful and might even be resisted by nurses. The skills of the supervisor, not only in facilitating the process of uncovering personal knowledge, but also in managing the hurt and distress that might follow, are therefore of utmost importance. With an experienced and empathic supervisor, guided reflection can therefore give nurses access to material about themselves and their patients, which might otherwise remain unconscious.

Reflective writing, on the other hand, is more of an intellectual and analytical process, a process of creation rather than of personal discovery. It might not give access to personal knowledge in the same way that guided reflection can, but, as Jasper demonstrates, it can develop critical thinking, cognitive (rather than emotional) understanding, and higher order conceptual skills by providing 'evidence of the thought processes behind the decision making, or the way that alternatives are considered and evaluated before nursing action is taken'.

Just as guided reflection can help nurses to generate and explore their body of personal knowledge, so reflective writing can help to generate experiential knowledge by processing and making sense of nurses' accumulation of experiences around specific care issues. Thus, by writing about their various experiences of, say, working with dying patients, they are able to explore commonalities and differences, to evaluate the effects of different interventions, to match different care interventions to different situations, and ultimately to transform a collection of disparate experiences into a coherent body of experiential knowledge. Furthermore, Jasper argues that reflective writing, or 'writing to learn', can achieve a level of analytical understanding that is not possible through other means of expression. Thus, Jasper claims, the reflective portfolio is 'a working dynamic document that a nurse uses creatively to explore issues, define problems, plan action, gather information, create strategies, test alternatives, and evaluate them in practice'.

Both of these techniques, guided reflection and reflective writing, are employed mainly to uncover theoretical knowledge or 'knowing that', whether it is knowledge about themselves, their patients, or their patients' families. In the chapter that follows, Scholes expanded the discussion by exploring the world of practical 'knowing how' through an examination of the non-verbal behaviour of nurses working with deeply unconscious patients. Echoing Johns, Stilwell and Barker, she argues that 'the capacity to presence, connect with the ... patient, is ... the very notion of advanced nursing practice.' However, whereas Johns was concerned primarily with the personal and emotional 'knowing that' of advanced practice, Scholes is interested in the tacit 'knowing how' expressed through the actions of the practitioner. Her choice of nurses working with unconscious patients provides a particularly pure example of how nurses might build a non-verbal therapeutic relationship, since there is no verbal dialogue (at least, not in the accepted meaning of the notion of dialogue as a two-way verbal interaction) between nurses and patients to confuse the issue.

Scholes' method was to video-record nurses at work and later to engage them in a reflective dialogue in front of a play-back of their video recording. In this way, the nurses were able to articulate the intricacies of their non-verbal interactions, and so uncover the practical know-how not usually available to them; indeed, know-how, for Benner, is unavailable to *anyone*, because she claimed that it does not exist in a tangible, accessible form. To take an example from Scholes' findings, she described how the nurses unconsciously scanned the various monitors at the patient's bedside at regular intervals, enabling them to respond immediately to any changes. They had always assumed that they *intuitively* knew when to look at the monitors, and it was only after seeing themselves on a video recording that they realized they had unconsciously been following the rule of scanning at regular intervals.

The importance of becoming aware of this unconscious knowledge, whether it is theoretical 'knowing that' or practical 'knowing how', is not only to improve practice, but to be able to pass it on to others. As Scholes points out (echoing Barker's appeal for advanced practitioners to develop 'conceptual maps' of their practice, which can then be passed on to others): 'Perhaps one of the features of advanced practitioners is their capacity to find innovative approaches to transfer these skills to others and to find ways to articulate the epistemology of practice in a meaningful and understandable language to their colleagues.'

This, argues Rolfe in the final chapter, is precisely the problem faced by the educationalist working with advanced practitioners. He claims that the aim of the educationalist is not to pass on knowledge, but, as Scholes so eloquently expressed it above, to enable the practitioners to 'find ways to articulate the epistemology of practice in a meaningful and understandable language to their colleagues'.

In many ways, this final chapter pulls together a number of the themes developed throughout the book, since, in order to design an educational programme for advanced practitioners, we must first have a clear understanding of who they are, what they do, and how they do it. Rolfe therefore returns to the view of advanced practice that he developed in his earlier chapter, and which is supported by many other of the writers in this book, by distinguishing between the processed based advanced practitioner and the skills based specialist practitioner. This distinction, which he illustrated in a table, develops a number of the differences highlighted by Frost in Part 1 between the expanded role and the extended role, and by Manley and Fulbrook in their research studies.

The course that Rolfe goes on to describe is constructed around the model of clinical supervision described by Johns, the techniques of reflective portfolio writing suggested by Jasper, and the detailed exploration of practice outlined by Scholes, and meets many of Frost's criteria for the education of advanced practitioners. First, it is practice centred, and, as Frost maintains, able to 'inform and be informed by good practice'. Secondly, it is predominantly concerned with extracting theory *from* practice and applying it back *to* practice, thereby conforming to Frost's stricture of 'an understanding of the relationship between theory and practice in ways that support the student in questioning and challenging concepts and conventional models'. Thirdly, it is concerned with the development of problem solving skills and the skills of analysis, synthesis and self-evaluation, addressing Frost's claim that the purpose of locating nursing education in universities is to develop the 'higher order skills of thinking and reasoning'. Most importantly, the course acknowledges the experience and knowledge that the students bring with them, and aims not to add directly to that knowledge and experience, but to enable the students to discover ways of adding to it themselves. It is, then, truly concerned with lifelong learning, with learning how to learn, and with learning not just from books but from practice, not just from others but from themselves.

Furthermore, as we have seen, *advanced* practitioners are also concerned with *advancing* practice, both their own and that of their colleagues. By coming to understand not only *what* they do, but also *how* they do it, advanced practitioners are able to pass on their know-how to others, thereby fulfilling the United Kingdom Central Council for Nursing,

Midwifery and Health Visiting criterion of 'advancing clinical practice, research and education to enrich nursing practice as a whole' (UKCC, 1994).

Reference

United Kingdom Central Council for Nursing, Midwifery and Health Visiting. (1994). *The Future of Professional Practice – the Council's Standards for Education and Practice Following Registration*. London: UKCC.

Advancing practice:
a guide for the perplexed

Introduction

This book is intended to be *a practitioners' guide*, and, like any guidebook, its intention is not to instruct but to suggest, to point out gently a number of possible routes. The reader who is looking for precise instructions on how to become an advanced practitioner will not find them here, or, we suspect, in any text. Indeed, we would suggest that, having read this far, anyone looking for such instructions has failed to grasp the essence of the role of the advanced practitioner as it has been described in the previous 17 chapters.

Similarly, the reader hoping to find a precise account of what advanced practice *is* (as opposed to what the advanced practitioner *does*) is also likely to be disappointed, since, as we noted in the Preface, this book does not claim to present a single coherent argument for a new model, neither is it a cookbook of recipes for doing advanced practice, nor an attempt by a group of academics to tell practitioners (yet again!) what to do. Rather, it is suggesting that one of the characteristics of advanced practitioners is precisely that they do not need academics (or managers, for that matter) to direct their practice.

The perplexed reader might be asking at this point: 'So what, then, was the point of the book; how can it help me to develop my practice?'

In reply, we would argue, first, that it has presented a number of different perspectives on advanced practice and the role of the advanced practitioner, from academics and managers as well as from practitioners themselves. These accounts do not all agree, and neither would we expect them to do so: sometimes they are describing similar roles from different viewpoints; sometimes they are describing roles that, at first glance, look very different; sometimes they are roles that already exist; and sometimes they are visions of what could or should be.

This in itself is not enough, and so the second function of this book has been to attempt to make some sense of this diversity of views in the commentary that accompanies each of the four parts. We have tried not to fall into the trap that we described in the Preface, the trap of attempting to define advanced practice in terms of its outcomes. Rather, we have sought, as Rorty (1989) suggested, to begin to establish a language in which advanced practitioners and those, like ourselves, with an interest in seeing advanced practice grow and flourish, can begin to talk to each other.

At first glance, the sceptical reader might claim that we have failed miserably at this task, and that we have fallen at the first hurdle by failing even to establish a terminology for advanced practice; indeed, that we have not even resolved the issue of what the advanced practitioner should be called. To raise that objection is to believe that the primary need for a common language is to describe and categorize what is, rather than to enable communication about what might be. We are also very aware that to give something a name not only describes what it has become at this point in time, but that it also determines what it might become in the future, and rather like butterfly collecting, the act of pinning it down also kills it. A role that is called the 'nurse consultant' is likely to evolve differently from a role called the 'specialist nurse' or one called the 'lecturer–practitioner', simply because the different names raise different expectations in the mind of the reader. We believe that the role that is beginning to emerge from the writings in this book is still far too young to have its future imposed on it in such a crude way.

Our approach in the commentaries to this book has therefore taken two diverse routes. First, we have tended largely to ignore the superficial differences such as those in terminology, in pursuit of an understanding of the essences that lie behind the diversity of names that a variety of writers have given to the phenomenon of advanced practice. Secondly, we have also focused on highlighting the deeper contradictions in the different perspectives, rather than attempting a facile 'synthesis' of a variety of conflicting views.

For example, it is interesting to note that the term 'advanced practice' is most often defined not by what it is, but by what it is not. Thus, some writers have contrasted it with 'advancing practice', some with 'specialist practice', and some with 'basic practice'. Rather than seeking to arrive at a common consensus of the term 'advanced practice', we have sought to explore the tensions inherent in the above dichotomies. What, for example, is the writer saying about his or her understanding of *advanced* practice when he or she contrasts it with *advancing* practice? Does the writer who sets up advanced practice in opposition to specialist practice see it in the same way as the writer who compares it to basic practice? Clearly, the differences in terminology can tell us far more than the similarities; we cannot synthesize until we have first analysed.

Emerging themes

Nevertheless, a number of common issues are beginning to emerge. First, there is the near unanimous agreement that our current understanding about the role of advanced practitioner and the nature of advanced practice is a mess, and that the history of advanced practice, in terms of previously developed roles, writings, research and policies, tells us little about the future or futures of advanced practice. The past provides us with a range of possibilities, but it does not help us to decide between them. It offers no imperative, moral, practical or otherwise. It suggests what we *could* do, but not what we *should* do. Furthermore, not only is there little agreement on what the role is, but there is also dispute over whose task it is to *define* what the role is. This difficulty cannot be overstated, since it allows us to dismiss the views of another without even bothering to find out what those views are, simply because that person is thought not to be qualified to express an opinion.

These problems have been compounded by the fact that a number of diverse roles have been developed with similar titles but very different functions and philosophies. This has led not just to confusion, but to a very fundamental problem for researchers, which was discussed in the commentary to Part 2 of this book, namely the problem of bootstrapping. In the absence of any solid ground on which to base their studies, researchers are having to pull themselves up by their own bootstraps. We might, for example, attempt to understand (or even define) what is meant by advanced practice by asking advanced practitioners themselves, but, *which* advanced practitioners do we ask? In order to identify our sample, we must first answer the very research question that we wish that sample to consider. Similarly, we might wish to identify existing advanced practitioner roles in order to study and understand them, but who decides on the criteria for identifying such roles? In order to learn from advanced practitioners what it is they do, we must first decide what it is *we* think they do. In choosing to study, say, the advanced practitioner movement in the USA, we are already imposing limits and constraints on what the role is.

Despite these problems, there is a surprising degree of consensus on the constituent components of the role. Many contributors to this book would agree that the role of an advanced practitioner includes the subroles of practitioner, consultant, educator and researcher. The subrole of manager is rather more contested, with a number of writers agreeing that the advanced practitioner should have a degree of input into policy and decision making, but should stop short of a fully-fledged management subrole. There is also fairly general agreement that these subroles should be integrated into practice, and that, when the advanced practitioner nurses, he or she is somehow carrying out a number of these subroles simultaneously, delivering nursing care, being an educator, conducting or implementing research, and possibly doing a number of other things at the same time. In a very real and practical sense, then, the advanced practitioner is acting as a role model for more junior staff, as well as being available to them for consultation and advocating for them through management and/or policy decisions.

Clearly arising from this is the issue of autonomy, particularly the question of where the advanced practitioner stands in relation to multidisciplinary colleagues, managers, employers and professional bodies. Autonomy relates not only to practice, where it is linked to other issues, such as those of safety and boundary setting, but also to the autonomy further to develop one's own role, which, in turn, raises the issues of role expansion and role extension, the 'medicalization' of nursing roles, and the perceived abdication of the United Kingdom Central Council for Nursing Midwifery and Health Visiting (UKCC) from taking the lead in driving advanced practice forward.

All of the above issues have been aired in the preceding chapters, but the main focus of the discussion of autonomy has been on the use of clinical judgement by the advanced practitioner. This issue has moved the focus of the book from a discussion of what advanced practitioners do to a discussion of how they do it, which is possibly the key to the whole vexed question of how to characterize advanced practice. It also suggests solutions to a number of other problems raised, including those of the art and science of practice, the integration of subroles, the question of hierarchical levels of practice, and the 'advanced versus advancing practice' debate.

The centrality of clinical judgement is apparent from the observation that the issue appears to surface in almost every chapter, often in a partially disguised form (for example, as 'know-how', as problem solving, as decision making, or as reflection), and usually against the grain of whatever is being discussed. For example, in one of the studies reported in the research section, the respondents effectively rejected the criteria for advanced practice imposed by the researcher to suggest that advanced practice was, in fact, much more related to a high level of clinical decision making. Several contributors related this to Benner's notion of intuitive expertise, but others emphasized the need for advanced practitioners to articulate consciously the decisions on which their practice is based, to provide 'conceptual maps', as one writer put it, or 'to articulate the epistemology of practice in a meaningful and understandable language', in the words of another.

The reason for this need by advanced practitioners to articulate their clinical decision making or professional judgement is related to their role as autonomous practitioners with responsibility for consultancy and education. First, if advanced practitioners are to practice in an autonomous way, then they must be able to justify their clinical decisions to their seniors; and, secondly, if they are to act as consultants, they must be able to communicate the underlying processes of their professional judgements to their juniors. By arguing, as Part 4 attempted to do, that the conscious articulation of practice (as opposed to Benner's 'intuitive grasp' based on tacit knowledge), pursued through clinical supervision, through reflective writing and through other reflective techniques, is a hallmark of advanced practice, we also manage to resolve the 'advanced versus advancing practice' debate. Thus, in order to advance practice, both their own and that of their colleagues, nurses must first be practising at an advanced level in which they have conscious access to their own decision making processes. As was pointed out in the Introduction, all nurses occasionally (often inadvertently) make advances in practice, but advanced practitioners are specially prepared nurses who advance practice on an everyday basis as part of their role.

Guidelines for advancing practice

Having revisited some of the main issues encountered in the book, we are now perhaps in a position to offer some of the promised guidelines for advanced or would-be advanced practitioners who wish to develop their role further.

Role definition

Neither the history of advanced practice development nor the UKCC guidelines will provide much help in defining your role unless you already have a fairly clear idea of what it is you want. The former gives some suggestions about what you *could* do, the latter, to a limited extent, sets the boundaries of what you *might* do, but neither tell you what you *should* do.

Advanced practitioner roles tend to develop individually in response to specific local needs, so look to what is already happening locally, to your trust's philosophy, to other roles currently being supported, to the particular needs within both your specialism and your geographical area, and to your own strengths, interests and beliefs.

Ground the role firmly in practice. You should be an expert in your own field of nursing who can act as a role model and a consultant to others. No one respects a non-practising 'expert', and, for this reason, the majority of your time should be spent in the clinical setting. You should be able not only to practice what you preach, but to preach what you practice.

Your role might include a number of subroles, perhaps those of researcher, educator and manager, but, as an advanced practitioner, you will be expected to integrate and demonstrate them within a practice setting. You should not aim sometimes to be a practitioner, sometimes to be a teacher, sometimes to be a manager and sometimes to be a researcher; you should be a practitioner who sometimes teaches, sometimes manages and sometimes researches *as part of your practice*, as circumstances demand.

Advanced practice roles will survive only if they are based on a sound foundation of a partnership with managers and educationalists. Both parties are absolutely essential to the role: managers to set and define the boundaries of your practice and of your clinical autonomy; and educationalists to facilitate the development of that practice and to enable you to push constantly at its boundaries. However, the partnership *must* be a partnership of equals. Managers and educationalists are, by definition, not expert practitioners; that is your role in the partnership. Thus, clinical role boundaries and educational needs and objectives must be negotiated and jointly agreed by expert practitioners, expert managers and expert educationalists.

It is also worth considering as part of your negotiations exactly where you want to be located within the organization. Are you negotiating a new post with a new title, possibly with a new pay scale, possibly jointly between nursing and education? Are you negotiating a new role within an existing post, possibly with extended responsibilities, possibly with informal links to education and management; or are you simply looking for recognition of a role that you already carry out, either formally or informally?

Educational considerations

Most writers agree that advanced practitioners should be educated at least to master's level, although the rationale underpinning that agreement tends to vary considerably. What is far less clear, however, is what that education should include. Some academics have argued that, as a clinical role, education for advanced practice should focus on advanced clinical skills and knowledge, often categorized according to specialism, whereas others have built courses around the subroles of education, management and research. However, the notion of advanced practice advocated here would suggest that neither of these syllabus models is entirely adequate. First, it is assumed that advanced practitioners would already be experts in their own clinical field and would therefore already possess many of the skills and much of the knowledge offered in a specialist clinical degree. Secondly, the subroles of education, management and research are implicitly integrated into the practice role. The advanced practitioner does not *specifically* need to know how to lecture formally or how to conduct formal research, although these skills and their underpinning knowledge bases are, of course, useful to most nurses.

We are therefore assuming that, as a potential advanced practitioner, you would bring with you to a master's course a well-developed and up-to-date specialist knowledge base and at least a smattering of management, education and research skills, but that what you might be lacking is the ability, first, to integrate them all in your practice consciously and intelligently, and, secondly, to articulate and critically appraise your extensive store of experiential knowledge through reflective techniques such as clinical supervision and reflective writing. You should therefore seek out a course where the emphasis is on critical reflection in a clinical nursing context, on facilitating learning as a partnership between expert colleagues from clinical practice and education, and on developing the higher-order cognitive skills of thinking and reasoning and of lifelong learning. In the absence of such a course locally, consider registering for a master/doctor of philosophy, preferably with a focus on practice rather than research, for example, through action research or practitioner based enquiry.

Do remember, however, that all of the above guidelines are merely pointers, and that the truly defining characteristic of advanced practitioners is that they are able to think for themselves, rather than rely on the directives of others.

Reference

Rorty, R. (1989). *Contingency, Irony and Solidarity*. Cambridge: Cambridge University Press.

Index

U.W.E.L. LEARNING RESOURCES